# MEDICAL MYCOLOGY

## Other Books by Dr. D.R. Arora
- Textbook of Microbiology, 5/e
- Medical Parasitology, 5/e
- Textbook of Microbiology for Dental Students, 4/e
- Microbiology for Nursing & Allied Sciences, 2/e
- MCQs in Microbiology and Parasitology (With Explanations)
- Exam-Oriented Microbiology (Questions and Answers)
- Essentials of Microbiology for B.Sc. Nursing Students
- Practical Microbiology
- Practical Microbiology for Dental Students
- Microbiology for Medical Laboratory Technology Students

# MEDICAL MYCOLOGY

## Second Edition

### Dr. D.R. Arora M.D., Ph.D., M.N.A.M.S.

*Ex*-Professor & Head, Department of Microbiology,
Postgraduate Institute of Medical Sciences, Rohtak, Haryana (India), and
Maharaja Agarsen Medical College, Agroha, Haryana (India)

*Ex*-Professor & Head, Department of Microbiology,
Medical Superintendent, and Dean Faculty of Allied Health Sciences,
SGT University, Gurugram, Haryana (India)

*Ex*-W.H.O. Fellow; and Visiting Professor, University of Mauritius

Lead Assessor and Member, Accreditation Committee,
National Accreditation Board for Testing and Calibration Laboratories (NABL),
Gurugram, Haryana (India)

Principal Assessor, National Accreditation Board for Hospitals &
Healthcare Providers (NABH), New Delhi (India)

Assessor, National Accreditation Board for
Education and Training (NABET), New Delhi (India)

### Dr. Brij Bala Arora M.D.

*Ex*-Senior Professor & Head, Department of Pathology,
Postgraduate Institute of Medical Sciences, Rohtak, Haryana (India)

*Ex*-Director-Principal and Senior Professor & Head,
Department of Pathology, SGT Medical College, Budhera,
Gurugram, Haryana (India)

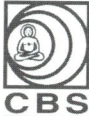

## CBS Publishers & Distributors Pvt. Ltd.

New Delhi • Bengaluru • Chennai • Kochi • Kolkata • Mumbai
Hyderabad • Nagpur • Patna • Pune • Jharkhand • Uttarakhand

ISBN: 978-93-87964-92-1

**First Edition:** 2014
Reprint: 2015
**Second Edition:** 2019
Reprint: 2020

Copyright © Dr. D.R. Arora

All rights reserved. No part of this book may be reproduced or transmitted in any form or by any means, electronic or mechanical, including photocopying, recording, or any information storage and retrieval system without permission, in writing, from the author.

Published by **Satish Kumar Jain** and produced by **Varun Jain** for
**CBS Publishers & Distributors Pvt. Ltd.,**
4819/XI Prahlad Street, 24 Ansari Road, Daryaganj, New Delhi - 110002
delhi@cbspd.com, cbspubs@airtelmail.in • www.cbspd.com
Ph.: 23289259, 23266861, 23266867 • Fax: 011-23243014

*Corporate Office:* 204 FIE, Industrial Area, Patparganj, Delhi - 110 092
Ph: 49344934 • Fax: 011-49344935
E-mail: publishing@cbspd.com • publicity@cbspd.com

*Branches:*
- *Bengaluru:* 2975, 17th Cross, K.R. Road, Bansankari 2nd Stage, Bengaluru - 70 • Ph: +91-80-26771678/79 • Fax: +91-80-26771680
  E-mail: cbsbng@gmail.com, bangalore@cbspd.com
- *Chennai:* No. 7, Subbaraya Street, Shenoy Nagar, Chennai - 600030
  Ph: +91-44-26681266, 26680620 • Fax: +91-44-42032115
  E-mail: chennai@cbspd.com
- *Kochi:* Ashana House, 39/1904, A.M. Thomas Road, Valanjambalam, Ernakulum, Kochi • Ph: +91-484-4059061-65
  Fax: +91-484-4059065 • E-mail: cochin@cbspd.com
- *Kolkata:* 6-B, Ground Floor, Rameshwar Shaw Road, Kolkata - 700014
  Ph: +91-33-22891126/7/8 • E-mail: kolkata@cbspd.com
- *Mumbai:* 83-C, Dr. E. Moses Road, Worli, Mumbai - 400018
  Ph: +91-9833017933, 022-24902340/41 • E-mail: mumbai@cbspd.com

*Representatives:*

- Hyderabad: 0-9885175004
- Patna: 0-9334159340
- Jharkhand: 0-9811541605
- Nagpur: 0-9021734563
- Pune: 0-9623451994
- Uttarakhand: 0-9716462459

*Printed at:*
Neekunj Print Process, Delhi (India)

*Dedicated to the Sweet Memories of  
Our Loving Daughter,  
Dr. Hina Arora*

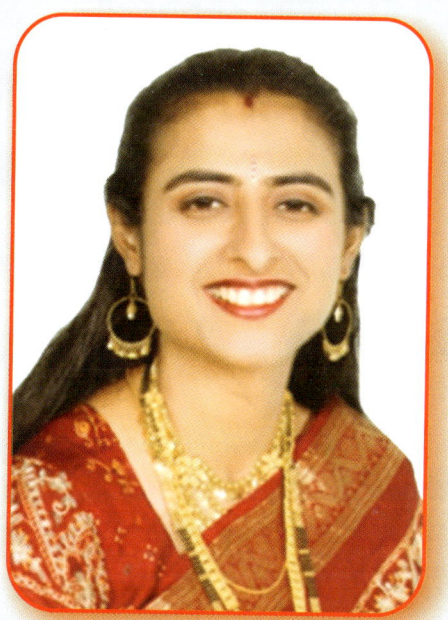

**Dr. Hina Arora**
BDS, IDES 2001
09-04-1976 to 02-11-2009

# Preface to the Second Edition

Due to the widespread use of antibacterial antibiotics, immunosuppressive drugs, drugs used in cancer therapy and acquired immunodeficiency syndrome there is tremendous increase in fungal infections. Second edition of Medical Mycology broadens the reader's knowledge and provides current information regarding the emerging (as well as established) pathogens that are being encountered, and new methods for the laboratory diagnosis of mycoses. Molecular studies of medically important fungi have brought recent changes in the field of mycology including taxonomy and nomenclature of some of the fungi. The same have been incorporated in the book. Although molecular methods have a role to play, relatively few isolates require or merit molecular identification, and molecular assays will not replace the need for knowledge of fungal morphology.

The book has been thoroughly revised. Fungal morphology, cultivation, identification, pathogenesis, pathology and laboratory diagnosis of mycoses have been described in detail. As in earlier edition, the book is divided into seven sections. These are general topics, superficial mycoses, subcutaneous mycoses, systemic mycoses, opportunistic mycoses, miscellaneous mycoses, and appendices. The text has been presented in a lucid manner for the readers to help them thoroughly imbibe the basics of the subject. A picture speaks more than a thousand words. Keeping this in mind all diagrams are coloured, uncomplicated and clear as also the pictures of gross and histopathological sections. Every chapter ends with essay type and multiple choice questions with answers, and references for further reading. The book is user-friendly and easy to understand.

I am deeply indebted to Dr. Paramjit S. Gill, M.D., Professor, Department of Microbiology, Postgraduate Institute of Medical Sciences, Rohtak (Haryana) for contributing a chapter on "Introduction, taxonomy and classification of fungi" and Dr. Seema Gupta, M.D., Assistant Professor, Department of Pharmacology and Therapeutics, Government Medical College, Jammu (J&K); and Dr. Vikram Gupta, M.D., Consultant Physician, Jammu (J&K) for contributing a chapter on "Antifungal drugs". Thanks are also due to Dr. Gill for meticulously drawing all figures.

I am grateful to Mr. B.M. Singh for meticulous proof-reading and valuable professional help and support. Thanks are also due to Mr. Anurag Trivedi for designing the book. I honestly acknowledge the most sincere and dedicated support and advice of Mr. Dharmvir.

This book will be highly useful to M.B.B.S., M.Sc., M.L.T. and M.D. microbiology students. It is also hoped that it will serve as a resource for teachers of microbiology and medical professionals engaged in the treatment of mycoses. The readers are requested to send suggestions for the improvement of the book which will be incorporated in subsequent editions. Shortcomings, if any, may please be communicated at draroradr@rediffmail.com

D.R. Arora

# Preface to the First Edition

During the last few decades there has been a rise in the global incidence and prevalence of fungal diseases. With increasing numbers of people taking advantage of the ease of worldwide travel, mycoses that were previously regarded as geographically limited can now be seen in any part of the world. Furthermore, in recent years, the number of fungi recognized as human pathogens has risen. Fungi that were considered as nonpathogenic are being recovered as opportunistic invaders. The widespread use of antibacterial antibiotics, immunosuppressive drugs and the drugs used in cancer therapy have resulted in a presumptive increase in mycoses.

Fungi are ubiquitous, capable of colonizing almost any environment, and generally, play an invaluable part in decomposition and recycling of organic matter. All fungi are heterotrophic and must exist as saprophytes or parasites. However, relatively few of the estimated quarter of a million species are pathogens of humans or other warm-blooded animals.

The book is divided into seven sections. These are general topics, superficial cutaneous mycoses, subcutaneous mycoses, systemic mycoses, opportunistic mycoses, miscellaneous mycoses and appendices. The text is presented in a simple and lucid manner. It is illustrated with coloured and computer-drawn figures, and clinical and photomicrographs. Essay type and multiple choice questions have been given at the end of each chapter.

We are deeply indebted to Dr. Seema Gupta, M.D., Assistant Professor, Department of Pharmacology and Therapeutics, Government Medical College, Jammu (J&K) and Dr. Vikram Gupta, M.D., Consultant Physician, Jammu (J&K) for contributing a chapter on "Antifungal drugs", and Dr. Paramjit S. Gill, Associate Professor, Department of Microbiology, Postgraduate Institute of Medical Sciences, Rohtak (Haryana), for contributing a chapter on "Introduction, taxonomy and classification of fungi". Thanks are also due to Dr. Gill for meticulously drawing all figures and proof-reading. We are grateful for valuable professional help and support provided by the staff at CBS Publishers & Distributors. We honestly acknowledge the most sincere and dedicated support and advice of Mr. Dharmvir. We are also thankful to the teachers who, after reading the chapter "Medical mycology" in our book "Textbook of Microbiology", encouraged us to write a full textbook on medical mycology.

This book will be highly useful to M.B.B.S., M.Sc. and M.D. microbiology students. It is also hoped that it will serve as a resource for teachers of microbiology and other specialities and medical professionals engaged in the treatment of mycoses. The readers are requested to send suggestions for the improvement of the book which will be incorporated in subsequent editions. Shortcomings, if any, may please be communicated at draroradr@rediffmail.com.

**D.R. Arora**
**Brij Bala Arora**

# Contents

*Preface to the Second Edition* ............................................................................................................... vii
*Preface to the First Edition* ................................................................................................................. viii

## SECTION 1
## General Topics            1–38

| | | |
|---|---|---|
| Chapter 1 | Introduction, Taxonomy and Classification of Fungi ............................................... | 3 |
| Chapter 2 | Epidemiology and Laboratory Diagnosis of Mycoses .............................................. | 16 |
| Chapter 3 | Antifungal Drugs ........................................................................................................ | 27 |

## SECTION 2
## Superficial Cutaneous Mycoses            39–58

| | | |
|---|---|---|
| Chapter 4 | Pityriasis versicolor, Tinea nigra and Piedra .......................................................... | 41 |
| Chapter 5 | Dermatophytoses ........................................................................................................ | 47 |

## SECTION 3
## Subcutaneous Mycoses            59–91

| | | |
|---|---|---|
| Chapter 6 | Mycetoma .................................................................................................................... | 61 |
| Chapter 7 | Sporotrichosis ............................................................................................................. | 73 |
| Chapter 8 | Chromoblastomycosis ................................................................................................ | 77 |

| | | |
|---|---|---|
| Chapter 9 | Phaeohyphomycosis | 82 |
| Chapter 10 | Lobomycosis | 89 |

## SECTION 4
## Systemic Mycoses    93–117

| | | |
|---|---|---|
| Chapter 11 | Histoplasmosis | 95 |
| Chapter 12 | Blastomycosis | 103 |
| Chapter 13 | Coccidioidomycosis | 109 |
| Chapter 14 | Paracoccidioidomycosis | 114 |

## SECTION 5
## Opportunistic Mycoses    119–177

| | | |
|---|---|---|
| Chapter 15 | Candidiasis | 121 |
| Chapter 16 | Cryptococcosis | 134 |
| Chapter 17 | Pneumocystosis | 141 |
| Chapter 18 | Penicilliosis marneffei | 146 |
| Chapter 19 | Aspergillosis | 150 |
| Chapter 20 | Mucormycosis | 159 |
| Chapter 21 | Hyalohyphomycosis | 170 |

## SECTION 6
## Miscellaneous Mycoses    179–198

| | | |
|---|---|---|
| Chapter 22 | Oculomycosis | 181 |
| Chapter 23 | Adiaspiromycosis | 187 |
| Chapter 24 | Rhinosporidiosis | 190 |
| Chapter 25 | Mycotoxicoses | 194 |

## SECTION 7
## Appendices    199–223

| | | |
|---|---|---|
| Appendix A | Culture Media | 201 |
| Appendix B | Laboratory Procedures | 206 |
| Appendix C | Staining Methods | 210 |
| Appendix D | Glossary | 217 |
| Appendix E | Overview of Medical Mycology | 222 |

*Index* ........ 225

# SECTION 1

# GENERAL TOPICS

**Chapter 1** Introduction, Taxonomy and Classification of Fungi
**Chapter 2** Epidemiology and Laboratory Diagnosis of Mycoses
**Chapter 3** Antifungal Drugs

# SECTION 1

# GENERAL TOPICS

# Introduction, Taxonomy and Classification of Fungi

Fungi (singular, fungus) are a group of eukaryotic organisms which multiply both sexually and asexually by production of spores. The word *'fungus'* is derived from Latin meaning 'mushroom', which, in turn, is derived from Greek word *'spongos'* meaning 'sponge' which refers to the morphology of mushrooms. The term *'mycology'* is derived from Greek words *'mykes'* (mushroom) and *'logy'* (study) which means study of fungi. **Medical mycology** is the study of morphology, pathogenesis, diagnosis and treatment of fungal infections in human beings.

Fungi are eukaryotic, which means, each cell possesses well defined nucleus with nuclear membrane, mitochondria, Golgi apparatus and endoplasmic reticulum. They can be *distinguished from other eukaryotes* by a rigid cell wall composed of chitin, β-glucans, mannan, as well as other polysaccharides, proteins and lipids. Within the cell wall, the cytoplasm is bounded by a cytoplasmic membrane in which the predominant sterol is not cholesterol, as in humans, but ***ergosterol***. Fungi differ from bacteria and other prokaryotes in many ways (Table 1.1).

In 1835, Augustino Bassi observed that muscardine, a disease of silkworm was caused by a fungus, *Baeuveria bassiana*. Shortly thereafter, in 1841, the mycologic etiology of favus was identified by David Gruby. Raymond Jacques Adrien Sabouraud (1864–1938), a dermatologist and mycologist was named as the **'Father of Mycology'** for his pioneering and extensive work on fungal scalp infections (mainly ringworm) and their treatment.

Fungi are ubiquitous, capable of colonizing almost any environment, and generally play an invaluable part in the decomposition and recycling of organic matter. About 1.5 million species of fungi are known. Most of them are found as saprophytes in the soil and on decaying plant material, and about 600 species are known to cause human disease.

Fungi are now considered as significant cause of morbidity and mortality as they have emerged as important etiological agents of ***opportunistic infections*** in patients with haematological malignancies undergoing chemotherapy, transplant recipients, patients with acquired immunodeficiency syndrome, severe burns, prematurity, and autoimmune diseases. Risk factors like admission to intensive care unit, diabetes, chronic liver and renal diseases are added to the list. Even immunocompetent hosts may occasionally acquire invasive

---

\* This chapter has been contributed by Dr. Paramjeet S. Gill, Professor, Department of Microbiology, Postgraduate Institute of Medical Sciences, Rohtak (Haryana) – 124001.

# SECTION 1 : General Topics

**Table 1.1.** Distinguishing features of fungi and bacteria

| Features | **Fungi** (Eukaryotic) | **Bacteria** (Prokaryotic) |
|---|---|---|
| Cell wall composition | Rigid, multi-layered, chitin, β-glucans, mannan, polysaccharides, proteins and lipids | *Gram-positive:* Peptidoglycan and teichoic acid<br>*Gram-negative:* Lipopolysaccharides, proteins, lipoprotein and peptidoglycan<br>*Acid-fast:* Lipids, proteins, polysaccharides |
| Cell membrane | Ergosterol (except in *Pneumocystis*) | Phospholipids and proteins |
| Cytoplasmic contents | Mitochondria, Golgi apparatus and endoplasmic reticulum | Lack mitochondria, Golgi apparatus and endoplasmic reticulum |
| Nucleus | True nucleus with nuclear membrane and paired chromosome | Single, circular piece of DNA present in cytoplasm attached to mesosome, no nuclear membrane and nucleolus |
| Ribosomes | 40S + 60S = 80S | 30S + 50S = 70S |
| Replication/Reproduction | Mitosis and meiosis | Binary fission |
| Spores | Method of **reproduction** (sexual and asexual) | Method of **preservation** |
| Morphology | *Yeast:* unicellular, *Mold:* multicellular | Coccal, bacillary, filamentous and spirochaetal forms |

fungal infections by direct introduction of fungi through indwelling devices, trauma or due to large inoculums of spores entering through respiratory tract.

The endemic mycoses prevalent in Asian countries include histoplasmosis, penicilliosis, blastomycosis, and sporotrichosis. Coccidioidomycosis has been occasionally reported as imported mycosis. Among opportunistic mycoses, invasive candidiasis is the commonest disease followed by aspergillosis and mucormycosis. In certain centres, cryptococcosis has been reported at high rate. Other opportunistic fungal infections such as fusiriosis and scedosporiosis are occasionally reported.

## MORPHOLOGY OF FUNGI

Broadly, fungi are divided into two morphological forms:
- Yeasts
- Molds

*Yeasts are unicellular fungi reproducing asexually by budding (blastoconidia) or by formation of transverse septum known as fission. Fungal spores germinate to produce multicellular branching filamentous structures known as hyphae. All molds are composed of branching hyphae.*

Although, all fungi exist in yeast or mold form but traditionally fungi are divided into four morphological groups:

### 1. Yeasts

Yeasts are round, oval or elongated unicellular fungi. These organisms remain in the yeast form at both, room temperature (25°C) and body temperature (37°C). Most of them reproduce by an asexual process called budding in which the cell develops a protuberance which enlarges and eventually separates from the parent cell (Fig. 1.1A). The buds are termed blastoconidia. Some reproduce by fission. They form moist or mucoid colonies. *Saccharomyces cerevisae* and *Cryptococcus neoformans* are the examples of nonpathogenic and pathogenic yeasts respectively.

### 2. Yeast-like

In some yeasts, like *Candida*, the bud remains attached to the mother cell and elongates, followed by repeated budding forming chains of elongated cells known as **pseudohyphae**. *C. albicans* and *C. dubliniensis* also produce germ tubes. **Germ tubes are the beginning of true hyphae** and appear as filaments that are not constricted at their points of origin on the parent cell. **If the filaments are constricted at their points of origin on the parent** cell, they are pseudohyphae, not germ tubes (Fig. 1.1B and C). True hyphae appear as filaments that are not constricted at their points of origin on the parent cell.

### 3. Molds

In molds, spores germinate to produce branching filaments called **hyphae** (singular, hypha). They are 2–10 μm in diameter. They may be septate or nonseptate (coenocytic). Cells in septate hyphae communicate with each other through pores present in the septa, whereas in nonseptate hyphae, the cells communicate freely as the protoplasm of the cells is continuous (Fig. 1.1D and E). However, sparse crosswalls or septa may occur. Where septa occur, they are not perforated but serve to isolate reproductive structures or vacuolated regions in the mycelium. The hyphae continue to grow (Fig. 1.1F) and branch to form tangled mass of growth called **mycelium** (plural, mycelia).

In the culture medium, the part of the mycelium which projects above the surface is called **aerial mycelium** and the part growing in the medium is called **vegetative mycelium**. Vegetative mycelium is responsible for absorbing water and nutrients from the medium. Spore or conidia-bearing fruiting bodies arise from aerial mycelium. Therefore, the latter is also known as reproductive mycelium. Molds reproduce by means of spores, produced often in large numbers, by an asexual process (involving mitosis only) or as a result of sexual reproduction (involving meiosis, preceded by fusion of the nuclei of two haploid cells). Dermatophytes, *Aspergillus*, *Penicillium*, *Mucor* and *Rhizopus* are the examples of molds.

### 4. Dimorphic fungi

Many fungi pathogenic to man like *Histoplasma capsulatum*, *Sporothrix schenckii*, *Blastomyces dermatitidis*, *Coccidioides immitis*, *Paracoccidioides brasiliensis*, and *Penicillium marneffei* have a yeast form in the host tissue and *in vitro* at 37°C on enriched media, and hyphal (mycelial) form *in vitro* at 25°C–30°C.

*If a single mycelium is capable of reproducing sexually, it is known as* **homothallic**, *and if two mycelia are required to reproduce sexually, they are known as* **heterothallic** *fungi.*

Yeasts are the most common fungi isolated in the clinical laboratory. They are ubiquitous in our environment and also live as inhabitants in our bodies, so it is often difficult to determine the clinical significance of an isolate. Implication of yeast as the etiologic agent of infection often requires repeated recovery from the site and direct microscopic demonstration of the yeast in infected tissue. The yeasts and yeast-like organisms are considered opportunistic pathogens, causing disease in patients:

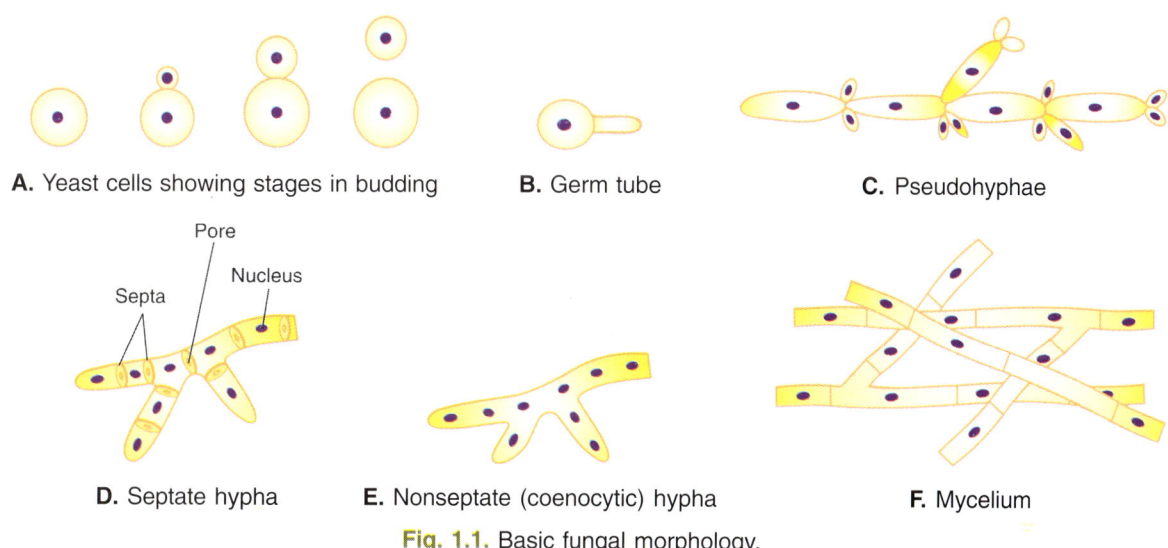

**A.** Yeast cells showing stages in budding  **B.** Germ tube  **C.** Pseudohyphae

**D.** Septate hypha  **E.** Nonseptate (coenocytic) hypha  **F.** Mycelium

**Fig. 1.1.** Basic fungal morphology.

- with a breakdown of the body's immune system;
- on prolonged treatment with antibiotics, corticosteroids or cytotoxic drugs;
- with intravascular catheters;
- with diabetes mellitus; or
- who are intravenous abusers.

## REPRODUCTION IN FUNGI

Reproduction in fungi may be asexual or sexual (Fig. 1.2).

### Asexual reproduction

Asexual reproduction is a result of mitosis which involves budding or fission, resulting in the production of spores. The spores possess haploid nuclei (polidity $n$). These spores may be present endogenously within **sporangium** and are called **sporangiospores**, or exogenously as conidia.

### Sexual reproduction

The sexual stage is characterized by several features that are unique to the kingdom Fungi. Most fungal mating types are morphologically indistinguishable and so, they are not referred to as male or female. In the case of sexual reproduction, compatible mating types fuse in a process that involves **plasmogamy** (fusion of cell membranes, and not the nuclei; polidity

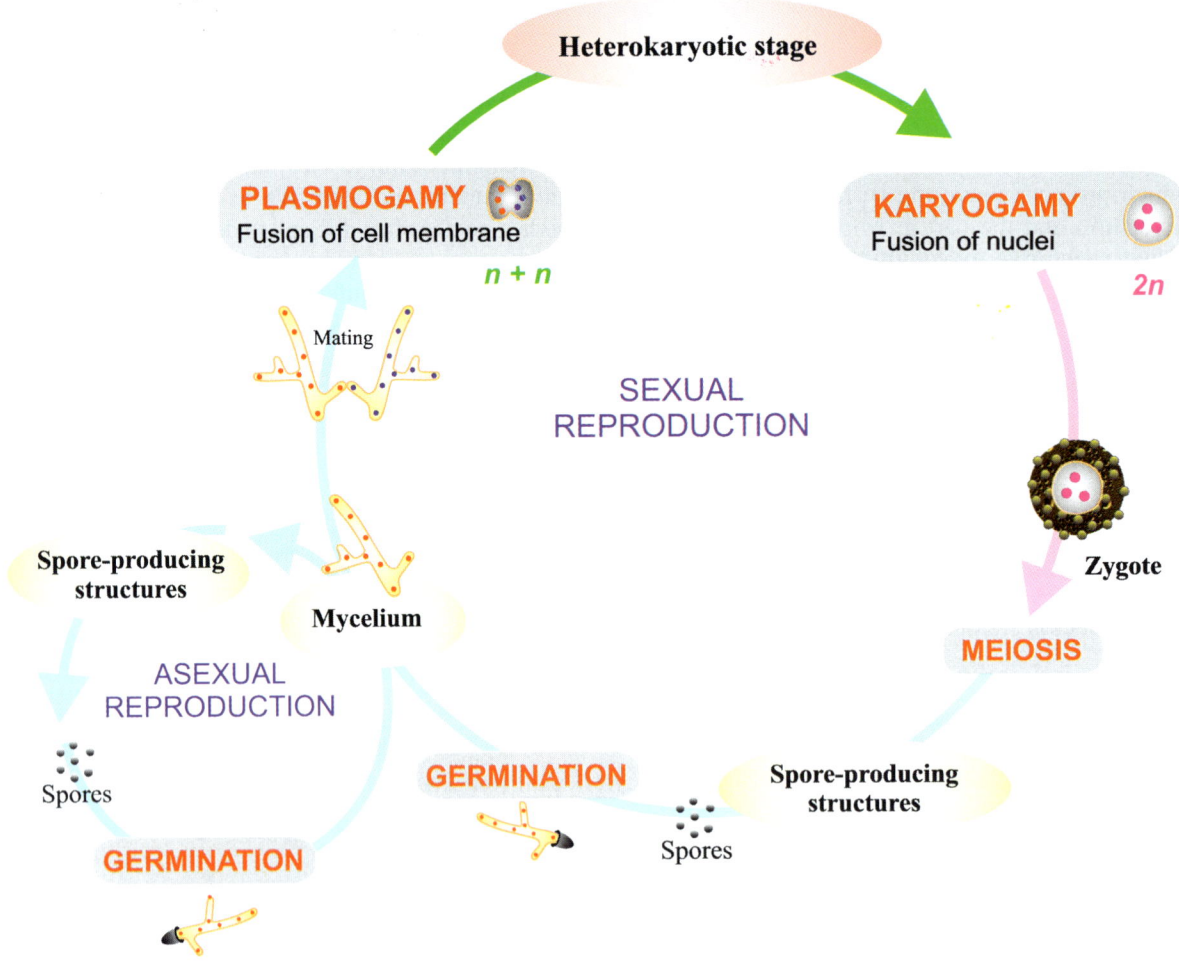

Fig. 1.2. Life cycle of fungi.

is $n + n$). This fusion produces a **heterokaryon** (a mycelium with multiple nuclei from the two mating types; found in the fungi of the order Mucorales) or **dikaryon** (a mycelium with two nuclei from the two mating types; these are found in Ascomycetes and Basidiomycetes), which can divide in the growing mycelium for a prolonged period. The dikaryotic state can last for months, or even years, while the fungus continues to grow and proliferate in its environment. When environmental conditions are suitable, two haploid nuclei fuse (**karyogamy**) to form a highly transient diploid state (polidity becomes $2n$). Meiosis follows, almost immediately, in a specialized spore-producing structure, and genetically distinct haploid spores (polidity $n$) are produced.

The asexual state of fungi is termed the **anamorphic** state, while the sexual state is termed **teleomorphic** state, e.g., *Histoplasma capsulatum* (anamorph) and *Ajellomyces capsulatus* (teleomorph).

## SPORES, CONIDIA AND CONIDIOGENESIS

**Spores** are the basic unit of fungal reproduction. They may arise from sexual reproduction (meiosis, meiospores), e.g., zygospores, ascospores and basidiospores, or they may arise from asexual reproduction (mitosis, mitospores). The asexual spores are called *conidia*. The term 'conidia' is derived from the Greek word for dust, *konia*. Sporangiospores contained within a sporangium in Mucorales, and microconidia and macroconidia in dermatophytes are the examples of asexual spores. The conidia are developed from the conidiogenous cells, conidiophores and conidiomata.

Three types of conidia may form from the vegetative mycelium:

- **Blastoconidia:** These are the budding forms characteristically produced by yeasts.
- **Chlamydoconidia:** These are formed from preexistent cells in the hyphae, which become thickened and often enlarged. Chlamydoconidia may be found within (**intercalary**), or at the tip (**terminal**) of the hyphae. This type of conidiation is characteristic of *Candida albicans*.
- **Arthroconidia:** These are also formed from preexistent cells in the hyphae, which become enlarged and thickened. On maturity, these conidia are released by lysis of adjacent cells. This type of conidiation is characteristic of the mold form of *Coccidioides immitis* and *Geotrichum* spp.

### Method of conidiogenesis

It is mainly of two types – **blastic** and **thallic** (Fig. 1.3).

### Thallic conidiogenesis

In this, a septum appears in the hypha before the conidium is initiated. It occurs in molds.

### Blastic conidiogenesis

In this, firstly the new conidium is initiated; it swells or thickens, and then is cut off by a septum. It can occur both in molds and yeasts.

When the wall of the conidium is continuous with the cell that produced it, it is called either holothallic (when thallic) or holoblastic (when blastic).

When only the inner walls of the conidium-bearing cell are involved in conidiogenesis, it is called enterothallic and enteroblastic.

Enterothallic types are rare, and enteroblastic types are probably the most common of all and are represented by the ubiquitous phialide. Multiple conidia are produced **serially** in enteroblastic, whereas they are produced **simultaneously** in rest of the three conidiogenesis types.

Fungi showing different types of conidiogenesis are as follows:

1. Holoblastic – *Trichocladium*
2. Enteroblastic – *Acremonium*, *Bipolaris*, *Penicillium*
3. Holothallic – *Geotrichum*
4. Enterothallic – *Coccidioides*

## CLASSIFICATION OF FUNGI

Robert H Whittaker, an American biologist, in 1969 grouped fungi in a separate kingdom in his Five-Kingdom System, i.e. Monera, Protista, Fungi, Plantae and Animalia. **Kingdom Fungi** includes terrestrial organisms like molds, yeasts and mushrooms, which do not have chlorophyll. Kingdom is the highest taxonomic category. It includes phyla, classes, orders, families, genera and species. The

# SECTION 1 : General Topics

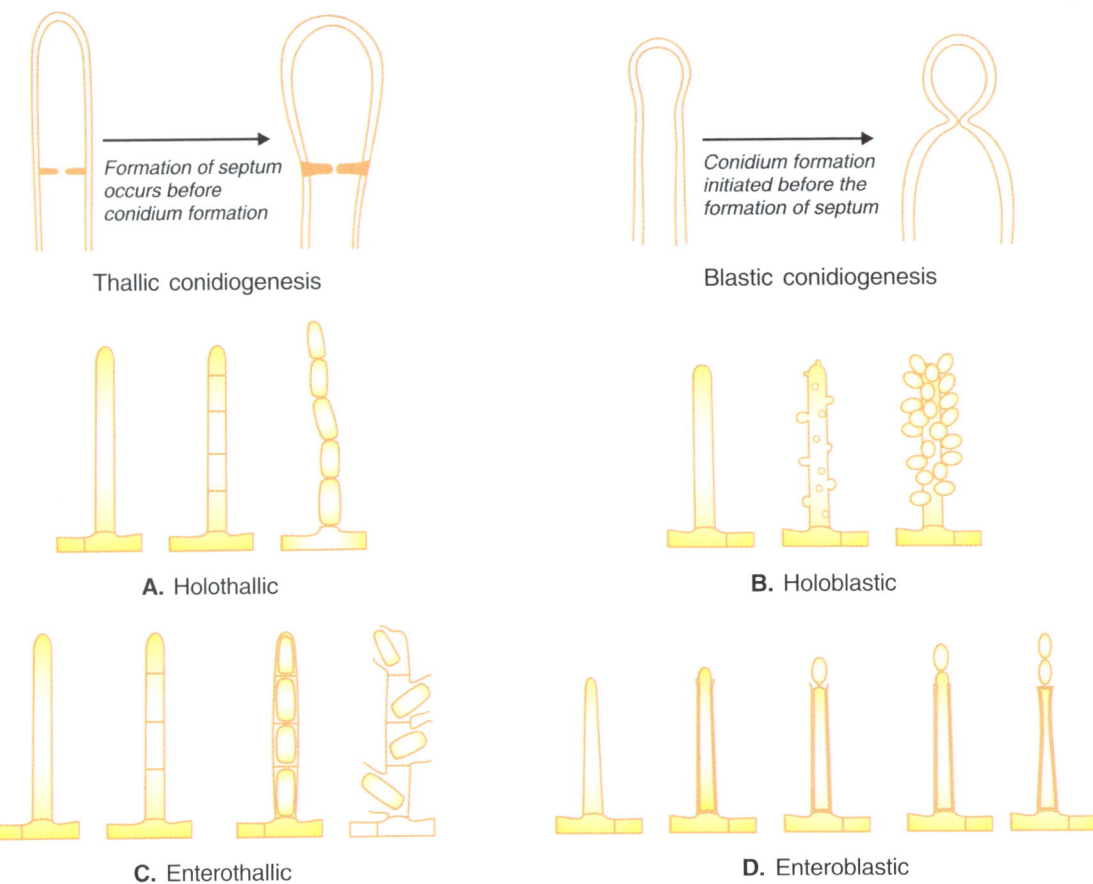

**Fig. 1.3.** Types of conidiogenesis.

endings that are used for various taxonomic levels in the kingdom Fungi are given below:

| | |
|---|---|
| *Kingdom* | Fungi |
| *Phylum* | -mycota |
| *Class* | -mycetes |
| *Order* | -ales |
| *Family* | -aceae |
| *Genus* | — |
| *Species* | — |

King Phillip Can Order Five Green Shirts. (Mnemonics to remember hierarchy of taxonomy)

The classification of kingdom Fungi 2007 is the result of a large scale collaborative research effort. It includes seven phyla within the kingdom Fungi, out of which Ascomycota and Basidiomycota are contained within a subkingdom Dikarya.

The name of a fungus is binomial composed of a generic name and a specific epithet subject to international code of Botanical Nomenclature. The names are usually derived from Latin or Greek and they are often descriptive of the fungus, source of isolation or derived from names of persons. The generic name is always capitalized while the species name is not capitalized – even if it is derived from a name of a country or a person. The names are always underlined when written and italicized when printed. The name of the author who described the species may be indicated after the binomial (e.g., *Aspergillus fumigatus* Fresenius).

## TAXONOMIC CLASSIFICATION

Fungi belong to the kingdom Fungi. The largest category of fungi pathogenic for humans belong to

Holomorph (whole fungus) = Teleomorph (sexual state) + Anamorph (asexual state)

### Dual naming of fungi

*Fungi are classified primarily based on the structures associated with sexual reproduction, which tend to be evolutionarily conserved. However, many fungi reproduce only asexually, and cannot be easily placed in a classification based on sexual characters; some produce both asexual and sexual states. These problematic species are often members of the Ascomycota, but may also belong to the Basidiomycota.*

*As per the Article 59 of the **International Code of Botanical Nomenclature (ICBN)**, mycologists are allowed to give separate names to asexual state (anamorph) and sexual state (teleomorph) of a fungus but this practice will be discontinued as of January 1, 2013, as the International Botanical Congress held in Melbourne in July 2011 made a change in the International Code of Nomenclature for Fungi that adopted the principle **"one fungus, one name"**. In cases where names are available for both anamorph and teleomorph states of the same fungus, the holomorph either takes the teleomorph name, or it can under some circumstances take the anamorph name only if it is subsequently epitypified with a teleomorph.*

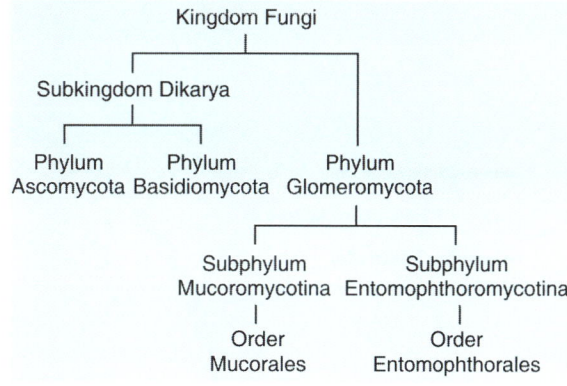

**Fig. 1.4.** Classification of kingdom Fungi.

– their **nonseptate** or **coenocytic hyphae**; and
– formation of **heterokaryotic** zygosporangium, in contrast to Ascomycota and Basidiomycota in which dikaryotic asci and basidia are produced respectively.

There are two types of sexual spores – **zygospores** and **oospores**. Two different haploid mating types are often required for sexual reproduction in the fungi. First, gametangia begin to form on hyphae of different mating types (Fig. 1.5). The gametangia then fuse to form the **heterokaryotic** state resulting in the development of heterokaryotic zygosporangium. The zygosporangium develops a rough and thickened cell wall, which renders it resistant to harsh conditions. When conditions become favorable for **zygospore** germination, the nuclei fuse (karyogamy) and a diploid state is briefly formed. Meiosis immediately follows and millions of haploid zygospores are formed in the sporangium by mitosis. The zygosporangium germinates and releases the spores and the cycle begins again.

**Oospore** result from fertilization of a specialized female structure (**oogonium**) which arises as a side hypha from the main mycelium and contains one or more ova by the sperm or nucleus of a nearby male structure (**antheridium**) (Fig. 1.6). The fertilization tube of the antheridium penetrates the wall of the oogonium and the male nucleus is discharged into the ovum. A thick wall is formed around this zygote and the **oospore** is formed.

the subkingdom Dikarya. It has two phyla – Ascomycota and Basidiomycota. The fungal pathogens previously classed in the phylum Zygomycota are now placed in phylum Glomeromycota, subphyla Mucoromycotina and Entomophthoromycotina. These subphyla contain orders Mucorales and Entomophthorales respectively (Fig. 1.4).

### Glomeromycota

These are most primitive classes of fungi. They are fast growing, widely distributed, terrestrial fungi which are largely saprobic on plant debris and soil. Many species are common environmental contaminants, often causing food spoilage, a few are pathogens of plants, insects, and more rarely of humans. They can be differentiated from other classes of fungi by:

The asexual spores are produced inside a swollen structure called **sporangium** (plural, sporangia) by

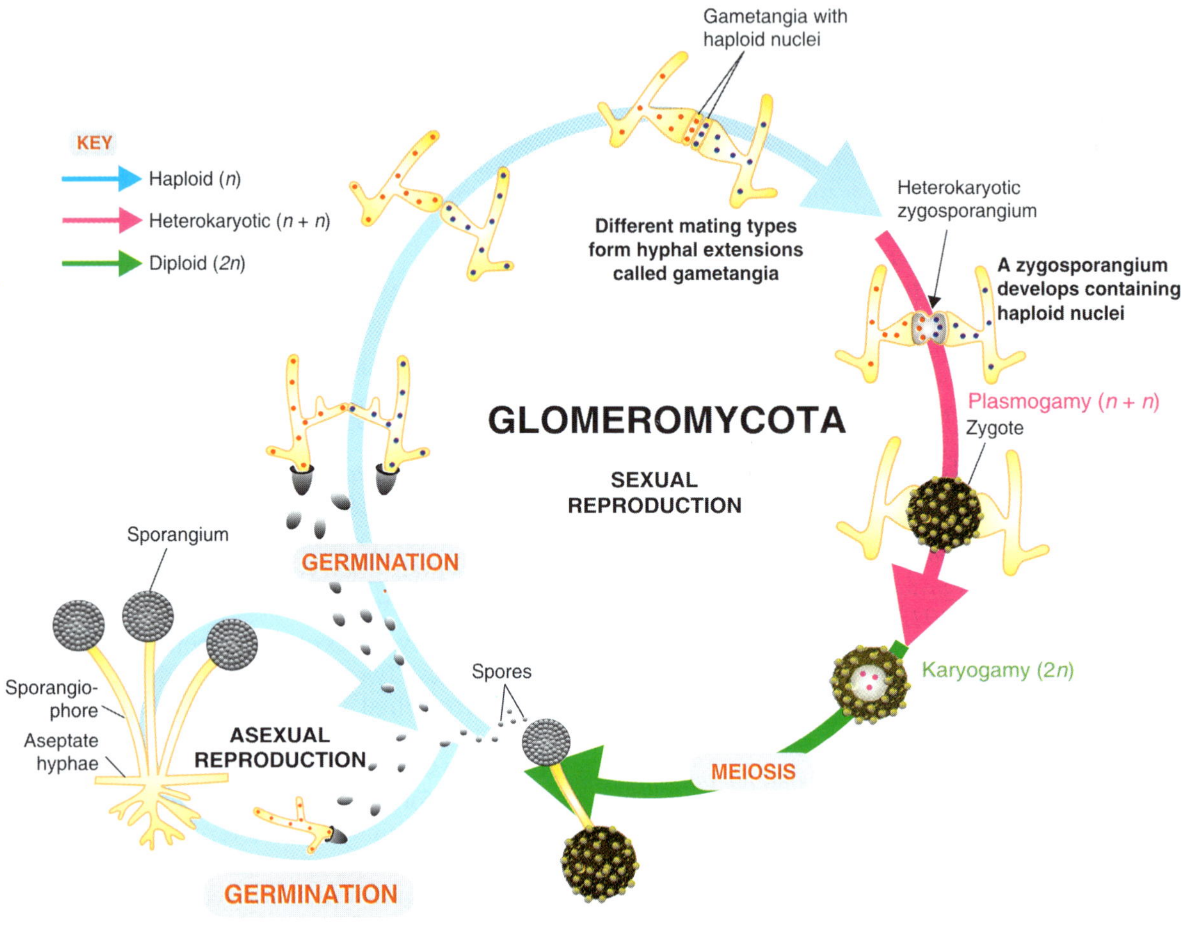

# SECTION 1 : General Topics

**Fig. 1.5.** Life cycle of Glomeromycota.

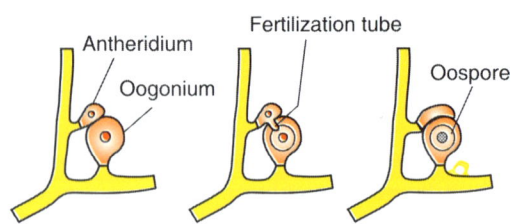

**Fig. 1.6.** Formation of oospores in Mucoromycota.

formation of cleavage planes. They develop on the end of branches or hyphae called **sporangiophores** (Fig. 1.5). The spores are known as **sporangiospores** (endoconidia). The sporangium ruptures, dispersing the sporangiospores and leaving the thin-walled sporangium in place.

### Ascomycota

Ascomycota are the largest, most biologically and morphologically diverse group of fungi.

- The defining morphological character of the phylum Ascomycota is the production of two to eight sexual spores in a microscopic sac-like cell called an **ascus**. Hence, they are sometimes referred to as "**sac fungi**."
- In addition, most Ascomycota bear their asci in macroscopic fruiting bodies called **ascocarps**.
- Ascomycota are also capable of producing enormous amounts of asexual spores called **conidia**, which allow them to propagate without having to undergo sexual recombination.

10

## Introduction, Taxonomy and Classification of Fungi

In the sexual part of the life cycle (Fig. 1.7), two compatible haploid hyphae become intertwined and form an **ascogonium** and an **antheridium**. A very fine hypha, called trichogyne emerges from *ascogonium*, and merges with *antheridium*. The ascogonium acts as a "female" and accepts nucleus from the antheridium after plasmogamy has occurred. The resultant dikaryon is then capable of forming an ascocarp. Asci begin to form on the surface of the ascocarp at the tips of the dikaryotic mycelium, and karyogamy occurs to form the highly transient diploid nucleus. The diploid nucleus immediately undergoes meiosis, yielding four, genetically distinct, haploid nuclei. After an additional round of mitosis, eight haploid nuclei are formed within the ascus. These eight nuclei eventually develop into eight ascospores, which are released from the ascus on the surface of the ascocarp. Finally, haploid mycelia arise from the ascospores as the sexual cycle begins again.

In the asexual part of the life cycle, the haploid mycelium is capable of producing asexual spores (conidia) by segmentation of its hyphae. These segments will compartmentalize into conidia, and wind or water dispersal will follow.

The asexually reproducing phase of the Ascomycota life cycle was more or less ignored for many years in favour of teleomorph studies. But when we

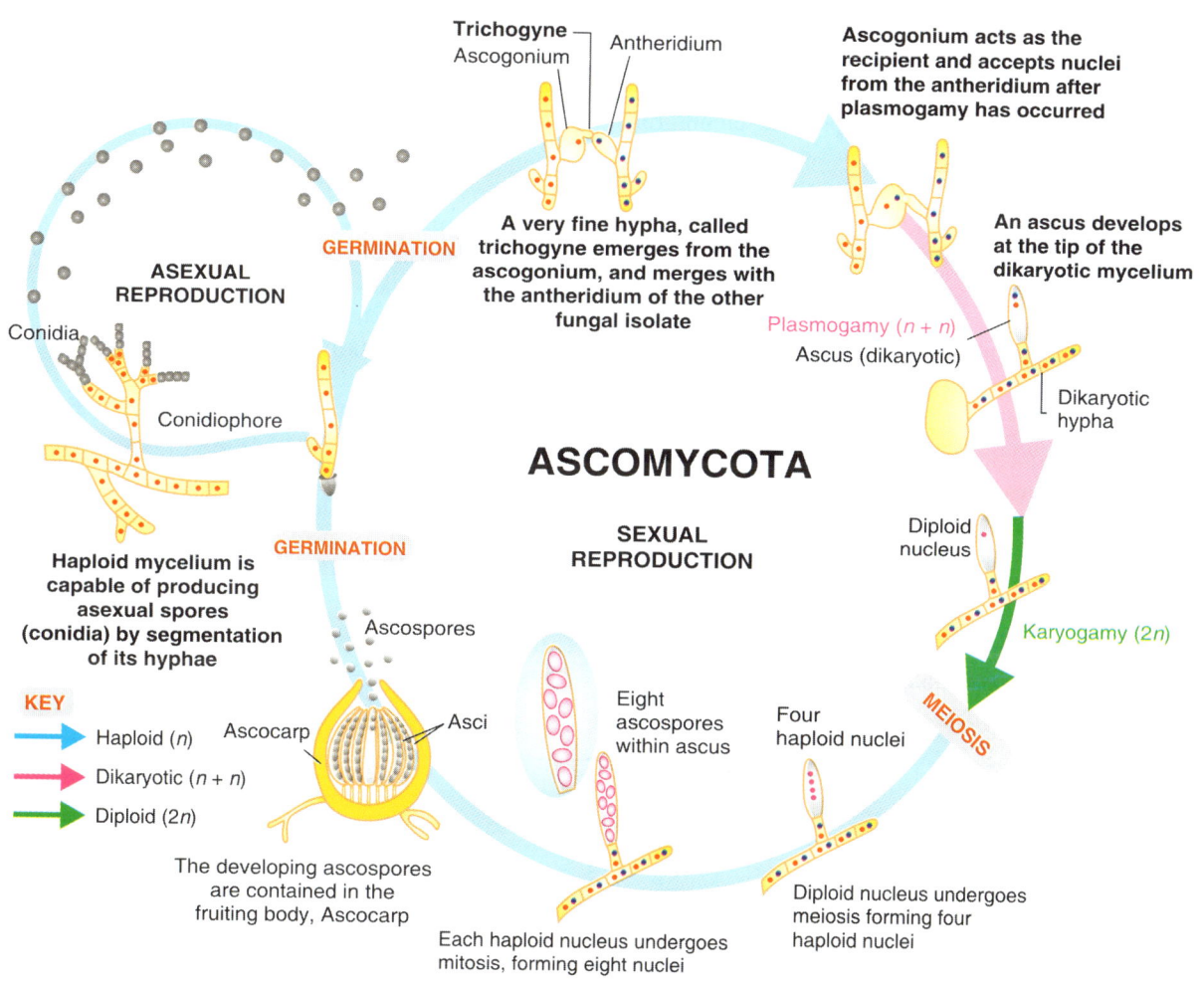

**Fig. 1.7.** Life cycle of Ascomycota.

consider that the anamorph is an important (and sometimes the only) phenotypic expression of many Ascomycota genotypes, we realize that it has much to tell us. Besides, one can get DNA and RNA from anamorphs just as easily as from teleomorphs, so we are beginning to understand the relationships of anamorphs better, even in many cases where no teleomorph is known.

Though they play essentially the same role in the life cycle, the anamorphs of Ascomycota differ from those of Glomeromycota in two very important respects:

1. While in Glomeromycota, sporangiospores originate by free-cell formation inside a sporangium, by cleaving from a single mass of cytoplasm, the conidia of Ascomycota originate either by budding or converted from a whole existing cell.
2. In Glomeromycota, anamorph and teleomorph often develop simultaneously (especially in homothallic species) and always share the same binomial. In Ascomycota, anamorph and teleomorph develop at different time.

## Basidiomycota

These fungi are unicellular or multicellular, sexual or asexual, and terrestrial or aquatic. These are characterized by:

– the production of **basidia** (singular, basidium), on which sexual spores are produced, and from which the group takes its name;
– a long-lived **dikaryon**, in which each cell in the thallus contains two haploid nuclei resulting from a mating event; and
– **clamp connections**, a kind of hyphal outgrowths that is unique to Basidiomycota.

Sexual reproduction (Fig. 1.8) is initiated by the fusion of two haploid hyphae of opposite mating types, and a dikaryon is often formed in which each cell contains two haploid nuclei, one from each partner. The hyphae develop **clamp connections** to ensure that each cell maintains the requisite two nuclei. Karyogamy occurs to form a diploid nucleus in each basidium. The paired nuclei eventually fuse within a terminal clavate or club shaped **basidium**, immediately followed by meiosis and each of four genetically distinct, haploid nuclei migrates into appendages and develops into basidiospores. **Basidiospores** are borne externally at the top of the basidium and each is discharged by hydrostatic forces from the tip of a narrow tapering sterigmata.

*Formation of clamp connection:* Clamp connections are formed by the terminal hypha during elongation. Before the clamp connection is formed this terminal segment contains two nuclei. Once the terminal segment is long enough it begins to form the clamp connection. Simultaneously, each nucleus undergoes mitotic division to produce two daughter nuclei (two red and two blue). As the clamp continues to develop it uptakes one of the daughter nuclei (red) and separates it from its sister nucleus. While this is occurring the remaining nuclei (blue) begin to migrate from one another to opposite ends of the cell. Once all these steps have occurred, a septum forms, separating each set of nuclei (Fig. 1.8).

Medically important fungi belonging to three phyla are given in Table 1.2.

## CLASSIFICATION OF MYCOSES

Infection caused by a fungus is known as **mycosis** (plural, mycoses). It can be divided into four categories:

Table 1.2. Medically important fungi

| Phylum | Fungi |
|---|---|
| Glomeromycota | *Mucor, Rhizopus, Absidia, Rhizomucor, Apophysomyces, Cunninghamella, Saksenaea, Conidiobolus, Syncephalastrum, Basidiobolus* |
| Ascomycota | *Candida, Pneumocystis, Histoplasma, Blastomyces, Paracoccidioides, Emmonsia, Trichophyton, Microsporum, Arthroderma, Epidermophyton, Chrysosporium, Fusarium, Aspergillus, Penicillium, Pseudallescheria, Scedosporium, Chladophialophora, Fonsecaea, Exophiala, Hortaea, Rhinocladiella, Bipolaris, Alternaria* |
| Basidiomycota | *Cryptococcus, Trichosporon, Malassezia* |

# Introduction, Taxonomy and Classification of Fungi

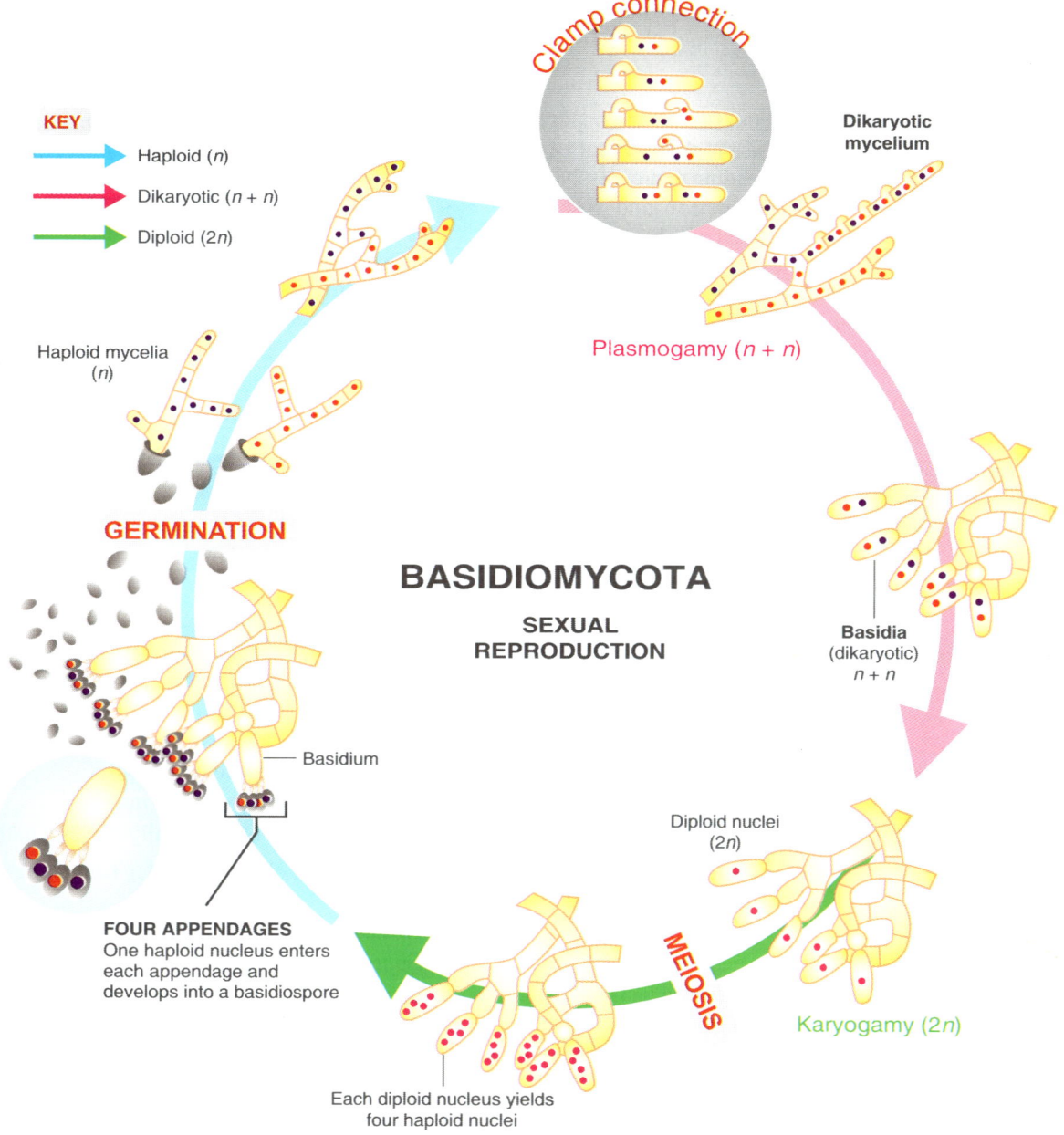

Fig. 1.8. Life cycle of Basidiomycota.

## I. Superficial mycoses

These are strictly surface infections involving skin, hair, nail and mucous membrane. These include:

- Infection of skin, hair and nail caused by dermatophytes.
- Infection of skin, nail and mucous membrane caused by *C. albicans*.
- Infection of skin caused by *Malassezia furfur* (pityriasis versicolor) and *Hortaea werneckii* (tinea nigra).

- Infection of hair caused by *Piedraia hortae* (black piedra) and *Trichosporon* spp. (white piedra).

### II. Subcutaneous mycoses

Mycoses of the skin, subcutaneous tissues and bones result from the inoculation of saprophytic fungi of the soil or decaying vegetation leading to progressive local disease with tissue destruction and sinus formation. The lesion may spread via lymphatics. These occur mainly in the tropics and subtropics. The principal subcutaneous mycoses are mycetoma, chromoblastomycosis, sporotrichosis and rhinosporidiosis.

### III. Systemic mycoses

Systemic mycoses are caused by inhalation of airborne spores produced by the fungi which are present as saprophytes in soil and on plant material. From the lungs the fungus may disseminate to CNS, bone and other internal organs. Systemic mycoses include blastomycosis, histoplasmosis, coccidioidomycosis and paracoccidioidomycosis.

### IV. Opportunistic mycoses

The opportunistic mycoses are infections attributable to fungi that are normally found as human commensals or in the environment. Virtually any fungus can serve as an opportunistic pathogen, and the list of those identified as such becomes longer each year. The most common opportunistic mycoses include aspergillosis, penicilliosis, mucormycosis, candidiasis, cryptococcosis and pneumocytosis.

## PATHOGENESIS

Our understanding of the pathogenesis of fungal infections is limited. Relatively few fungi are sufficiently virulent to be considered **primary pathogens**. Primary pathogens are capable of initiating infection in a normal, apparently immunocompetent host. These include *Blastomyces dermatitidis*, *Coccidioides immitis*, *Histoplasma capsulatum*, and *Paracoccidioides brasiliensis*. These fungi possess virulence factors that allow them to actively breach host defences that ordinarily restrict the invasive growth of other microbes.

Healthy immunocompetent individuals have a high innate resistance to fungal infection, despite the fact that they are constantly exposed to the infectious forms of various fungi present as part of the normal commensal flora (endogenous) or in the environment (exogenous). Important opportunistic fungal pathogens include *Candida* spp., *Cryptococcus neoformans*, and *Aspergillus* spp.

 **Important Questions**

1. Discuss classification of fungi.
2. Tabulate differences between fungi and bacteria.
3. Write short notes on:
   (a) Taxonomic classification of fungi
   (b) Morphological classification of fungi
   (c) Classification of mycoses.

### Multiple Choice Questions

1. Fungi possess:
   (a) a well-defined nucleus.
   (b) mitochondria.
   (c) endoplasmic reticulum.
   (d) All of the above.
2. Which of the following statements is **incorrect** about fungi?
   (a) They are prokaryotic organisms.
   (b) They are devoid of chlorophyll.
   (c) They possess well-defined nuclei.
   (d) They reproduce both sexually and asexually.
3. Fungi have been classified under Kingdom:
   (a) Plantae.
   (b) Animalia.
   (c) Fungi.
   (d) Protista.
4. Genus *Rhizopus* belongs to which of the following phyla?
   (a) Ascomycota.
   (b) Glomeromycota.
   (c) Basidiomycota.
   (d) None of the above.
5. *Penicillium marneffei* is a:
   (a) yeast.
   (b) yeast-like.
   (c) mold.
   (d) dimorphic fungus.

6. Which of the following fungi **does not** possess ergosterol in their plasma membrane?
   (a) *Candida albicans*.
   (b) *Pneumocystis jiroveci*.
   (c) *Blastomyces dermatitidis*.
   (d) *Histoplasma capsulatum*.

7. During sexual reproduction the hyphae develop clamp connections in which of the following fungal phyla?
   (a) Basidiomycota.
   (b) Ascomycota.
   (c) Glomeromycota.
   (d) Deuteromycota.

8. Which of the following scientists is known as "Father of Mycology"?
   (a) Emmons.
   (b) Sabouraud.
   (c) Conant.
   (d) David Gruby.

9. Which of the following fungal diseases is communicable?
   (a) Dermatophytosis.
   (b) Aspergillosis.
   (c) Histoplasmosis.
   (d) Sporotrichosis.

10. Which of the following is **not** true of fungi?
    (a) Eukaryotic.
    (b) Heterotrophic.
    (c) Photosynthetic.
    (d) Mitochondria present.

11. The soil-dwelling mold produces conidia, which when inhaled germinate in the lung as a budding yeast. The fungus is said to be:
    (a) allergenic.
    (b) dimorphic.
    (c) opportunistic.
    (d) thermophilic.

## ANSWERS TO MCQs

1. (d), 2. (a), 3. (c), 4. (b), 5. (d), 6. (b), 7. (a), 8. (b), 9. (a), 10. (c), 11. (b).

## Further Reading

1. Bowman B, Taylor JW, White TJ. Molecular evolution of the fungi: human pathogens. *Mol Biol Evol* 1992; 9: 893–904.
2. Odds FC. Fungal dimorphism. *J Mycol Med* 1998; 8: 55–6.
3. Reis E, Hearn VM, et al. Structure and function of the fungal cell wall. *J Med Vet Mycol* 1992; 30 (Suppl. 1): S143–56.
4. de Hoog GS, Bowman B, et al. Molecular phylogeny and taxonomy of medically important fungi. *Med Mycol* 1998; 36 (Suppl. 1): S52–6.
5. Guarro J, Gene J, Stchigel AM. Developments in fungal taxonomy. *Clin Microbiol Rev* 1999; 12: 454–500.
6. Kwon-Chung KJ. Phylogenetic spectrum of fungi that are pathogenic to humans. *Clin Infect Dis* 1994; 19 (Suppl. 1): S1–7.
7. Prillinger H, Lopandic K, et al. Phylogeny and systematics of the fungi with special reference to the ascomycota and basidiomycota. *Chem Immunol* 2002; 81: 207–95.
8. Taylor J, Jacobson D, Fisher M. The evolution of asexual fungi: reproduction, speciation and classification. *Annu Rev Phytopathol* 1999; 37: 197–246.

# CHAPTER 2

# Epidemiology and Laboratory Diagnosis of Mycoses

## EPIDEMIOLOGY

### Infection in the community

The usual reservoir from which a fungus infects humans is a site in nature where the fungus is growing as saprophyte. Human mycoses are poorly communicable from person to person. Mycoses are often endemic but rarely epidemic. Endemicity occurs in areas where a fungus is more frequent in the environment.

Over the past three decades, the incidence of both nosocomial and community-associated fungal infections has increased dramatically. Factors which have contributed to the increase in fungal infections include a growing population of immunosuppressed or immunocompromised patients whose mechanisms of host defence have been impaired by primary disease states (e.g., AIDS, cancer) and the use of new and aggressive medical and surgical therapeutic strategies, including broad-spectrum antibiotics, cytotoxic chemotherapies, and organ transplantation.

### Venereal transmission

Venereal transmission of blastomycosis and histoplasmosis has been reported. With both these mycoses, vulvovaginal and endometrial lesions have resulted from sexual intercourse with a partner who had disseminated disease. Penile lesions have been present in some, but not all, patients suggesting that fungus can be transmitted in seminal fluid.

### Transplacental transmission

There is no well-documented example of transplacental transmission of any mycosis.

### Infection in the hospital

Patients susceptible to invasive aspergillosis are particularly congregated in oncology, transplantation, and intensive care units of hospitals. Protection against airborne *Aspergillus* conidia can be afforded by high efficiency air filtration, such as occurs in a laminar flow room.

Prevention of candidiasis involves different principle because the usual reservoir is the patient's own body. Decreasing the concentration of *Candida albicans* in the gastrointestinal tract is commonly attempted in the patients with severe and prolonged neutropenia. Such patients are prone to develop haematogenously disseminated candidiasis from numerous small ulcers caused by *Candida* species in the stomach, oesophagus, and intestine. Despite massive oral doses of nystatin, more than a ten- or hundred-fold reduction in *Candida* colonies per gram of stool has proved difficult; prevention of disseminated candidiasis by nystatin has not been convincingly demonstrated.

### Infection in the laboratory

Many ubiquitous fungi, such as *Candida* and *Aspergillus*, can be handled with biosafety level 1 precautions. Working with the mold forms of *Coccidioides immitis* and *Histoplasma capsulatum* requires special precautions. Biosafety levels 3 and 2 should be observed when handling *Coccidioides immitis* and *Histoplasma capsulatum* respectively.

### Precautions with infected laboratory animals

Urine of animals infected with *Cryptococcus neoformans*, *Histoplasma capsulatum* and *Coccidioides immitis* may contain the fungus and contaminate the cage.

### Laboratory-acquired mycoses

Accidental cutaneous inoculation of fungi may occur in laboratory workers as a result of needle sticks, scalpel cuts, or scratches containing infectious material. Local cutaneous granulomata due to the agents of cryptococcosis, blastomycosis, coccidioidomycosis, or histoplasmosis generally resolve spontaneously. Laboratory workers may acquire clinical ringworm while working with dermatophytes or handling guinea pigs experimentally infected with *Trichophyton mentagrophytes*. These lesions are unlikely to resolve spontaneously and usually require treatment.

## LABORATORY DIAGNOSIS OF MYCOSES

Laboratory diagnosis of mycoses depends on:

- Recognition of the pathogen in tissue by microscopy.
- Isolation of the causal fungus in culture.
- Use of serological tests.
- Detection of fungal DNA by the polymerase chain reaction.

Successful laboratory diagnosis of mycoses is dependent not only upon the mycologic expertise of the clinical laboratory workers but also heavily upon the quality of the specimens provided for laboratory analysis. Specimens for the diagnosis of mycoses include skin scrapings, oral scrapings, vaginal scrapings, corneal scrapings, hairs, nails, bone marrow, blood, cerebrospinal fluid, urine, sputum, bronchial lavage specimens, mycetoma grains, pus and tissue.

Specimen should be collected under aseptic conditions, i.e., after appropriate cleaning and decontamination of collection site in a leak-proof sterile container and processed as soon as possible. Anaerobic transport media or anaerobic containers should never be used for fungi. Specimens that contain normal bacterial flora should be transported as soon as possible because bacterial overgrowth can inhibit slower-growing fungi as well as inhibit fungal viability.

If the lesion has a definite edge, the material should be taken from the active margin, otherwise a general scraping is adequate. When blisters are present, a pair of fine scissors may be used to cut off a blister roof for microscopic examination and culture; such samples are often packed with hyphae. The scrapings should be collected and transported in folded paper, which keeps the specimen dry, thus preventing contamination. Hairs to be examined for the presence of black or white piedra may be simply cut off at skin level. If dermatophytosis is suspected, the hairs should be removed with roots intact; cut hairs are unsuitable.

Isolation of the pathogen in culture from nail material is more difficult to achieve than for skin and hair samples. In the majority of nail infections, the material for examination is taken from the distal end of the nail, despite the fact that the infection is advancing proximally. The hyphae at the distal end of the nail are less likely to be viable. Debris from under the nail is a fruitful source of material, which may be scraped out using the flat end of a dental probe. The mouth or vagina may be sampled using a blunt scalpel or by using swabs. Scraping from the external ear canal may be supplemented with swab samples.

When thrush is suspected, the lesions should be scraped gently with a wooden spatula and material transferred to a clean glass slide for wet mount microscopy. With oral lesions, a tongue depressor works well. With vaginal smears, the cervical cytology spatula is useful. Procedure for collection of sputum, bronchial brushing, biopsy and bronchial lavage fluid, cerebrospinal fluid, urine, prostatic secretions and exudates is given in Table 2.1.

Culturing the centrifuged sediment from 50–100 ml urine may yield *Cryptococcus neoformans*, *Blastomyces dermatitidis*, *Histoplasma capsulatum* and *Coccidioides immitis* in the presence of disseminated infection, even without clinical evidence of genitourinary infection.

**Table 2.1.** Procedure for collection of specimen for fungus culture

| Specimen | Procedure |
|---|---|
| Sputum | The first early-morning sample should be collected after vigorously rinsing mouth with water followed by coughing of sputum into a sterile, screw-capped container. |
| Bronchoscopy | Bronchial brushing, biopsy or broncho-alveolar lavage fluid should be transported promptly to the laboratory in a sterile, sealed container. |
| Cerebrospinal fluid (CSF) | As much CSF as possible should be used for the culture of fungi. If processing is to be delayed, the sample should be left at room temperature in an adequate fluid culture medium in which fungal elements can survive until subcultured. |
| Urine | Mid-stream urine specimen should be collected aseptically in sterile screw-capped container. If a delay in processing beyond 2 hours is anticipated, the urine sample should be refrigerated at 4°C to inhibit overgrowth of rapidly growing bacteria. |
| Prostatic secretions | The bladder is first emptied, followed by prostatic massage. Secretions should be inoculated directly into appropriate fungal culture media. If secretions are not obtained then 5–10 ml of urine be collected and processed. |
| Exudates | The skin over pustular lesions should be disinfected and exudates aspirated using a sterile needle and syringe. Hair, nails, and skin scrapings may be stored up to 72 hours at room temperature before culture, and they may be shipped by mail. |

The clinical information is very important in guiding the laboratory in terms of specimen processing and interpretation of results. This is especially important when dealing with specimens from non-sterile sites such as sputum, bronchial washings and skin. Furthermore, it alerts the laboratory personnel that they may be dealing with potentially dangerous pathogen such as *Coccidioides immitis*. If delay in processing is unavoidable, the specimen for fungal culture may be stored at 4°C for a short time. Specimens not likely to contain contaminating microorganisms, e.g., **spinal fluid should not be refrigerated**. Causative agents of mycoses can be identified by following methods:

## I. Direct microscopic examination of specimens

The direct microscopic examination of clinical specimen may be as simple as placing a drop of liquid specimen onto a clean glass slide and examining it with light microscope, or it may involve more complex procedures, including staining of tissue. Although, the Gram stain performed in the routine microbiology laboratory often gives the first evidence of infection with yeast, other direct stains give more specific information concerning a mold infection. The types of direct examination used in identification of fungal infections include wet preparation such as KOH preparation, KOH with calcofluor white, India ink, and tissue stains such as periodic acid-Schiff (PAS) stain, Gomori methenamine silver (GMS) stain, Giemsa stain, and haematoxylin and eosin (H&E) stain.

### *KOH preparation*

A 10–20% solution of KOH is useful for detecting fungal elements in skin, hair, nails, and tissue. In this procedure, KOH is mixed in equal proportions with the specimen on a slide and the specimen material is teased with two inoculating needles. A coverslip is placed over it and heated gently. Preparation with KOH clears the tissue and cellular debris from all types of clinical specimens without damaging the fungal cells. This clearing process requires only 5–10 minutes, after which one can observe the fungal morphology as well as the pigment of the fungal cell wall under a phase-contrast or bright-field microscope, using low-power followed by high-power objectives.

Nail specimens take longer to clear, but if small pieces and debris are taken, they will usually soften within 10 minutes. In those instances, where the nails do not soften satisfactorily, the slide may be put in a 37°C incubator for one hour, and the material then be flattened. In contrast to skin and nail samples, infected hairs are very delicate, and if heated or left in mounting fluid for more than a few minutes tend to disintegrate, obscuring the characteristic arrangement of the arthroconidia. They should, therefore, be examined as soon as possible after mounting.

Reaction of KOH with pus, sputum, and skin may produce artifacts that superficially resemble hyphae or budding forms of fungi. Therefore, experience is required in interpreting the results. Moreover, crystals can form on standing, so that reading of the smear becomes difficult.

With KOH preparation, a definitive diagnosis of blastomycosis, paracoccidioidomycosis, coccidioidomycosis, mycetoma, phaeohyphomycosis, lobomycosis or rhinosporidiosis can be made. Tentative diagnosis can be derived from the presence of fungal elements compatible to the etiologic agents of aspergillosis, mucormycosis, dermatophytosis, candidiasis, sporotrichosis, or cryptococcosis. To confirm such a diagnosis, however, culture proof is necessary.

### KOH with calcofluor white

A drop of 0.1% calcofluor white solution (fluorescent reagent) can be added to the KOH preparation prior to placing coverslip over it. Calcofluor white binds to polysaccharide present in the chitin of the fungus or to cellulose. Fungal elements fluoresce apple green or blue-white, depending on the combination of filters used. The actual fungal structure must be seen before a positive preparation is reported.

### India ink

India ink preparations may be used for detecting encapsulated yeast *Cryptococcus neoformans* in cerebrospinal fluid (CSF). A drop of India ink is mixed with a drop of centrifuged deposit of CSF, and the preparation is examined under high power. With the negative stain, budding yeast surrounded by a large clear area against a dark background is presumptive evidence of *C. neoformans*. White blood cells and other artifacts may resemble encapsulated organisms; therefore, careful examination is necessary.

The morphologic characteristics of fungi seen on direct microscopic examination include budding yeasts, hyphae and pseudohyphae. *Rhizopus*, *Mucor* and *Lichtheimia* (*Absidia*) characteristically show broad, ribbon-like, nonseptate hyphae. Dematiaceous fungi show darkly pigmented yeast-like and hyphal forms.

### Tissue stains

The diagnosis of fungal diseases should preferably be established on the basis of histopathologic evidence combined with cultural evidence, because detection of fungi in tissue and confirmation of tissue invasion are required in diagnosing many opportunistic fungal infections. For example, isolation of common fungi such as *Aspergillus*, *Penicillium*, and *Rhizopus* species from sputum does not establish pulmonary infection by these fungi unless there is also histopathological evidence. Moreover, certain mycoses, e.g., rhinosporidiosis, lobomycosis, and *Pneumocystis jirovecii* infection can only be diagnosed by histologic studies since growth conditions of the fungi causing these infections have not been defined.

Histopathologic procedures are rapid and relatively inexpensive. Because of the size, characteristic morphology, and staining properties of many fungi, histopathologic studies often yield a presumptive diagnosis. There are several mycoses in which etiologic agents can be identified to the generic level because the morphologic characteristics are distinctive to the genus involving several species, e.g., aspergillosis and candidiasis.

**Haematoxylin and eosin (H&E) stain** used routinely in the pathology laboratory is often not adequate for detecting fungal elements. Many fungi stain poorly and some fungi do not stain at all with H&E. However, with this stain the tissue response can be demonstrated better than with any special stain and the innate colour of the fungal elements, whether dematiaceous or hyaline, can be determined.

No specific inflammatory reaction is characteristic of any particular mycotic agent. A single etiologic agent can elicit more than one type of tissue response and many different fungi can cause identical tissue responses. H&E procedure stains *Leishmania donovani*, *Toxoplasma gondii*, and *Trypanosoma cruzi*, which can be confused with *Histoplasma capsulatum*. This problem can be avoided by using special stains for fungi.

Special stains used in the histologic section for detection of fungal elements are Gomori methenamine silver (GMS), Gridley fungus (GF), periodic acid-Schiff (PAS), Giemsa, Mayer's mucicarmine and alcian blue stains.

- **The GMS staining procedure** provides better contrast between the fungi and background tissue. This procedure results in the brownish black coloration of all forms of viable and non-viable fungal cells. Extracellular capsule and intracellular details are not visible by this method. The GMS stain is the best special fungal stain for screening and H&E is the best for studying the tissue response to etiologic agents.
- **The GF stain** colours fungal cells purplish red with a yellow background. Mucin and elastic tissue are also stained purplish red. Non-viable fungi at the time of fixation may not be stained.
- **The PAS stain** is one of the most widely used stains for fungal histopathology. Aldehydes produced by the oxidation of fungal polysaccharide react with periodic acid and colour the fungi pinkish red. In old caseous foci of histoplasmosis, yeast cells may be stained by GMS but not by PAS.
- **Giemsa stain** is used primarily to detect *Histoplasma capsulatum* in blood or bone marrow.
- **Mayer's mucicarmine and alcian blue procedures** stain the mucopolysaccharide capsule of *Cryptococcus* spp. red and blue respectively. These stains, therefore, are useful in differentiating cryptococci from the other fungi of similar size and appearance, although, these stains are not specific for cryptococci. *Rhinosporidium seeberi* and some cells of *Blastomyces dermatitidis* are also variably stained with mucicarmine. *R. seeberi*, however, produces endoconidia within the large spherules and should not be mistaken for *C. neoformans*.
- **Acid-fast staining** is useful for detecting *Nocardia* spp. and for differentiating them from other aerobic actinomycetes. *Nocardia* spp. exhibit partial acid-fastness. Some of the filaments stain red with carbol-fuchsin staining, while others may appear blue because of a counterstain effect. *Nocardia asteroides* and *Streptomyces* spp. are used as positive and negative controls respectively.

Applications and limitations of staining techniques for demonstrating fungi and related pathogens in tissue sections are given in Table 2.2.

### Disadvantages of special stains

1. They mask the innate colour of fungal elements, making it impossible to determine whether a fungus is hyaline or phaeoid. Such a determination may be crucial to the diagnosis of a mycosis caused by pigmented fungi, e.g., phaeohyphomycosis, chromoblastomycosis, and black grain eumycotic mycetomas. Therefore, duplicate H&E stained or unstained tissue sections, should always be examined to look for brown pigmentation of fungal cell walls.
2. They do not allow adequate study of the host reaction to fungal invasion. To avoid this limitation, H&E can be used as the counterstain for the GMS procedure. This combination of stains (GMS-H&E) readily colour fungal elements brownish-black while staining background tissue components as expected. Thus it is possible simultaneously to detect the fungus and to evaluate the host's inflammatory response and its relationship to the fungus. When only a single unstained section from a suspected lesion is available for examination, GMS-H&E is the best stain combination for attempting to make a diagnosis. Tissue sections stained with Giemsa, PAS, and GF procedures can be decolorized in acid alcohol after the coverslip has been removed and then restained with GMS.

## II. Culture

For some of the superficial mycoses such as pityriasis versicolor and, to a lesser degree, black piedra, white piedra and tinea nigra, the appearance of the fungal elements observed on direct examination is so

**Table 2.2.** Applications and limitations of staining techniques for demonstrating fungi and related pathogens in tissue sections

| Stain/Method | Applications | Limitations |
|---|---|---|
| Haematoxylin and eosin (H&E) | • Tissue response can be demonstrated better than with any other stain.<br>• Innate colour of the fungal elements whether phaeoid (pigmented) or hyaline, can be determined.<br>• Haematoxylin stains nuclei of most yeast-like cells.<br>• Some fungi, e.g., the aspergilli and Mucorales are haematoxylinophilic and are readily delineated with H&E. | • Does not stain many fungi or stain poorly. Even in the instance of poor staining careful examination often reveals the outlines of unstained fungal elements, which suggest the existence of fungal infection.<br>• Inadequate to screen for sparse fungal elements. |
| Gomori methenamine silver (GMS) | • Provides better contrast between the fungi and background tissue.<br>• This procedure results in the brownish black coloration of all forms of viable and non-viable fungal cells. | • GMS may overstain fungi and obscure internal details.<br>• Does not allow proper study of host response. |
| Gridley's fungus (GF) | • Colours fungal cells purplish red with a yellow background.<br>• Mucin and elastic tissue are also stained purplish red. | • Non-viable fungi at the time of fixation may not be stained.<br>• Does not allow proper study of host response.<br>• Fungi stained with GF stain tend to fade with prolonged storage. |
| Periodic acid-Schiff (PAS) | • Colours the fungi pinkish red. | • In old caseous foci of histoplasmosis, yeast cells may be stained by GMS but not by PAS. |
| Mayer's mucicarmine, and Alcian blue staining | • Stain mucopolysaccharide capsular material of *Cryptococcus neoformans*. | • Not specific for *Cryptococcus neoformans*. They may also stain *Rhinosporidium seeberi* and some cells of *Blastomyces dermatitidis*. |
| Gram stain (Brown and Brenn) | • Demonstrates Gram-positive filaments of actinomycetes, e.g., *Actinomyces, Nocardia, Actinomadura*, etc.<br>• Demonstrates causative agents of botryomycosis.<br>• Some fungi, especially the yeast forms of *Candida* spp. and the conidia of *Aspergillus* spp. are usually Gram-positive. | • Do not selectively stain most fungi (those that do stain are Gram-positive). |
| Modified Ziehl-Neelsen stain | • Useful to detect *Nocardia asteroides, N. brasiliensis* and *N. otitidiscaviarum*.<br>• As the *Nocardia* spp. are weakly acid-fast and non-alcohol-fast in tissue sections, these filamentous bacteria can be distinguished from the agents of actinomycosis with modified Ziehl-Neelsen stain that uses a weak aqueous solution consisting of 0.5 or 1% sulphuric acid for decolourization. The nocardiae are weakly acid-fast, whereas the agents of actinomycosis are not acid-fast.<br>• The cytoplasm of certain fungi with yeast-like tissue forms, especially *Blastomyces dermatitidis* and *Histoplasma Capsulatum* var. *capsulatum* is also variably acid-fast. | • Most fungal cells and the agents of actinomycosis are not acid-fast. |

*(Contd.)*

| Stain/Method | Applications | Limitations |
|---|---|---|
| Calcofluor white | • Stains cell walls of most fungi including *Pneumocystis jirovecii*. | • Requires a fluorescence microscope.<br>• May not stain degenerated fungi. |
| Fluorescent monoclonal antibody treatment | • Examination of respiratory specimen for *Pneumocystis jirovecii*. | • Sensitive and specific method for detecting the cysts of *Pneumocystis jirovecii*. Does not stain trophozoites or trophic forms. |

characteristic that culture is not strictly necessary for the diagnosis of infection. On the other hand, for otomycosis, culture is essential, as the range of organisms that cause infection is enormous, and the specific identification of the pathogen will have profound effect on the therapy selected. In case of dermatophyte infections, on direct examination of skin and nail scrapings different species are indistinguishable. Generally, all the dermatophyte species are believed to respond similarly to the major systemic and topical antifungals available, and treatment is initiated on the basis of direct examination. However, this may not be true with some of the more recent antifungals developed.

Optimal recovery of medically important fungi from clinical specimens is related to multiple factors. The first is the specimen itself, which must be freshly collected and appropriate for the mycotic infection being considered. In general, there are fewer fungal cells at the site of an infection than there are bacterial cells in a bacterial infection. Therefore, enough specimen must be cultured to ensure optimal recovery. **Fluids**, e.g., peritoneal fluid, pericardial fluid and CSF in volumes of >1–2 ml should be concentrated by centrifugation and the sediment should be inoculated on the culture media. Alternatively, the specimen may be filtered through a 0.45 µm pore size membrane filter, and the filter can then be cultured. Most fungi will not survive the 2% NaOH treatment used for recovery of mycobacteria.

Most pathogenic fungi are easy to grow in culture. **Sabouraud dextrose agar** (SDA) is most commonly used. This may be supplemented with chloramphenicol (50 mg/l) to minimize bacterial contamination and cycloheximide (500 mg/l) to reduce contamination with saprophytic fungi. Cycloheximide should not be added to all media because the growth of *Cryptococcus* spp., *Candida* spp., *Trichosporon* spp., *Aspergillus* spp., Mucorales, hyalohyphomycetes, yeast phase of *Histoplasma capsulatum*, *Blastomyces dermatitidis* and *Paracoccidioides brasiliensis* are completely or partially inhibited by it. Chloramphenicol is likely to prevent the growth of aerobic actinomycetes; therefore, if *Nocardia* or any other filamentous bacteria are suspected, it is necessary to inoculate media lacking it. Special (differential) media may be used for isolation and to help rapid identification when the identity of a particular fungus is strongly suspected. For example, *C. neoformans* develops black colonies on **bird seed agar**.

Specimens for the isolation of fungi are inoculated on slants or agar plates. For isolating discrete colonies, culture plates are more useful than slants, because the plates have a larger surface area. However, the plates are more susceptible to laboratory contamination and must be taped with an oxygen-permeable tape. When slants are used, the culture tube should be large enough (2 × 15 cm) to provide a wide surface area for growth. The screw caps should be left loosened during incubation to permit an adequate supply of oxygen.

Many fungal pathogens have an optimum growth temperature below 37°C. For molds, the temperature of incubation should be 25–30°C, and for *Candida* spp., the temperature of incubation should be 37°C. With some dimorphic pathogens, enriched media such as **brain-heart infusion agar** or **blood agar** are used to promote growth of yeast phase. Many fungi grow relatively slowly and cultures should be retained for at least 2–4 weeks before being discarded.

Growth of *Candida*, *Aspergillus*, *Mucor* and *Rhizopus* species appears within 24–72 hours. Therefore, fungal cultures should be examined for growth daily for the 1st week, three times for the 2nd week, twice for the 3rd week, and once for the 4th week rather than being evaluated once at the end of 4 weeks. Plates must be opened inside a certified biological cabinet to prevent contamination of plate and exposure of personnel to potentially dangerous fungi. Tubed media have a smaller surface area but offer maximum safety and resistance to dehydration and contamination.

It is important to use media with and without inhibitory agents. Specimens from normally sterile sites can be inoculated on media without inhibitory substances. Selective media should be tested with strains known to be sensitive and resistant to the inhibitory agent in the media, while the differential media should be evaluated with fungi that produce both positive and negative reactions.

Once an organism has grown, it is examined for characteristic gross and microscopic structures, so that identification can be made. Pigment on the reverse side of the colony or in aerial mycelium is noted. For microscopic examination **slide mounts** should be made in **lactophenol cotton blue** (LPCB). On occasion, a **slide culture** may be prepared (see Appendix A), when the initial isolate fails to show conidial morphology. Many molds begin as white mycelial growths, coloration occurs at the time of conidiation or sporulation. Characteristics that should be observed are septate versus nonseptate hyphae, hyaline or dematiaceous hyphae, and the types, size, shape, colour and arrangement of conidia. Identification of medically important fungi is given in Table 2.3.

## III. Serological tests

Positive fungal cultures can be difficult to obtain – the yield being low, growth often slow, and taking biopsy from a deep infected site may be difficult or impossible. Therefore, serological tests have been developed for the diagnosis of fungal infections. Tests for antibody have an established diagnostic use in coccidioidomycosis, paracoccidioidomycosis, aspergillosis, blastomycosis, and in some patients with histoplasmosis.

Serological tests have been developed commercially for detecting cryptococcal and *Candida* antigens. Detection of polysaccharide cryptococcal antigen in serum and cerebrospinal fluid by latex agglutination is a method of choice for the rapid diagnosis of meningitis and disseminated infection caused by *C. neoformans*. The most widely used is the assay for the detection of *Histoplasma* antigen. This test has proven useful for the detection of antigenemia in patients having disseminated disease, particularly those with acquired immunodeficiency syndrome.

Serological tests for the detection of fungal antibodies and fungal antigens are given in Table 2.4.

### Molecular testing

- **In situ hybridization:** One of the simplest approaches used has been in situ hybridization using specific nucleic acid probes for identification of organisms in patient specimens.
- **Polymerase chain reaction:** Amplification assays using the polymerase chain reaction allow for the detection of small amounts of target DNA in clinical specimens. Specific primers with or without specific probes have been used with some success. Assays have been developed to detect DNA of *Candida*, *Aspergillus*, *Fusarium*, *Cryptococcus*, *Histoplasma*, *Blastomyces*, *Paracoccidioides*, *Pneumocystis jirovecii* and *Penicillium marneffei*.

## MICROBIOLOGICAL SAFETY CABINETS

Microbiological safety cabinets provide a barrier between the worker and the infective material and are designed to prevent infection by splashing or aerosol.

### Class 1

These cabinets are open-fronted. These rely on the walls, glass upper front and integral tray to contain spills and splashes. An inward airflow provides a protection factor of at least $1.5 \times 10^5$; this factor represents the number of particles which, if liberated into the air of the cabinet, will not escape into the room. The air-borne particles are contained within the cabinet and filtered from the exhaust air through a HEPA (high efficiency particulate air) filter.

Table 2.3. Identification of medically important fungi

| Hyaline | | | Mold colonies | | Dematiaceous | | Yeast colonies | Yeast-like colonies |
|---|---|---|---|---|---|---|---|---|
| Growth in < 3 days | Growth in 3–5 days | Growth in > 5 days | Growth in 3–5 days | Growth in > 5 days | Growth in 3–5 days | Growth in > 5 days | Growth in 2–5 days | Growth in 2–5 days |
| Hyphae broad and nonseptate **Mucorales** • *Mucor* • *Rhizopus* • *Lichtheimia (Absidia)* • *Syncephalastrum* • *Cunninghamela* | Hyphae hyaline and septate **Agents of hyalohyphomycosis** Conidia in chains: • *Aspergillus* • *Penicillium* • *Paecilomyces* • *Scopulariopsis* Conidia in clusters: • *Acremonium* • *Fusarium* • *Trichoderma* • *Gliocladium* Conidia borne singly: • *Scedosporium apiospermum* • *Scedosporium prolificans* • *Chryosporium* • *Spedonium* | Hyphae hyaline and slender Colonies often granular and pigmented; hyphae hyaline and septate **Dermatophyte** • *Trichophyton* spp. • *Microsporum* spp. • *Epidermophyton floccosum* | Hyphae hyaline and slender Growth on cycloheximide agar Yeast forms when incubated at 37°C **Dimorphic fungi:** • *Blastomyces dermatitidis* • *Coccidioides immitis* • *Histoplasma capsulatum* • *Sporothrix schenckii* • *Paracoccidioides brasiliensis* | Dark colony; black reverse; hyphae yellow-pigmented and septate **Agents of phaeohyphomycosis** Conidia have both transverse and longitudinal septa: • *Alternaria* spp. Conidia divided by transverse septa only: • *Curvularia* spp. • *Bipolaris* spp. • *Exserohilum* spp. | Dark colony; black reverse; hyphae yellow-pigmented and septate **Agents of chromoblastomycosis** **Cladosporium-type sporulation:** • *Cladophialophora carrionii* • *Cladophialophora bantiana* **Phialophora-type sporulation:** • *Phialophora verrucosa* **Acrotheca-type sporulation:** • *Fonsecaea pedrosoi* • *Fonsecaea compacta* **Agent of mycetoma** **Phialophora-type sporulation:** • *Exophiala jeensemei* | Smooth, pasty or mucoid colonies **Yeast and yeast-like** • *Candida albicans* • *Cryptococcus neoformans* • *Rhodotorula* • *Malassezia furfur* | Yeast-like colonies with low aerial mycelium **Arthroconidia produced:** • *Geotrichum candidum* • *Trichosporon* spp. |

# Epidemiology and Laboratory Diagnosis of Mycoses

**Table 2.4.** Serological tests for detection of fungal antibodies and fungal antigens

| Tests for detection of fungal antibodies | Tests for detection of fungal antigens |
| --- | --- |
| • Immunodiffusion<br>• Counter immuno-electrophoresis<br>• Whole cell agglutination<br>• Complement fixation<br>• Enzyme-linked immuno-sorbent assay (ELISA) | • Latex agglutination<br>• ELISA |

*Class 2*

These cabinets are also open-fronted, but are designed to prevent air-borne contamination of the work materials and reduce exposure of the operator to particles dispersed within the cabinet. These objectives are achieved by recirculating filtered air over the work area while maintaining an inflow of air through the working aperture. Some of the air is exhausted through a HEPA filter.

*Class 3*

These cabinets are totally enclosed and separate the operator from the work by an airtight barrier. These are scavenged by air entering and leaving through HEPA filters, the air pressure in the cabinet being kept less than that in the room.

Biosafety level 2 (BSL 2) practices are recommended for handling and processing clinical specimens, identifying isolates, and processing animal tissues suspected of containing pathogenic fungi. BSL 2 is also sufficient for mold cultures of *Blastomyces dermatitidis*, *Histoplasma capsulatum*, *Cryptococcus neoformans*, *Penicillium marneffei*, *Sporothrix schenckii*, *Bipolaris* spp., *Cladophialophora bantiana*, *Wangiella dermatitidis*, *Exserohilum* spp., *Fonsecaea pedrosoi*, *Ochroconis gallopava*, and *Scedosporium prolificans*.

BSL 3 conditions should be observed when working with mold-form cultures identified as *Coccidioides* spp. and *Histoplasma capsulatum*.

 **Important Questions**

1. Discuss in detail laboratory diagnosis of mycoses.
2. Discuss briefly staining techniques used for identification of fungi in tissue sections. Give merits and demerits of each.
3. Discuss applications and limitations of staining techniques for demonstrating fungi and related pathogens in tissue sections.

## Multiple Choice Questions

1. Which of the following fungi is potentially dangerous to the laboratory workers?
   (a) *Candida albicans*.
   (b) *Cryptococcus neoformans*.
   (c) *Coccidioides immitis*.
   (d) *Trichophyton rubrum*.

2. India ink preparation may be used for detecting
   (a) *Cryptococcus neoformans*.
   (b) *Candida albicans*.
   (c) *Trichosporon*.
   (d) *Geotrichum*.

3. For the culture of molds the temperature of incubation should be
   (a) 20–22°C.
   (b) 25–30°C.
   (c) 30–32°C.
   (d) 35–37°C.

4. Which of the following statements is **incorrect** for haematoxylin and eosin staining for the diagnosis of fungal infections?
   (a) Tissue response can be demonstrated better than with any other stain.
   (b) Does not stain many fungi or stain poorly.
   (c) Innate colour of the fungal elements whether phaeoid or not can be determined.
   (d) Adequate to screen for sparse fungal elements.

5. How will you process CSF specimen for the diagnosis of fungal infection?
   (a) Centrifuge and place a drop of sediment in India ink preparation and examine under microscope.
   (b) Centrifuge and inoculate sediment on Sabouraud dextrose agar.
   (c) Inoculate a drop of sediment on bird seed agar.
   (d) All the above.

## ANSWERS TO MCQs

1. (c), 2. (a), 3. (b), 4. (d), 5. (d).

### Further Reading

1. Alexander BD. Diagnosis of fungal infection: new technologies for the mycology laboratory. *Transpl Infect Dis* 2002; 4 (Suppl. 3): 32–7.
2. Balajee SA, Sigler L, Brandt ME. DNA and the classical way: identification of medically important molds in the 21st century. *Med Mycol* 2007; 45: 475–90.
3. Chakrabarti A, Kaur R, Das S. Molecular methods in diagnosis and epidemiology of fungal infections. *Indian J Med Microbiol* 2000; 18: 146–52.
4. de Repentigny L, Kaufman L, et al. Immunodiagnosis of invasive fungal infections. *J Med Vet Mycol* 1994; 32 (Suppl. 1): S239–52.
5. Fussl R. Diagnosis of fungal infections. Mycoses 1997; 40 (Suppl. 2): S13–5.
6. Guanzli C, Meihua F, Weida L. Study on detection and identification of pathogenic fungi by PCR. *J Clin Dermatol* 2000; 29: 264–6.
7. Harrington BJ, Hageage GJ. Calcofluor white: a review of its uses and applications in clinical mycology and parasitology. *Lab Med* 2003; 34: 361–7.
8. Kappe R, Seeliger HP. Serodiagnosis of deep-seated fungal infections. *Curr Top Med Mycol* 1993; 5: 247–80.
9. Lindsley MD, Hurst SF, et al. Rapid identification of dimorphic and yeast-like fungal pathogens using specific DNA probes. *J Clin Microbiol* 2001; 39: 3505–11.
10. Makimura K, Murayama SY, Yamaguchi H. Detection of a wide range of medically important fungi by polymerase chain reaction. *J Med Microbiol* 1994; 40: 358–64.
11. Pincus DH, Orenga S, Chatellier S. Yeast identification: past, present and future methods. *Med Mycol* 2007; 45: 97–121.
12. Verweij PE. Advances in diagnostic testing. *Med Mycol* 2005; 43 (Suppl. 1): S121–4.
13. Yeo SF, Wong B. Current status of nonculture methods for diagnosis of invasive fungal infections. *Clin Microbiol Rev* 2002; 15: 465–84.

# CHAPTER 3

# Antifungal Drugs

Fungal infections (mycoses) are widespread and there has been a steady increase in the incidence of serious secondary systemic fungal infections since 1970s. The major contributory factors which predispose patients to invasive fungal infections are the use of broad-spectrum antibiotics, corticosteroids, anti-cancer/immunosuppressive drugs, denture, in-dwelling catheters and implants, and emergence of AIDS. As a result of breakdown of host defence mechanisms, saprophytic fungi easily invade the living tissue. Elderly people, diabetics, burn wound victims and pregnant ladies are particularly at risk of developing fungal infections such as candidiasis.

Fungi are also important nosocomial pathogens causing severe morbidity and mortality in hospitalized patients with a combination of a variety of risk factors and immunosuppression. Systemic infections caused by *Candida* spp. other than *C. albicans*, *Aspergillus* spp., and other filamentous fungi (molds) are being reported more frequently. As fungal infections became an important public health problem and resistance to established antifungal agents began to emerge, pharmaceutical companies developed new agents with either a broader spectrum or different targets of activity.

Unlike the development of antibacterial agents, to date relatively few drug targets in fungi have been exploited in the development of currently available antifungal agents. Antibacterial agents have taken advantage of multiple targets available in bacteria that are not present in mammalian cells. Fungi have similarities to mammalian cells that have made the search for antifungal targets difficult. Nevertheless, hosts and fungal cells do have some significant differences, and effective therapeutic agents have been discovered or developed to exploit them.

To date three targets – plasma membrane sterols, nucleic acid synthesis and cell wall constituents, have been exploited with varying degree of success. There is poor penetration of drugs in tissues because fungi infect relatively poorly vascularized areas. Furthermore, slow growth of fungi and granulomatous response of host tissue also decrease drug penetration into the target sites. In addition, poor absorption from gastrointestinal tract demands the use of parenteral route entailing an increased toxicity of these drugs.

The number of agents available to treat fungal infections has increased by 30% since 2000. The greater number of medications now available allows for therapeutic choices; however, differences in anti-

---

* This chapter has been contributed by Dr. Seema Gupta, M.D., Associate Professor, Department of Pharmacology and Therapeutics, Government Medical College, Jammu (J&K), and Dr. Vikram Gupta, M.D., Consultant Physician, Jammu (J&K).

fungal spectrum of activity, bioavailability, formulation, drug interactions and side effects necessitate a detailed knowledge of each drug class.

## Classification of antifungal drugs

Fungal infections have been divided into two distinct classes, systemic and superficial. Therefore, the majority of the antifungal agents are discussed under two main headings – systemic and topical, although this division is becoming arbitrary as many antifungal agents may be used both systemically and topically, and many superficial infections can be treated either systemically or topically (Table 3.1).

**Table 3.1.** Systemic and topical antifungal drugs

**A. SYSTEMIC ANTIFUNGAL DRUGS**
1. **Antibiotics**
   - Polyene: Amphotericin B*
   - Heterocylic benzofurans: Griseofulvin
2. **Azoles**
   - Imidazoles: Clotrimazole*, Ketoconazole
   - Triazole: Fluconazole, Itraconazole, Voriconazole, Posaconazole
3. **Echinocandins:** Capsofungin, Anidulafungin, Micafungin
4. **Allylamines:** Terbinafine*
5. **Antimetabolite:** Flucytosine

**B. TOPICAL ANTIFUNGAL DRUGS**
1. **Polyene antibiotics:** Nystatin, Hamycin, Natamycin
2. **Azoles:** Clotrimazole, Miconazole, Econazole, Oxiconazole
3. **Allylamines:** Butenafine, Naftifine, Amorolfine
4. **Other topical agents:** Tolnaftate, Undecylenic acid, Ciclopirox olamine, Benzoic acid, Salicylic acid and Sodium thiosulphate

* Used topically as well

## SYSTEMIC ANTIFUNGAL DRUGS

### ANTIBIOTICS

#### Amphotericin B

It is an amphoteric polyene macrolide which remains the most effective antifungal agent for severe systemic mycoses. It is a fungicidal antibiotic without antibacterial activity. It is derived from culture of aerobic actinomycete, *Streptomyces nodosus*. Discovered by Gold in 1956, it truly represents a gold standard in the treatment of fungal infections.

### Mechanism of action

Ergosterol, a key component of the fungal cell membrane, is critical to the integrity of the membrane and functions by regulating membrane fluidity and symmetry. It is not present in mammalian cells and thus it is an ideal target for antifungal activity.

Amphotericin B binds to ergosterol in the cell membrane of fungi and thus increases its permeability and induces cell lysis. It has probably more than one mechanism of action but its most important property is probably its ability to form large pores in the cell membrane. This causes gross disturbances in ion balance, including loss of intracellular $K^+$.

In addition to direct antifungal activity, amphotericin B stimulates release of cytokines such as tumour necrosis factor and interleukin-1 from mammalian phagocytic cells and also stimulates release of macrophage superoxide ion, all of which augment antifungal activity. Cholesterol, present in host cell membranes, closely resembles ergosterol. The polyenes bind to it as well, though with lesser affinity. Thus, the selectivity of action of polyenes is low, and amphotericin B is one of the most toxic systemically used antibiotics.

**Resistance** may develop from changes in ergosterol structure and decreased amounts of ergosterol in the fungal cell membrane which makes it less susceptible to the drug.

### Antifungal spectrum

It has broad-spectrum of activity against *Candida* spp., *Cryptococcus neoformans*, *Coccidioides immitis*, *Histoplasma capsulatum*, *Blastomyces dermatitidis*, *Paracoccidioides brasiliensis*, *Sporothrix schenckii*, *Aspergillus* spp., *Penicillium marneffei*, and the Mucorales. It has limited activity against the protozoa *Leishmania brasiliensis* and *Naegleria fowleri*. It has no antibacterial activity.

### Pharmacokinetics

It is not absorbed from gastrointestinal tract which makes intravenous administration necessary. It can be given orally for intestinal amoebiasis. Administered intravenous as a suspension made with the help of deoxycholate, it gets widely distributed in the body, but penetration in CSF is poor. Therefore, only intrathecal administration can be effective for treatment of fungal meningitis.

It binds to sterols in tissues and to lipoproteins in plasma and stays in the body for long periods. The terminal elimination $t_{1/2}$ is 15 days. About 60% of amphotericin B is metabolized in the liver. Excretion occurs slowly both in urine and bile, but urinary concentration of active drug is low.

### Uses

1. Amphotericin B is the most effective drug for various types of systemic mycoses, viz, disseminated candidiasis, cryptococcal meningitis, coccidioidomycosis, histoplasmosis, blastomycosis and extracutaneous sporotrichosis.
2. It can be applied locally for oral, vaginal and cutaneous candidiasis and otomycosis.
3. It is the most effective drug for resistant cases of kala-azar and mucocutaneous leishmaniasis.

### Adverse effects

Amphotericin B is highly toxic.

(a) **Acute reaction:** This consists of chills, fever, aches and pain all over the body, nausea, vomiting and dyspnoea lasting for 2–5 hours.
(b) **Long-term toxicity:** Nephrotoxicity is the most important complication which can manifest as hypokalemia and renal tubular acidosis. It can be minimized by adequate hydration. The lipid based amphotericin B formulations have shown lower incidence of nephrotoxicity. Most patients develop slowly progressive anaemia which is due to bone marrow depression. It is largely irreversible. CNS toxicity occurs only on intrathecal injection leading to headache, vomiting, nerve palsies, etc.

### Drug interactions

1. Amphotericin B has synergistic effect with flucytosine in the treatment of systemic candidiasis and cryptococcosis.
2. It should not be co-administered with other drugs with nephrotoxic potential.

### Griseofulvin

It is a narrow spectrum antifungal agent isolated from cultures of *Penicillium griseofulvum*. It is a fungistatic drug. It acts by interacting with fungal microtubules and interfering with mitosis. It can be used to treat dermatophyte infection of skin or nails when local treatment is ineffective but treatment needs to be very prolonged.

### Pharmacokinetics

The absorption of griseofulvin from gastrointestinal tract is erratic. Fatty meals and microfining the drug particles can improve its oral absorption. It is metabolized in the liver with plasma $t_{1/2}$ of 24 hours. Griseofulvin gets deposited in keratin forming cells of skin, hair and nails. It is especially concentrated and retained in tinea infected cells. Because it is fungistatic and not fungicidal, the newly formed keratin is not invaded by fungus, but the fungus persists in already infected keratin, till it is shed off. Therefore, the duration of treatment is dependent upon the site of infection, thickness of infected keratin and its turnover rate. It has largely been superseded by other drugs.

### Adverse effects

Toxicity of griseofulvin is low. It may cause allergic reactions, headache and gastrointestinal disturbances.

## AZOLES

The azoles were introduced in 1980s and have become the most widely used antifungal agents presently. The azole antifungals include two broad classes, imidazoles and triazoles, according to the number of nitrogen atoms in the azole ring. Both the classes have same antifungal spectrum and mechanism of action. Clotrimazole, econazole, miconazole and oxiconazole from the imidazoles are used topically, while ketoconazole is used both orally and topically. Triazoles especially fluconazole and itraconazole have largely replaced ketoconazole for systemic mycoses because of better efficacy, longer $t_{1/2}$, fewer side effects and drug interactions.

### Spectrum of activity

The azoles are a group of fungistatic agents which have broad-spectrum antifungal activity against common fungal pathogens, e.g., *Candida* spp., *Cryptococcus neoformans*, *Blastomyces dermatitidis*, *Histoplasma capsulatum*, *Coccidioides immitis*, *Paracoccidioides brasiliensis*, *Sporothrix schenckii*, *Aspergillus* spp. and dermatophytes. *Candida krusei* and agents of mucormycosis are resistant. These drugs also have antiprotozoal effect against *Leishmania major*.

## Mechanism of action

These cause blockades of fungal cytochrome P450 mediated synthesis of ergosterol from lanosterol, thus inhibiting fungal growth. These inhibit the fungal cytochrome P450-3A enzyme, lanosine 14-β-demethylase, which is responsible for converting lanosterol to ergosterol, the main sterol in the fungal cell membrane. The fluidity of the membrane is altered due to ergosterol depletion which interferes with the action of membrane associated enzymes. The net effect is an inhibition of replication.

There is, however, cross reactivity with human cytochrome P450 enzymes which explains their potential for inhibition of steroid synthesis in humans and for various interactions with other hepatically metabolised drugs. Development of fungal resistance to azoles has been noted among *Candida* spp. infecting advanced AIDS patients

## Ketoconazole

It was the first successful orally used azole antifungal agent in 1980. It is available in both oral and topical formulations. It is an effective broad-spectrum antifungal drug, useful in both dermatophytosis and deep mycoses. However, for systemic mycoses, ketoconazole has been superseded by fluconazole and itraconazole due to their improved pharmacokinetics, tolerability and efficacy. Topical formulations of ketoconazole are useful for treating seborrheic dermatitis. It is widely distributed in tissues but concentration in CSF and urine are low. It is not effective in fungal meningitis. The most common side effects are nausea, vomiting, anorexia, headache, paresthesia, hair loss, rashes, gynaecomastia, oligospermia and menstrual irregularities. It has a greater potential for drug interactions which is one of its main limitations.

## Fluconazole

Fluconazole possesses the most desirable pharmacological properties including high bioavailability, low degree of protein binding, wide distribution into body tissues and long half-life. It displays a high degree of water-solubility and good CSF penetration. Oral bioavailability is not affected by food or gastric pH. It can be administered orally as well as intravenously. It is indicated for the treatment of cryptococcal meningitis, systemic and mucocutaneous candidiasis in both normal and immunocompromised patients, coccidioidal meningitis and histoplasmosis. Generally, recommended dosages of fluconazole are 50–400 mg once daily for either oral or intravenous administration. It is ineffective in aspergillosis and mucormycosis. Side effects are nausea, vomiting, abdominal pain, rash and headache.

## Itraconazole

It has a broader spectrum of activity than ketoconazole and fluconazole. It is fungistatic and is effective in immunocompromised patients. Oral absorption is enhanced by food and gastric acid. It gains extensive distribution in all tissues, but penetration into CSF is poor. It is used for the treatment of histoplasmosis, blastomycosis, sporotrichomycosis, paracoccidioidomycosis and chromoblastomycosis. It affords some relief in aspergillosis.

## Voriconazole

It has potent broad-spectrum activity against various fungi. It is used for difficult to treat fungal infections like invasive aspergillosis, disseminated infections caused by fluconazole-resistant *Candida* and *Fusarium* infections. It has become the azole of choice in aspergillosis. It is available for oral and intravenous administration. Pharmacokinetics, indications and adverse effects of commonly used azoles – ketoconazole, fluconazole, itraconazole and voriconazole are given in Table 3.2.

## Posaconazole

Posaconazole is a novel lipophilic antifungal triazole with broad range of activity against *Candida* spp., *Aspergillus* spp. and Mucorales. After oral adminis-

**Table 3.2.** Pharmacokinetics, indications and adverse effects of ketoconazole, fluconazole, itraconazole and voriconazole

| Drug | Pharmacokinetics | Indications | Adverse effects |
|---|---|---|---|
| Ketoconazole | • Oral bioavailability 75%<br>• Protein binding 99%<br>• CSF penetration < 10%<br>• Elimination $t_{1/2}$ 7–10 hours | • Replaced by fluconazole and itraconazole for most fungal infections | • Hepatotoxicity, gastro-intestinal disturbances, pruritis, gynaecomastia and adverse drug interactions |
| Fluconazole | • Oral bioavailability > 80%<br>• Protein binding 11%<br>• Excellent CSF penetration > 70%<br>• Elimination $t_{1/2}$ 22–35 hours | • Fungal meningitis (cryptococcosis, coccidioidomycosis)<br>• Candidiasis (deep and superficial)<br>• Prophylaxis in immuno-compromised host | • Nausea, headache, pain abdomen, exfoliative skin lesions (in AIDS patients), hepatitis (rare), and drug interactions seen only at higher doses > 400 mg |
| Itraconazole | • Oral bioavailability > 70%<br>• Protein binding > 99%<br>• Poor CNS penetration < 1%<br>• Elimination $t_{1/2}$ 24–42 hours | • Non-meningeal infections (e.g., histoplasmosis)<br>• Reserved for oropharyngeal candidiasis in case of unresponsiveness to fluconazole | • GIT disturbances, headache, dizziness, allergic skin reactions and drug interactions |
| Voriconazole | • Oral bioavailability 96%<br>• Protein binding 56%<br>• Elimination $t_{1/2}$ 6 hours | • Invasive aspergillosis<br>• Initial treatment of candidiasis | • Transient abnormal vision, skin rash and hepatotoxicity (rare) |

tration, it is absorbed within three to five hours. It is predominantly eliminated through the liver, and has a half life of about 35 hours. Oral administration of posaconazole taken with a high-fat meal exceeds 90% bioavailability. Posaconazole has been approved by USFDA and other regulatory authorities for the treatment of oropharyngeal candidiasis and for the prophylaxis of invasive aspergillosis and *Candida* infections in severely immunocompromised patients. It is generally well tolerated.

## ECHINOCANDINS

The echinocandins comprise a ring of six amino acids linked to a lipophilic side chain.

### Mechanism of action

All echinocandins have the same mechanism of action but differing pharmacologic properties. They act by inhibiting the synthesis of 1,3-β-glucan, a glucose polymer, a vital component of cell wall that is necessary for maintaining the structure of cell walls of fungi. Fungal cells lose integrity in the absence of this polymer and lysis quickly follows.

### Antifungal spectrum

They are fungicidal against some yeasts (most species of *Candida*, but not against *Cryptococcus*, *Trichosporon* and *Rhodotorula*), fungistatic against some molds (*Aspergillus*, but not *Fusarium* and *Rhizopus*), and modestly or minimally active against dimorphic fungi (*Blastomyces* and *Histoplasma*). In vitro resistance can be conferred in *C. albicans* by mutation in one of the genes that encodes 1,3-β-glucan synthase. Azole-resistant isolates of *C. albicans* remain susceptible to echinocandins.

The first approved echinocandin was caspofungin, and later micafungin and anidulafungin were approved. All these preparations so far have low oral bioavailability, so must be given intravenously only. Echinocandins have now become one of the first line of treatment for *Candida*, and even as antifungal prophylaxis in haematopoietic stem cell transplant patients.

### Adverse effects

These include fever, headache, nausea, vomiting, diarrhoea, abdominal pain, itching, and pain and redness around injection site. Altered liver enzyme levels are also reported. Compared to amphotericin

B, caspofungin seems to have a relatively low incidence of side effects.

## ALLYLAMINES

The allylamines are a group of synthetic antifungal compounds effective in the topical and oral treatment of dermatophytoses. The various drugs included in this group are terbinafine, butenafine, naftifine and amorolfine.

### Terbinafine

It is the most commonly used antifungal drug from the allylamine group.

*Mechanism of action*

It acts by preventing ergosterol synthesis of fungal cell by inhibiting the key fungal enzyme squalene epoxidase with resultant ergosterol deficiency and squalene accumulation which results in cell death. Ergosterol is the principal sterol in the membrane of susceptible fungal cells. It is orally and topically active drug against dermatophytes and *Candida*. It is less effective against cutaneous and mucosal candidiasis. In contrast to azoles which are primarily fungistatic, terbinafine is fungicidal. Shorter courses of therapy are required and relapse rates are low. It is available as oral and cream formulation. It is applied topically as 1% cream or administered orally 250 mg once a day. It does not seem to affect cytochrome P450 system and has demonstrated no significant drug interaction.

*Adverse effects*

Side effects of oral terbinafine are gastric upset, rashes and taste disturbance. Some cases of hepatic dysfunction, haematological disorder and severe cutaneous reactions are reported. Topical terbinafine can cause erythema, itching, dryness, irritation, urticaria and rashes.

Butenafine, naftifine and amorolfine are discussed under topical antifungal agents.

## ANTIMETABOLITE

### Flucytosine

Flucytosine is a fluorinated pyrimidine analog that is used orally to treat severe fungal infections. To exert its effect, flucytosine is taken up in susceptible fungi by the transport enzyme cytosine permease. Once inside the fungal cell, flucytosine rapidly undergoes intracellular conversion to 5-fluorouracil via cytosine deaminase, and subsequently converted to 5-fluorouridine triphosphate, which is incorporated into fungal RNA and interferes with protein synthesis. 5-Fluorouracil intermediate also inhibits thymidylate synthetase, and interferes with DNA synthesis. Mammalian cells do not convert flucytosine to fluorouracil which is responsible for the fungal selectivity of this drug.

*Antifungal spectrum*

It has narrow spectrum of activity. It is active against *Cryptococcus neoformans*, *Candida* spp., and chromoblastomycosis. It is fungistatic in action.

*Therapeutic uses*

It is primarily used in the treatment of cryptococcal meningitis and serious systemic candidiasis in combination with amphotericin B. Drug resistance develops rapidly due to altered drug permeability. For this reason amphotericin B and flucytosine are given in combination due to their synergistic effects.

*Pharmacokinetic*

It is absorbed rapidly and well from gastrointestinal tract. It is actively secreted and concentrated into the urine with an elimination $t_{1/2}$ of 2.5–6 hours. It has wide distribution including CSF.

*Adverse effects*

Flucytosine may depress the bone marrow and lead to leucopenia and thrombocytopenia. Patients are more prone to this complication if they have underlying haematological disorders. Other untoward effects include rash, nausea, vomiting and severe enterocolitis. Toxicity is more severe in patients with AIDS and when plasma concentration exceeds 100 μg/ml.

## TOPICAL ANTIFUNGAL AGENTS

Topical treatment is useful in many superficial fungal infections, i.e., those confined to the stratum corneum, squamous mucosa, or cornea. Such diseases include dermatophytosis, candidiasis, pityriasis versicolor, piedra, tinea nigra and fungal keratitis. A plethora of topical agents is available for the treatment of superficial mycoses. The systemic agents used for the treatment of superficial mycoses are discussed above.

## POLYENE ANTIBIOTICS

### Nystatin

Nystatin is a polyene macrolide antibiotic, obtained from *Streptomyces noursei*. It is similar to amphotericin B in antifungal action and other properties. However, it is too toxic for parenteral administration and is used only locally in superficial candidiasis including vaginal candidiasis and oral thrush. Given orally, it is not absorbed. It can be used for diarrhoea caused by *Candida* spp. Nausea and bad taste in mouth is the only side effect. It is effective (but less than azoles) in vaginal candidiasis and oral thrush. It is also used for corneal, conjunctival and cutaneous candidiasis in the form of an ointment. It is ineffective in dermatophytosis.

### Hamycin

Hamycin is isolated from *Streptomyces pimprina*. It is similar to nystatin, but more water soluble. Its use is restricted to topical application for oral thrush, cutaneous candidiasis, otomycosis by *Aspergillus* spp., vaginal candidiasis and *Trichomonas* vaginitis.

### Natamycin

Natamycin is isolated from *Streptomyces natalensis*. It is similar to nystatin. It has a broader spectrum of action, and is used only topically. A 1% ointment or 5% suspension have been used particularly in *Fusarium solani* keratitis. Vaginal keratitis and *Trichomonas* vaginitis are also amenable to natamycin.

## TOPICAL AZOLES

A number of topical azoles are available for the treatment of superficial mycoses such as clotrimazole, econazole, miconazole, oxiconazole, etc.

### Clotrimazole

It is the most commonly used azole for the treatment of superficial mycoses. It acts by interfering with amino acid transport into the fungus by an action on cell membrane. It is effective in the topical treatment of dermatophytosis, otomycosis and oral/cutaneous/vaginal candidiasis. The standard regimens for vaginal candidiasis are one 100 mg vaginal tablet once a day inserted at bedtime for 7 days or one 200 mg tablet once a day for 3 days. For oropharyngeal candidiasis, 10 mg troche of clotrimazole is allowed to dissolve in the mouth 3–4 times a day, or can be applied as lotion/gel. Local irritation occurs in some patients. However, no systemic toxicity is seen after topical use.

### Econazole

It is similar in activity to clotrimazole. It penetrates superficial layers of the skin and is highly effective in dermatophytosis, otomycosis and oral thrush. It is somewhat inferior to clotrimazole for the treatment of vaginitis. With the exception of local irritation in a few cases, no adverse effects have been reported.

### Miconazole

This imidazole derivative has a broad-spectrum of activity. Topical formulations are highly effective for the treatment of tinea, pityriasis versicolor, otomycosis, and cutaneous and vulvovaginal candidiasis. No systemic adverse effects are seen, however, it may lead to vaginal irritation and even pelvic cramps.

### Oxiconazole

It is a new topical imidazole, effective in tinea and other dermatophytic infections, as well as vaginal candidiasis. In some cases local irritation may occur.

## TOPICAL ALLYLAMINES

### Butenafine

Butenafine is a benzylamine derivative of terbinafine with a mechanism of action similar to that of terbinafine. Efficacy in tinea cruris, tinea corporis and tinea pedis is similar to that of topical terbinafine. It displays superior activity against *C. albicans* than terbinafine. Butenafine achieves high concentrations in skin and remains in skin tissue for prolonged periods. It is mostly distributed in epidermis. A small amount is detectable also in dermis, probably due to transport via sebaceous glands and hair follicles. It exerts antiinflammatory as well as antifungal activity. This property is particularly beneficial in dermatophytic infections that are accompanied by a marked inflammatory reaction in the infected tissue.

### Adverse reactions

Topical butenafine is well tolerated and adverse reactions are rare. Mild burning sensation at the application site has been observed in some patients.

## Naftifine

Naftifine is a topically active allylamine antifungal drug. It is used as 1% cream for the topical treatment of tinea pedis, tinea cruris, and tinea corporis. Twice daily application is recommended. The drug is well tolerated although some patients may develop local irritation.

## Amorolfine

Amorolfine is a morpholine derivative which is used topically as an antifungal agent. It acts by inhibiting two separate enzymes, reductase and isomerase, in the pathway of ergosterol synthesis resulting in depletion of ergosterol in the fungal cytoplasmic membrane. It has a broad spectrum of activity, including dermatophytes, various filamentous and dematiaceous fungi, yeasts and dimorphic fungi. Its activity is fungicidal for most species. Amorolfine 5% nail lacquer is applied once or twice weekly for up to 6 months for the treatment of onychomycosis.

## MISCELLANEOUS TOPICAL AGENTS

## Tolnaftate

Tolnaftate is a thiocarbamate. It is effective in the treatment of cutaneous mycoses caused by dermatophytes and *Malassezia furfur*, but it is ineffective against *Candida*. It is available in a 1% concentration as a cream, gel, powder and topical solution. The preparations are applied locally twice a day. Symptomatic relief occurs early, but if applications are discontinued before the fungus bearing tissue is shed, relapses are common.

## Undecylenic acid

Undecylenic acid is primarily fungistatic. It is used topically in combination with its zinc salt. It is available as foam, ointment, cream, powder, soap, and liquid. Undecylenic acid preparations are used in the treatment of various dermatophytoses, especially tinea pedis. The preparations as formulated are usually not irritating to tissue, and sensitization to them is uncommon.

## Ciclopirox olamine

Ciclopirox olamine is broad-spectrum antifungal agent used for the treatment of superficial mycoses. It is fungicidal to *C. albicans*, *Epidermophyton floccosum*, *Microsporum canis*, *Trichophyton mentagrophytes*, *T. rubrum* and *Malassezia furfur*. After application to the skin, it penetrates superficial layers and reaches hair follicles and sebaceous glands, but systemic absorption is negligible. It can sometimes cause hypersensitivity. It is available as cream and lotion for the treatment of cutaneous candidiasis, and for tinea corporis, tinea cruris, tinea pedis, and pityriasis versicolor. It is available as 1% shampoo for the treatment of seborrheic dermatitis of the scalp, and 8% solution for the treatment of onychomycosis.

## Benzoic acid and Salicylic acid

An ointment containing benzoic acid and salicylic acid is known as Whitfield's ointment. It contains benzoic acid and salicylic acid in a ratio of 2 : 1 in which fungistatic action of benzoic acid is combined with the keratolytic action of salicylic acid. It is used mainly in the treatment of tinea pedis and sometimes it is also used to treat tinea capitis. Since benzoic acid is only fungistatic, eradication of infection occurs only after the infected stratum corneum is shed, therefore, medication is required for several weeks to months. The salicylic acid accelerates desquamation. Mild irritation may occur at the site of application

## Sodium thiosulphate

Sodium thiosulphate is weak fungistatic. It is active against *Malassezia furfur*. A 20% solution applied twice daily for 2–3 weeks is effective in pityriasis versicolor. However, normal pigmentation of skin takes longer to return.

Antifungal drugs used for the treatment of important superficial and systemic mycoses are given in Table 3.3.

## MECHANISMS OF RESISTANCE TO ANTIFUNGAL AGENTS

Expanded use of antifungal drugs has accelerated the development of resistance to these compounds. There are two types of resistance – **intrinsic resistance**, which is an inherited characteristic of a species or strain, and **acquired resistance**, which occurs when a previously susceptible isolate develops resistant phenotype, usually as a result of prolonged treatment with antifungals. In certain genera of fungi, some species are susceptible and other species are resistant to specific antifungals.

### Intrinsic azole resistance

*Candida krusei* is intrinsically resistant to azoles. In addition, many strains of *C. glabrata* are intrinsically resistant and other strains can quickly acquire resistance during therapy. Therefore, *C. krusei* and *C. glabrata* are increasing in frequency in oral and systemic candidiasis in patients that use azole drugs for treatment or prophylaxis.

### Acquired azole resistance

Acquired azole resistance in fungi develops when long-term azole therapy is used. Oral candidiasis was a common opportunistic infection in human immunodeficiency virus (HIV)-infected patients, occurring in over 90% of all patients with low CD4 counts. Azole drugs were commonly prescribed at relatively low doses for long-term suppressive therapy that was administered intermittently. Therefore, azole resistance in oral candidiasis became a significant problem. In addition to *C. albicans*, *C. dubliniensis* also has the ability to develop resistance to azole drugs.

Acquired resistance to azoles has also developed in isolates of *Cryptococcus neoformans* from AIDS patients who have been on maintenance azole therapy to prevent cryptococcal meningitis, and in isolates of *A. fumigatus* from patients who have received repeated treatment with itraconazole or voriconazole.

**Table 3.3.** Antifungal drugs used for the treatment of important superficial and systemic mycoses

| Mycoses | Drugs |
|---|---|
| **I. SYSTEMIC MYCOSES** | |
| Aspergillosis | Voriconazole, Amphotericin B, Caspofungin, Itraconazole, Posaconazole, Anidulafungin, Micafungin |
| Blastomycosis | Amphotericin B, Itraconazole, Fluconazole, Posaconazole, Voriconazole |
| Candidiasis | Amphotericin B, Fluconazole, Voriconazole, Caspofungin, Itraconazole, Posaconazole, Anidulafungin, Micafungin |
| **Coccidioidomycosis** | |
| Mild to moderate | Itraconazole, Fluconazole |
| Severe | Amphotericin B |
| Meningitis | Fluconazole, intrathecal Amphotericin B |
| **Cryptococcosis** | |
| Meningitis | Amphotericin B + Flucytosine followed by Fluconazole |
| Non-meningeal infection | Fluconazole, Amphotericin B |
| **Histoplasmosis** | |
| Moderate disease | Itraconazole, Fluconazole |
| Severe disease and meningitis | Amphotericin B |
| Mucormycosis | Amphotericin B, Posaconazole |
| Sporotrichosis | Itraconazole, Amphotericin B (extracutaneous) |
| Paracoccidioidomycosis | Amphotericin B, Fluconazole, Itraconazole, Posaconazole, Voriconazole |
| **II. SUPERFICIAL MYCOSES** | |
| **Candidiasis** | |
| Cutaneous | Amphotericin B, Clotrimazole, Ciclopirox, Econazole, Miconazole, Nystatin (Topical) |
| Oropharyngeal | Clotrimazole, Nystatin (Topical) Fluconazole, Itraconazole (Oral) |
| Vulvovaginal | Clotrimazole, Miconazole, Nystatin (Topical) Fluconazole (Oral) |
| Dermatophytosis (Ringworm infection) | Clotrimazole, Miconazole, Butenafine, Terbinafine, Naftifine (topical), and Itraconazole, Griseofulvin, Terbinafine (systemic) |

## Intrinsic amphotericin B resistance

Intrinsic resistance to amphotericin B has been seen in yeasts *C. krusei* and *C. lusitaniae*, and the molds *Aspergillus terreus* and *Scedosporium* spp.

## Acquired amphotericin B resistance

Acquired resistance to fungicidal amphotericin B is rare; it occurs mostly in yeasts from cancer patients who have received repeated doses of the drug to treat recurring systemic fungal infections.

## Mechanism of azole drug resistance

Mechanism of azole drug resistance in fungi may be due to overexpression of efflux pump. Drug resistance in fungi is not normally associated with gene amplification. Unlike studies with prokaryotes, studies with fungi have not yet identified any plasmids or episomes containing resistance markers. There is no report of transfer of drug resistance from one fungal isolate to another.

## Mechanism of nonazole drug resistance

### Flucytosine resistance

Up to 10% of clinical isolates of *C. albicans* have intrinsic resistance to flucytosine, and 30% of the susceptible isolates develop acquired resistance during drug therapy. Resistance can be associated with mutation.

### Amphotericin B resistance

Amphotericin B-resistant clinical isolates of *C. tropicalis* have been identified. This is due to greatly reduced levels of ergosterol in their plasma membranes, which decreases the binding ability of amphotericin B.

### Echinocandin resistance

Echinocandin-resistant clinical isolates are limited in number, because the echinocandins have not yet been in clinical use for as long as the other agents. The mechanism of resistance to the echinocandins that has been characterized in laboratory strains of *Candida albicans*, *C. glabrata*, *C. tropicalis*, *C. krusei* and *C. lucitaniae* is one of an altered glucan synthesis enzyme complex that shows a decreased sensitivity to inhibition by agents within the class.

Though lot of advancement has been made in the treatment of fungal infections but still there is a need for novel drugs due to the problem of drug resistance and toxicity with current drugs. Cytokine therapy (such as interferon-$\alpha$) and use of growth factors such as granulocyte macrophage-colony stimulating factor (GM-CSF) have been shown in animal studies to increase clearance of fungi and result in better clinical outcomes and are being evaluated in human disease. Development of an antifungal vaccine is also being considered with advances in antibody technology.

### Important Questions

1. Classify antifungal drugs. Discuss their mechanism of action and indications.
2. Write short notes on:
   (a) Systemic antifungal drugs
   (b) Topical antifungal drugs
   (c) Antifungal drug resistance.

### Multiple Choice Questions

1. Which of the following targets has/have been exploited in the development of antifungal drugs?
   (a) Plasma membrane sterols.
   (b) Nucleic acid synthesis.
   (c) Cell wall constituents.
   (d) All of the above.

2. Which of the following is systemic antifungal drug?
   (a) Nystatin.
   (b) Griseofulvin.
   (c) Hamycin.
   (d) Natamycin.

3. Amphotericin B is an:
   (a) amphoteric polyene macrolide
   (b) azole.
   (c) echinocandin.
   (d) antimetabolite.

4. Which of the following is the most toxic systemically used antifungal drug?
   (a) Griseofulvin.
   (b) Amphotericin B.
   (c) Flucytosine.
   (d) Fluconazole.

## Antifungal Drugs

5. Which of the following antifungal drugs can be used both orally and topically?
   (a) Clotrimazole.
   (b) Miconazole.
   (c) Ketoconazole.
   (d) Econazole.

6. Which of the following antifungal drugs is fungicidal?
   (a) Amphotericin B.
   (b) Griseofulvin.
   (c) Flucytosine.
   (d) Itraconazole.

7. Which of the following antifungal drugs can be used for the treatment of diarrhoea caused by *Candida* spp.?
   (a) Hamycin.
   (b) Natamycin.
   (c) Nystatin.
   (d) Miconazole.

8. Which of the following antifungal drugs is **not** fungicidal?
   (a) Undecyclinic acid.
   (b) Amphotericin B.
   (c) Amorolfine.
   (d) Ciclopirox olamine.

9. Amphotericin B can be used for the treatment of:
   (a) aspergillosis.
   (b) candidiasis.
   (c) blastomycosis.
   (d) All of the above.

10. Which of the following drugs can be used for the treatment of dermatophytosis?
    (a) Griseofulvin.
    (b) Clotrimazole.
    (c) Terbinafine.
    (d) All of the above.

11. Which of the following antifungal drugs acts by inhibiting synthesis of plasma membrane ergosterol?
    (a) Nystatin.
    (b) Amphotericin B.
    (c) Clotrimazole.
    (d) Ciclopirox olamine.

12. Flucytosine is used in combination with which antifungal drug for the treatment of cryptococcal meningitis?
    (a) Ketoconazole.
    (b) Amphotericin B.
    (c) Caspofungin.
    (d) Griseofulvin.

13. Which of the following antifungal drugs is an antimetabolite?
    (a) Griseofulvin.
    (b) Nystatin.
    (c) Voriconazole.
    (d) Flucytosine.

14. Griseofulvin is effective against dermatophyte infection of:
    (a) skin.
    (b) hair.
    (c) nail.
    (d) All of the above.

15. Which of the following azole antifungal drugs has the lowest protein binding?
    (a) Fluconazole.
    (b) Itraconazole.
    (c) Ketoconazole.
    (d) Miconazole.

16. Which of the following statements about amphotericin B is **not** correct?
    (a) It is active against yeast-like, dimorphic and filamentous fungi.
    (b) In high concentrations it is fungicidal.
    (c) It acts by binding to ergosterol of fungal cell membrane.
    (d) It is least toxic antifungal drug.

17. Which of the following antifungal drugs is obtained from *Streptomyces nodosus*?
    (a) Amphotericin B.
    (b) Nystatin.
    (c) Griseofulvin.
    (d) Flucytosine.

18. Flucytosine is effective against which of the following fungal infections?
    (a) Cryptococcosis.
    (b) Candidiasis.
    (c) Chromoblastomycosis.
    (d) All of the above.

## SECTION 1: General Topics

19. Nephrotoxicity is the most serious long-term toxicity of:
    (a) griseofulvin.
    (b) amphotericin B.
    (c) butenafine.
    (d) clotrimazole.

20. The absorption of which of the following drugs is greatly decreased in the absence of gastric acidity?
    (a) Flucytosine.
    (b) Fluconazole.
    (c) Nystatin.
    (d) Itraconazole.

21. Which of the following antifungal drugs enters the CSF in adequate concentration in cryptococcal meningitis in HIV-infected patients?
    (a) Miconazole.
    (b) Ketoconazole.
    (c) Fluconazole.
    (d) Clotrimazole.

22. Which of the following is the drug of choice for the treatment of aspergillosis?
    (a) Griseofulvin.
    (b) Ketoconazole.
    (c) Nystatin.
    (d) Voriconazole.

23. Which of the following azole antifungal drugs is most effective in the treatment of *Candida* bloodstream infection?
    (a) Clotrimazole.
    (b) Fluconazole.
    (c) Itraconazole.
    (d) Miconazole.

24. Which of the following statements is/are **true** about amphotericin B?
    (a) Acute adverse effects may include chills, fever, headache, nausea, loss of appetite.
    (b) Chronic adverse effects include kidney toxicity.
    (c) It binds to ergosterol in the cell membrane of fungi and thus increases its permeability and induces cell lysis.
    (d) All of the above.

25. Flucytosine combination therapy is preferred primary therapy with:
    (a) amphotericin B to treat cryptococcosis.
    (b) fluconazole to treat systemic candidiasis.
    (c) itraconazole to treat aspergillosis.
    (d) micafungin to treat mucormycosis.

26. For which disease is oral terbinafine therapy recommended?
    (a) Black piedra.
    (b) Oral thrush.
    (c) Pityriasis versicolor.
    (d) Dermatophyte infection (tinea unguim).

## ANSWERS TO MCQs

1. (d), 2. (b), 3. (a), 4. (b), 5. (c), 6. (a), 7. (c), 8. (a), 9. (d), 10. (d), 11. (c), 12. (b), 13. (d), 14. (d), 15. (a), 16. (d), 17. (a), 18. (d), 19. (b), 20. (d), 21. (c), 22. (d), 23. (b), 24. (d), 25. (a), 26. (d).

## Further Reading

1. Chris J Van Boxtel. Antimicrobial Agents. Drug Benefits and Risks. International Textbook of Clinical Pharmacology (Revised 2$^{nd}$ edition) 2008; 407–436.
2. George R. Thompson III, Jose Cadena, Thomas F. Patterson. Overview of Antifungal Agents. *Clinical Chest Med.* 2009; 30: 203–215.
3. John E. Bennett. Antifungal agents. Goodman & Gilman's the Pharmacological Basis of Therapeutics (12$^{th}$ ed.) 2011; 1571–1592.
4. William E. Dismukes. Introduction to Antifungal Drugs. *Clinical Infect. Dis.* 2000; 30: 653–657.

# SECTION 2

# SUPERFICIAL CUTANEOUS MYCOSES

**Chapter 4**  Pityriasis versicolor, Tinea nigra and Piedra
**Chapter 5**  Dermatophytoses

# CHAPTER 4

# Pityriasis versicolor, Tinea nigra and Piedra

## PITYRIASIS VERSICOLOR

Pityriasis versicolor is a mild, chronic superficial fungal infection of the stratum corneum characterized by white-brown or fawn-coloured discrete to confluent lesions covered with thin scales localized in upper trunk. It has a worldwide distribution, though it is more frequent in tropical climates. The incidence in temperate climates is much lower. It affects mainly young adults of both sexes. In tropical zones, it is also very common in infancy and even in babies.

It is caused by *Malassezia* species. The species most commonly associated with infection in humans are *M. globosa* and *M. sympodialis*, and to a lesser extent *M. furfur*, *M. obtusa*, *M. restricta* and *M. sloofiae*. These are common members of the normal skin flora and most infections are thought to be endogenous. The lesions may appear hypo- or hyper-pigmented, depending on the degree of pigmentation of the surrounding skin. In dark-skinned individuals, the lesions are hypopigmented and in light-skinned individuals these are pink to pale-brown. The commonest sites involved include chest, back, abdomen, neck and upper arms.

### Laboratory diagnosis

#### KOH preparation

Scales are scraped with a scalpel and placed in a drop of 10% KOH. It is heated gently, covered with coverslip and seen under microscope. Clusters of round or oval budding cells 2–8 µm in diameter along with short, curved and occasionally branched hyphae 2.5–4 µm in diameter can be seen (Fig. 4.1).

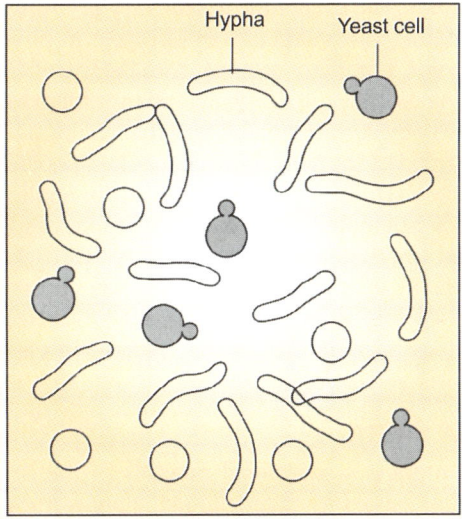

**Fig. 4.1.** *Malassezia* species.

#### Histopathology

In biopsy specimens, they can be seen with haematoxylin and eosin (H&E) stain but are best demonstrated by special stains for fungus, preferably periodic acid-Schiff (PAS).

### Fungus culture

The fungus can be isolated from skin scrapings by inoculating it on Sabouraud dextrose agar (SDA) containing chloramphenicol and cycloheximide. The etiologic agent, *Malassezia* species, grow only on medium that has been overlaid or supplemented with olive oil or another long chain fatty acid. Creamy colonies develop in 5–7 days at 30°C. Lactophenol cotton blue (LPCB) wet mount of the colonies shows yeast-like cells measuring 1.5–4.5 × 3–7 µm in diameter. These cells are unique in being round at one end and bluntly cut off at the other where wide budlike structures form singly on a broad base, but narrow in some species. Hyphal elements are usually absent, but sparse rudimentary forms may occasionally develop. Since *Malassezia* species are part of the normal flora of the skin, therefore, positive culture does not always indicate infection.

### Treatment

Topical azole antifungals work well in pityriasis versicolor. The usual time to recovery is 2–3 weeks. Terbinafine 1% cream is also effective in pityriasis versicolor. The major problem with the use of topical antifungals is the difficulty of applying cream to such a wide body surface area. A possible solution to this is provided by the development of a shampoo version of ketoconazole. A second approach is application of 2.5% selenium sulphide in a detergent base. It is applied to all affected areas and left overnight and washed off the next morning. Oral ketoconazole (a single 400 mg dose) and itraconazole (800–1000 mg given over 5 days) are very effective in cases of pityriasis versicolor.

## TINEA NIGRA

Tinea nigra is a superficial mycosis of the stratum corneum caused by traumatic inoculation from soil, wood or compost. No invasion of living tissue occurs. It is common in tropical regions of Central and South America, Africa and Asia. In Southeast Asia, this has been reported from Sri Lanka, India, southern China, Java, Sumatra and other adjoining countries. It is more common in females and the infection is more evident in young people and children.

It is characterized by single, discrete, painless, brown to black (due to an accumulation of melanin pigment produced by the fungus), non-scaly macules or patches affecting thickly keratinized sites such as palms and soles, and rarely other skin surfaces. Tinea nigra is so superficial that it can be scraped off with vigorous effort.

Tinea nigra must be differentiated from malignant melanoma and junctional nevus in order to prevent unnecessary excision. Melanoma and nevi are often slightly indurated, elevated, or both. A reddish hue in black or brownish-black lesion, which can be seen in melanoma, is rare in tinea nigra.

It is caused by *Hortaea (Phaeoannellomyces) werneckii*. This organism has also been described as *Exophiala werneckii*.

### Laboratory diagnosis

### KOH preparation

The diagnosis is made by scraping the stratum corneum and examination of 10% KOH wet mount. It shows darkly pigmented, branched, septate, narrow hyphae (1.5–3.0 µm wide) usually accompanied by elongated budding cells (1.5–5.0 µm in diameter).

### Histopathology

A biopsy specimen can be obtained painlessly from a patient with tinea nigra by carefully scraping off the stratum corneum with a scalpel blade. The organism stains well with special fungal stains, but the natural pigmentation can be best seen with H&E stain. Tissue reaction reveals mild to moderate hyperplasia and/or hyperkeratosis in the epidermis. A minimal mononuclear cell infiltrate may occur in dermis.

### Fungal culture

*H. werneckii* can be cultured on SDA with cycloheximide. It is incubated at 25–30°C. Growth usually appears in 2–3 weeks. The colony is at first yeast-like and white to grey but quickly changes to olive or greenish-black. Microscopic examination reveals budding yeasts with 0–1 septa and hyphae. Hyphae are up to 7 µm wide, becoming thick walled, olivaceous-black, and densely septate at maturation. Conidia are produced laterally from hyphae or from the poles of budding cells by annellidic conidiogenesis. Annellated zones are conspicuous and 1–2 μm wide, with clearly visible annellations. Conidia are initially hyaline and one-celled but soon become olivaceous. After liberation they inflate and develop transverse and occasionally oblique septa. Liberated cells are converted into budding cells or chlamydoconidia-like cells (Fig. 4.2).

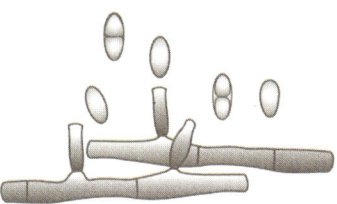

**Fig. 4.2.** Darkly pigmented, septate hyphae and budding cells of *Hortaea werneckii* in 10% KOH preparation.

## Treatment

Topical azole creams such as econazole and ketoconazole are effective. Topical application of keratolytic agents such as Whitfield's ointment or 5–10% salicylic ointment, and thiabendazole 2% in 90% dimethyl sulfoxide once a day for 14 days give good result.

## PIEDRA

Piedra, meaning stone in Spanish, is an asymptomatic fungal infection of the hair shaft, resulting in the formation of **nodules** of different hardness on the infected hair. The infection is also known as **trichomycosis nodularis**. There is little or no tissue reaction. The nodules are concretions of hyphae and fruiting bodies of the fungus from which fungal spores are released. Both sexes and people of all ages are equally affected. Two varieties of piedra are seen – black piedra and white piedra.

## Black piedra

It is caused by *Piedraia hortae*, an **ascomycetous fungus**. It occurs in humid wet tropical regions in the Americas and in Southeast Asia. The fungus is believed to exist in the soil and affects monkeys as well as man. It is characterized by the presence of discrete, black, gritty, hard nodules which are composed of a mass of fungus cells on the hair shaft. The nodules vary in size from microscopic to 1 mm or more in diameter, and are adherent to the hair shaft. Infection is normally restricted to scalp hair but may involve hairs of the beard, moustache and pubic hair with fungal activity limited to the cuticle. Humans as well as other primates are infected.

Black piedra is more frequent than white piedra. As nodules are gritty to feel metallic sound may be heard when hair are combed or brushed. The nodules cannot be pulled off the hair shaft. Multiple nodules may be present on a single hair, weakening the hair shaft and possibly resulting in breakage. Patients do not experience pruritis and they are otherwise asymptomatic. Black piedra can be distinguished from pediculosis, white piedra, tinea capitis and other similar conditions by examining individual hair in a KOH preparation using light microscope.

### KOH preparation

Crushing the nodule in 10% KOH reveals dark septate hyphae, held together by a cement-like substance, around the surface of the hair with round or oval asci containing 2–8 hyaline, nonseptate banana-shaped ascospores. The preparation should first be observed under the low power of objective to reveal the dark mass of compacted hyphae around the surface of the hair, and then examined under the high-power objective to observe the asci and ascospores. *P. hortae* produces sexual spores in its parasitic phase.

### Fungus culture

It grows on SDA at 25°C. Growth is slow. It matures in 21 days. Colonies are small, adherent, compact, somewhat raised, and dark greenish-brown to black and may be glabrous or covered with very short aerial hyphae. Reddish-brown to black diffusible pigment may form. Reverse is black. Microscopic examination shows closely septate, dark, and thick-walled hyphae with many intercalary chlamydoconidium-like cells. Asci may be produced in culture. The walls of the asci readily dissolve, releasing single-celled, curved ascospores (5–10 × 30–35 μm) that taper at the ends to form whiplike extensions (Fig. 4.3). Ascospores are more likely to be seen on direct microscopic examination of the specimen than on culture.

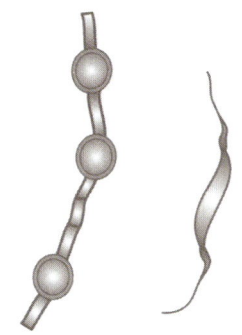

**Fig. 4.3.** *Piedraia hortae.*

### Treatment

Shaving or cutting the hair cures this condition. For prevention of recurrence, antifungal preparations such as benzoic acid ointment or a 1 : 2000 solution of mercury perchloride may be applied to the hair after shampooing.

### White piedra

White piedra is a superficial infection of the hair shaft of the scalp, face, axillary or pubic regions. It is characterized by white, yellow or green nodules composed of hyaline septate hyphae and arthroconidia. Nodules are adhered less firmly and are softer as compared to black piedra. These vary in size from microscopic to 1 mm in diameter, and can be easily detached from the hair. The fungus grows both within and outside the hair shaft, and the hair shaft may be weakened and break off. The infection occurs sporadically in North America, and Europe and more commonly in South America, Africa, and parts of Asia.

White piedra is caused by several *Trichosporon* species. It is considered as a **basidiomycetous yeast**. Genus *Trichosporon* is characterized by the production of true hyphae, pseudohyphae, arthroconidia and blastoconidia (budding yeast cells). This genus has undergone extensive taxonomic revision in 1992. Partial sequencing of the small and large subunits of the rRNA have clearly delineated numerous species. Some are soil borne and others are associated with animals and humans. Six species are of clinical significance – *T. ovoides*, *T. inkin*, *T. cutaneum*, *T. asteroides*, *T. asahii* and *T. mucoides*.

Infection of the scalp hair is caused by *T. ovoides* whereas *T. inkin* infects the pubic hair. *T. asteroides* and *T. cutaneum* have been associated with superficial skin lesions. *T. asahii* causes systemic infection with predilection for haematogenous dissemination. *T. mucoides* causes systemic infection with preference for central nervous system. The infection occurs in South America, Africa, Central and Eastern Europe, and Japan. The horse and certain species of monkey may be affected.

### Laboratory diagnosis

#### KOH preparation

Hair mounted in 10% KOH mount reveal intertwined hyphae around the shaft which fragment into arthroconidia or produce blastoconidia 2–8 μm in diameter. The mycelial elements are held together in a cement-like substance.

#### Fungus culture

On SDA, it forms cream-coloured, dry, wrinkled colonies within 48–72 hours upon incubation at room temperature. The fungus is composed of septate hyphae that fragment into oval or rectangular arthroconidia. Blastoconidia are also produced (Fig. 4.4). Most *Trichosporon* species are inhibited by cycloheximide, therefore, this antibiotic should be excluded from the culture medium.

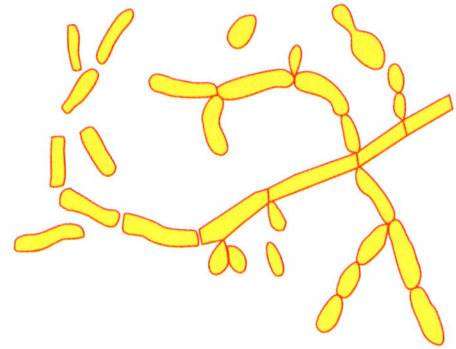

**Fig. 4.4.** Septate hyphae, oval or rectangular arthroconidia and blastoconidia of *Trichosporon* spp. in culture.

### Treatment

As in case of black piedra, shaving or cutting the hair may effect a cure.

# Pityriasis versicolor, Tinea nigra and Piedra

 **Important Questions**

Discuss causative agents, pathogenesis, clinical features, laboratory diagnosis and treatment of:
(a) Pityriasis versicolor
(b) Tinea nigra
(c) Black piedra
(d) White piedra.

## Multiple Choice Questions

1. Which of the following fungi causes pityriasis versicolor?
   (a) *Malassezia* species.
   (b) *Hortaea werneckii*.
   (c) *Piedraia hortae*.
   (d) *Trichosporon* spp.

2. Which of the following fungi causes tinea nigra?
   (a) *Malassezia* species.
   (b) *Hortaea werneckii*.
   (c) *Piedraia hortae*.
   (d) *Trichosporon* spp.

3. Which of the following fungi causes black piedra?
   (a) *Malassezia* species.
   (b) *Hortaea werneckii*.
   (c) *Piedraia hortae*.
   (d) *Trichosporon asteroides*.

4. Which of the following fungi causes white piedra?
   (a) *Malassezia* species.
   (b) *Hortaea werneckii*.
   (c) *Piedraia hortae*.
   (d) *Trichosporon* spp.

5. Which of the following fungi forms asci and ascospores *in vivo*?
   (a) *Malassezia* species.
   (b) *Hortaea werneckii*.
   (c) *Piedraia hortae*.
   (d) *Trichosporon* spp.

6. Which of the following is a lipophilic yeast-like fungus?
   (a) *Malassezia* species.
   (b) *Hortaea werneckii*.
   (c) *Piedraia hortae*.
   (d) *Trichosporon* spp.

7. Which of the following is an ascomycetous fungus?
   (a) *Malassezia* species.
   (b) *Hortaea werneckii*.
   (c) *Piedraia hortae*.
   (d) *Trichosporon* spp.

8. Which of the following is considered as a basidiomycetous yeast?
   (a) *Malassezia* species.
   (b) *Hortaea werneckii*.
   (c) *Piedraia hortae*.
   (d) *Trichosporon* spp.

9. Which of the following yeasts form/forms true hyphae?
   (a) *Candida albicans*.
   (b) *Trichosporon* spp.
   (c) *Geotrichum* spp.
   (d) All of the above.

10. Hard, gritty, discrete dark-brown to black nodules that adhere firmly to scalp hair or beard describe the superficial mycosis called:
    (a) black piedra.
    (b) white piedra.
    (c) tinea nigra.
    (d) pityriasis versicolor.

11. White to light brown nodules occur on hair shaft of the scalp, beard, or moustache, less commonly in the axilla or groin. Nodules are soft, and are not firmly adherent to the hair shaft. This is caused by:
    (a) black piedra.
    (b) white piedra.
    (c) tinea nigra.
    (d) pityriasis versicolor.

12. White-brown or fawn-coloured discrete to confluent lesions covered with thin scales localized to upper trunk describe the superficial mycosis called:
    (a) white piedra.
    (b) black piedra.
    (c) tinea nigra.
    (d) pityriasis versicolor.

### ANSWERS TO MCQs

1. (a), 2. (b), 3. (c), 4. (d), 5. (c), 6. (a), 7. (c), 8. (d), 9. (d), 10. (a), 11. (b), 12. (d).

**Further Reading**

1. Ashbee HR, Evans EGV. Immunology of diseases associated with *Malassezia* species. *Clin Microbiol Rev* 2002; 15: 21–57.
2. Ashbee HR. Update on genus *Malassezia*. *Med Mycol* 2007; 45: 287–303.
3. Ayhan M, Sancak B, et al. Colonization of neonate skin by *Malassezia* species: relationship with neonatal cephalic pustulosis. *J Am Acad Dermatol* 2007; 57: 1012–8.
4. Gaitanis G, Chasapi V, Velegraki A. Novel application of the Masson-Fontana stain for demonstrating *Malassezia* species melanin-like pigment-production *in vitro* and in clinical specimens. *J Clin Microbiol* 2005; 43: 4147–51.
5. Guillot J, Bond R. *Malassezia pachydermatis*: a review. *Med Mycol* 1999; 37: 295–306.
6. Guillot J, Gueho E, et al. Identification of *Malassezia* species: a practical approach. *J Mycol Med* 1996; 6: 103–10.
7. Gupta AK, Batra R, et al. Skin diseases associated with *Malassezia* species. *J Am Acad Dermatol* 2004; 51: 785–98.
8. Kaneko T, Makimura K, et al. Revised culture-based system for identification of *Malassezia* species. *J Clin Microbiol* 2007; 45: 3737–42.
9. Lin X, Yuping R, Guangping Z. Advances in nomenclature and taxonomy of the genus *Malassezia*. *J Clin Dermatol* 2000; 29: 310–2.

# CHAPTER 5

# Dermatophytoses

Dermatophytes are filamentous fungi that are able to digest and obtain nutrients from keratin (the primary component of skin, hair and nails) by unique enzymatic capacity (keratinase). Thus they invade the skin, hair and nails. They simply colonize the keratinized outermost layer of skin. **The living tissue is not invaded.** The disease caused by dermatophytes is known as **dermatophytosis**, **tinea** or **ringworm**. It is due to the host reaction to the enzymes released by the fungus during its digestive process. **It is a communicable skin disease.**

Hypersensitivity to fungus antigens may lead to secondary eruptions occurring in sensitized patients because of circulation of allergenic products from the primary site of infection. It is known as **dermatophytid** or **id reaction**. The infection of the skin caused by non-dermatophytic fungi and the cutaneous manifestations of systemic mycoses are known as **dermatomycosis**. Dermatophytosis is caused by 41 species of dermatophytes which belong to three genera (*Trichophyton*-24, *Microsporum*-16 and *Epidermophyton*-1).

As with a number of fungi, dermatophytes exhibit two phases in their life cycle – the **anamorph state** (imperfect or asexual) that is the state isolated in the laboratory, and the **teleomorph state** (perfect or sexual phase). The teleomorphs of only 23 dermatophytes of the genera *Trichophyton* and *Microsporum* have been described. Sexual state of *Epidermophyton* has not yet been described. The generic name of dermatophytes capable of reproducing sexually is *Arthroderma*.

Dermatophytes comprise three genera that can generally be differentiated by their conidium formation (Table 5.1 and Fig. 5.1). On the basis of their natural inhabits and host preferences, the dermatophytes can be classified into three groups (Table 5.2):

### 1. Geophilic species

They occur as saprophytes of keratinous material (e.g., hair, feathers, horns, hooves, nails, etc.) in soil and occasionally cause infection in man and animals.

### 2. Zoophilic species

Zoophilic dermatophytes are those whose natural hosts are animals but which may also infect man. These are thought to have developed the ability to hydrolyze keratinous debris in the soil and evolved into "keratinophilic fungi" that parasitize animal host. These fungi are primarily animal parasites. Man acquires infection by direct and indirect contact with domestic animals (cats and dogs) and occasionally with wild animals.

## SECTION 2 : Superficial Cutaneous Mycoses

**Table 5.1.** Generic characteristics of dermatophyte macroconidia

| Genus | Frequency | Size | Shape | Number of septations | Thickness of wall | Surface of wall | Manner of attachment |
|---|---|---|---|---|---|---|---|
| Microsporum | Very numerous (except *M. audouinii*) | 5–100 × 3–8 μm | Fusiform to obovate | 3–15 | Thick (except *M. gypseum* and *M. nanum*) | Rough | Singly |
| Trichophyton | Usually rare | 20–50 × 4–6 μm | Cylindrical, fusiform or clavate | 2–8 | Thin | Smooth | Singly |
| Epidermophyton | Numerous | 20–40 × 6–8 μm | Clavate, broadened and rounded at distal end | 2–6 | Both thin and slightly thick | Smooth | Singly or in clusters |

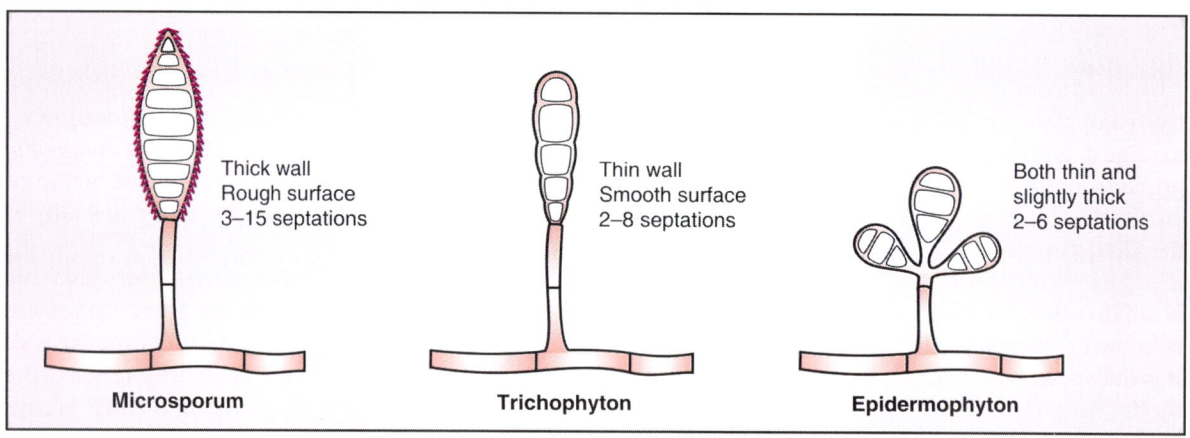

**Fig. 5.1.** Macroconidia in the three genera of dermatophytes.

**Table 5.2.** Grouping of dermatophytes on the basis of host preference and natural habitat

| Anthropophilic | Zoophilic (main animal host group) | Geophilic |
|---|---|---|
| • *Epidermophyton floccosum*<br>• *Microsporum* spp.<br>  – *M. audouinii*<br>  – *M. ferrugineum*<br>• *Trichophyton* spp.<br>  – *T. mentagrophytes*<br>  – *T. rubrum*<br>  – *T. schoenleinii*<br>  – *T. tonsurans*<br>  – *T. violaceum*<br>  – *T. sudanense*<br>  – *T. megninii*<br>  – *T. concentricum*<br>  – *T. violaceum* | • *Microsporum* spp.<br>  – *M. canis* (cats, dogs and horses)<br>  – *M. gallinae* (poultry)<br>  – *M. nanum* (pigs)<br>  – *M. persicolor* (rodents and other small mammals)<br>• *Trichophyton* spp.<br>  – *T. equinum* (horses)<br>  – *T. mentagrophytes* (rodents, rabbits and cavies)<br>  – *T. simii* (monkey)<br>  – *T. verrucosum* (cattle) | • *Microsporum* spp.<br>  – *M. gypseum*<br>  – *M. vanbreuseghemii*<br>  – *M. racemosum* |

### 3. Anthropophilic species

A few dermatophytes have become adapted to human hosts and are termed anthropophilic. These are believed to have evolved from zoophilic fungi and are confined to man as a host.

Zoophilic species tend to produce highly inflammatory reactions in humans and this may lead to a spontaneous cure. Anthropophilic species produce mild but chronic lesions. Although, the inflammatory responses of dermatophyte infection involve the dermis and the Malpighian stratum of the epidermis, the fungus itself is found growing within the stratum corneum of the epidermis, within and around the fully keratinized hair shaft, and in the nail plate and keratinized nail bed. **Within these keratinized tissues, fungus exists only as mycelium and arthroconidia. In this parasitic phase of fungal growth, there are no micro- or macroconidia and no specialized vegetative structures such as spiral or pectinate hyphae. Therefore, precise identification of the species of an infecting dermatophyte is generally impossible on direct microscopy of skin or nail.**

Dermatophytes are among the few fungal species that cause **contagious, directly host-to-host transmissible diseases of humans and animals**. The transmission of these fungi is usually carried out by arthroconidia that have formed in or on infected host tissue. These arthroconidia may be spread by direct skin contact or via fomites containing free arthroconidia, shed skin scales or hairs. Tissue invasion is normally cutaneous. Dermatophytes are usually unable to penetrate deeper tissues as a result of:

– nonspecific inhibitory factors in serum,
– a barrier formed of epidermal keratinocytes, and
– other immunological barriers.

Dermatophytes tend to grow in an annular fashion on the skin producing "ringworm" infection. The lesions are more or less raised with erythematous active area at the periphery and a relatively inactive zone at the centre of established lesions. The organisms can often only be isolated from the active, peripheral ring.

The *Trichophyton* spp. usually infect skin, hair and nails, *Microsporum* spp. infect skin and hair, and *Epidermophyton* spp. infect skin and nails. Many dermatophyte species produce two types of asexual spores – multicelled macroconidia and single-celled microconidia. Classification into three genera *Trichophyton*, *Microsporum* and *Epidermophyton* is based on the morphology of the macroconidia (Table 5.1 and Fig. 5.1), although the identification of the species is also based on the shape and disposition of the microconidia and the macroscopic appearance of the colonies. Clinically, ringworm can be classified depending on the site involved. Tinea corporis, tinea capitis, tinea barbae, tinea cruris, tinea manuum, tinea unguium and tinea pedis involve glabrous (non-hairy) skin of body, shaft of hair of scalp, beard and moustache, groin, hands, nail plates and feet respectively. Types of lesions and causative fungi are given in Table 5.3. Three types of hair infection can be seen in 10% KOH wet mounts:

**Table 5.3.** Types of lesions and causative dermatophytes

| Lesion | Causative dermatophytes |
|---|---|
| Tinea barbae | *T. verrucosum, T. mentagrophytes* |
| Tinea capitis | *T. tonsurans, T. canis* |
| Tinea favus | *T. schoenleinii* |
| Tinea corporis | Any dermatophyte |
| Tinea cruris | *T. rubrum, T. floccosum* |
| Tinea pedis and tinea manuum | *T. mentagrophytes, T. rubrum, Epidermophyton floccosum* |
| Tinea unguium | *T. rubrum* |

1. **Ectothrix:** In this, the arthroconidia are present on the surface of hair shaft (Figs. 5.2A and 5.3). Arthroconidia appear as a mosaic sheath around the hair or as chains on the surface of the hair shaft. In *M. canis*, *M. audouinii* and *M. ferrugineum* infections, colonized hairs fluoresce green under a Wood's lamp; other ectothrix infections are nonfluorescent.
2. **Endothrix:** In this the arthroconidia are present within the hair completely filling the hair shaft without a conspicuous external sheath of arthroconidia. This is caused by *T. tonsurans*, *T. violaceum* and *T. sudanense* (Fig. 5.2B). Hairs are Wood's lamp negative.

# SECTION 2 : Superficial Cutaneous Mycoses

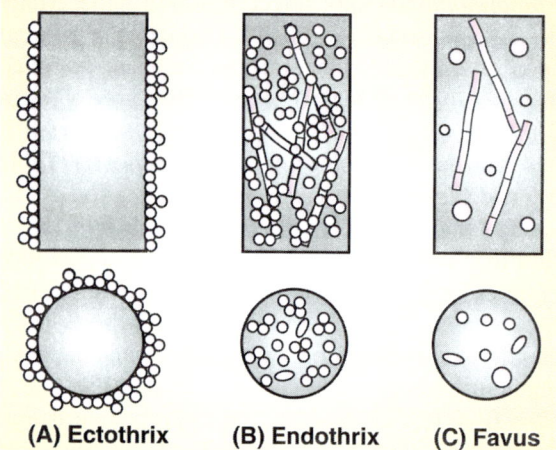

**Fig. 5.2.** Hair invasion of dermatophytes in longitudinal and transverse sections.

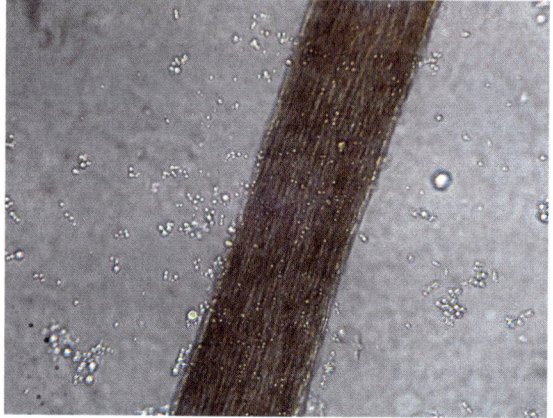

**Fig. 5.3.** Lactophenol cotton blue preparation of hair showing ectothrix (×400).

3. **Favus:** In this, there is sparse hyphal growth and formation of air bubbles or tunnels and fat droplets within the hair shaft. This is caused by *T. schoenleinii* (Fig. 5.2C).

The pattern of hair invasion affects the clinical appearance of the lesion.

- In endothrix infection the hair breaks off at, or just below, the mouth of the follicle to give what is described as a 'black dot' appearance.
- In ectothrix infection the hair usually breaks off 2–3 mm above the mouth of the follicle, leaving short stumps of hair.
- In favus, caused by *T. schoenleinii*, fungal growth within the hair is minimal. The hair remains intact, but intense fungal growth within and around the hair follicle produces a waxy, honeycomb-like crust on the scalp.

Dermatophytosis affects all ages, but children are at higher risk for tinea capitis and tinea corporis (ringworm of smooth skin). Other risk groups include diabetics, those receiving systemic corticosteroid therapy, and persons living with HIV or AIDS. Military troops in the tropics are at risk for tinea cruris and tinea pedis.

Person-to-person transmission is caused by sharing caps and combs, by walking barefoot in public shower rooms, and through exposure to kittens and puppies, which may harbour *M. canis* and cause dermatophytosis, particularly in children. Geophilic dermatophytes such as *M. gypseum* are acquired from soil, causing tinea corporis and tinea capitis.

## Laboratory diagnosis

### KOH preparation

The direct microscopic examination of a properly collected specimen is one of the most rapid and effective methods of detecting dermatophytes. Skin scrapings, hair stubs, and nail clipping or scrapings are collected into folded paper square for transport to the laboratory. The use of paper allows the specimen to dry out, which helps reduce bacterial contamination and provides conditions under which specimen can be stored for 12 months or more without appreciable loss of viability of the fungus. Nail samples should be collected by taking clippings from any discoloured, dystrophic or brittle parts of the nail and, importantly, by scraping material from underneath the nail. Scales from skin lesions should be collected by scraping outwards with a blunt scalpel from the edge of the lesions.

A drop of 10% KOH is placed on a slide, a small amount of specimen is added to the drop, a coverslip is placed over it and the preparation is gently heated. KOH softens and clears the specimen for easier detection of hyphae by digesting any proteinaceous debris and disrupting the keratin cellular sheets, thereby rendering the more biochemically resistant fungus more visible as colourless, septate branched

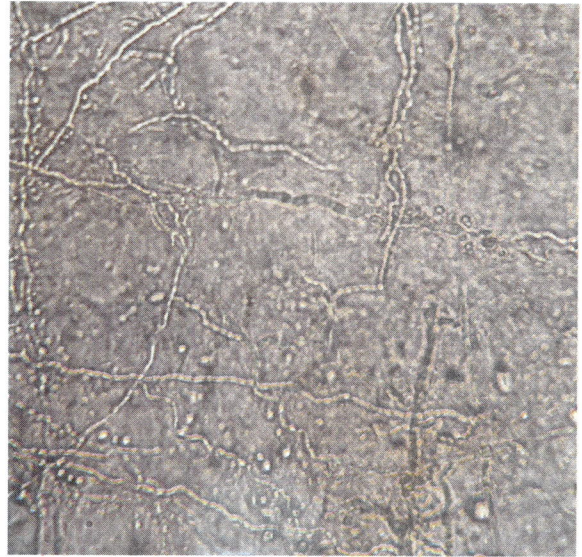

**Fig. 5.4.** KOH preparation of skin scrapings showing septate, branched and unbranched hyphae (×400).

hyphae (2–4 μm in diameter) that characteristically break up into chains of arthroconidia (Fig. 5.4).

In hairs, fungal elements may appear as arthroconidia on the outside (ectothrix invasion) of the hair shaft, or within the hair completely filling the hair shaft (endothrix), or they may appear as hyphae co-occurring, with bubbles and channels (favic invasion). Fungal hyphae must be differentiated from a variety of hypha-like artifacts such as cotton wool and synthetic fibres and from so-called mosaic fungus. The last artifact consists of cholesterol crystals deposited around the periphery of epidermal cells. It can be recognized by its regularity of outline and abrupt changes in width.

## Calcofluor white stain

Calcofluor white stain, a fluorescent dye, binds to chitin and cellulose in fungus cell wall and fluoresces on excitation by long-wave ultraviolet rays or short-wave visible light. This increases the sensitivity of the direct examination; however, this requires a fluorescence microscope. Calcofluor white can be combined with KOH for rapid clearance of the specimens. Although, background elements may also fluoresce, the fungal components are generally brighter and readily recognizable.

## Culture method

Culture is available adjunct to direct microscopy. The clinical specimen should be inoculated on Sabouraud dextrose agar (SDA) with cycloheximide and chloramphenicol, and dermatophyte test medium (DTM). Both these media contain cycloheximide to inhibit saprophytes contaminating molds, e.g., *Penicillium* and *Aspergillus*. DTM incorporates gentamicin, and chlortetracycline to inhibit bacteria and a phenol red indicator that changes colour from yellow to red within 14 days when the medium becomes alkaline as a result of growth of dermatophytes. However, many non-dermatophytes also turn this medium red giving false-positive results, and isolates often exhibit atypical colonial and microscopic characteristics when grown on DTM. It cannot be used to study pigment production because of the intense red colour of the indicator.

For isolation of dermatophytes, SDA slants are less liable to contamination and do not dry out so quickly as compared to cultures in petri dishes. These should be incubated at 25–30°C for a total of 4 weeks before being considered mycologically negative. However, majority of the cultures becomes positive within 1–2 weeks.

Dermatophyte isolates can be identified to genus/species by colonial morphology, colour, pigment production, microscopic examination (production of microconidia and macroconidia), cellophane tape mount, hair perforation test and urease test.

## Colony character and microscopic morphology

- **Trichophyton:** Colonies may be powdery, velvety or waxy with pigmentation characteristic of different species. Macroconidia are usually rare but microconidia are abundant. The latter are arranged in clusters along the hyphae or borne on conidiophores. Macroconidia have smooth, thin walls, and variable in shape (cylindrical, fusiform or clavate), vary in number of septa (2–8), and in size (20–50 × 4–6 μm) (Table 5.1). They are borne singly or in clusters. Some species possess special types of hyphae, i.e., **spiral hyphae**, **racquet hyphae** and **favic chandeliers** (Fig. 5.5). Fungi of this genus can infect skin, hair and nails. *T. rubrum* is the most common species infecting man.

## SECTION 2 : Superficial Cutaneous Mycoses

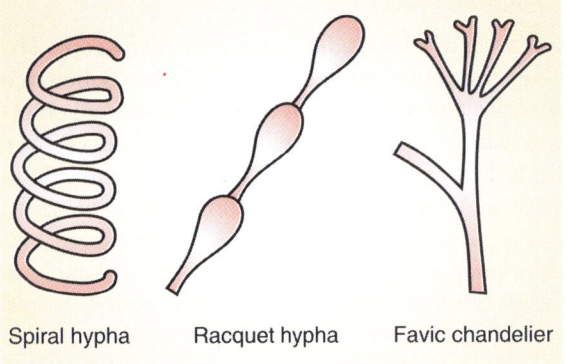

Spiral hypha   Racquet hypha   Favic chandelier

**Fig. 5.5.** Special types of hyphae in *Trichophyton* spp.

- **Microsporum:** Colonies of the fungi of this genus are cottony, velvety or powdery with white to brown pigmentation. Macroconidia are very numerous and microconidia are relatively scarce. The distinguishing characteristic is the macroconidium, which is typically thick-walled and rough (varying from minutely to strongly roughened). Macroconidia also vary in shape (fusiform to obovate), number of septa (3–15), size (5–100 × 3–8 µm) and thickness of the cell wall (Table 5.1 and Fig. 5.1). Microconidia are pyriform or clavate and are usually arranged singly along the sides of the hyphae. They infect skin and hair but not the nails.

- **Epidermophyton:** Colonies are powdery and greenish-yellow. Microconidia are absent and macroconidia are club-shaped. They have 2–6 septa, are 20–40 × 6–8 µm in size, thin- and slightly thick-walled and are borne singly or in clusters (Table 5.1 and Fig. 5.1). *E. floccosum* is currently the only recognized *Epidermophyton* species. It infects skin and nails but not the hair.

Salient characteristics of common dermatophytes are given in Table 5.4.

**Table 5.4.** Salient characteristics of common dermatophytes

| Species | Colony character | Microscopic morphology |
|---|---|---|
| T. mentagrophytes | Growth on SDA is relatively rapid, maturing in 6–10 days. Colony varies greatly; surface may be tan and powdery, becoming yellowish, or white and downy. Powdery form exhibits concentric and radial folds. Reverse is usually brownish tan but may be colourless, yellow, or red. | Hyphae are septate and at places spirally coiled (Figs. 5.5 and 5.6). Microconidia in powdery culture are round (4–6 µm in diameter) and clustered on branched conidiophores or, in fluffy strains, are smaller, fewer in number and tear-shaped. Macroconidia are sometimes present. They are thin-walled, club-shaped, spindle-shaped or long pencil-shaped. They are 4–8 × 20–50 µm in size, contain 1–6 cells and have narrow attachment to hyphae. |
| T. rubrum | Growth on SDA is relatively slow; matures within 14 days. The surface is granular or fluffy, white to buff. The reverse is deep red or purplish or occasionally brown, yellow-orange or colourless (Fig. 5.7). The pigment production is best seen on potato dextrose agar or corn dextrose agar. | Hyphae are septate. Tear-shaped microconidia (2–3.5 × 3–5.5 µm) usually form singly along the sides of the hyphae (Fig. 5.8). Macroconidia (4–8 × 40–60 µm) are narrow and thin-walled with parallel sides (pencil-like), and have 4–10 cells. They may be abundant, rare or absent. |
| T. tonsurans | Growth is slow; matures in 12 days. Colonies are white, tan, yellow or reddish brown with radial or concentric folds. The reverse is usually reddish brown. Pigment may diffuse into the medium (Fig. 5.9). | Hyphae are septate, with many teardrop or club-shaped microconidia formed along the hyphae or on short conidiophores. Intercalary and terminal chlamydoconidia are common in older cultures. Macroconidia are rare, irregularly shaped and slightly thick-walled. |

*(Contd.)*

## Dermatophytoses

| Species | Colony character | Microscopic morphology |
|---|---|---|
| T. schoenleinii | Grows slowly; matures within 15 days. Colony is white to tan, glabrous, waxy, heaped and folded. Growth is often submerged and splits the agar medium. Reverse is colourless or pale yellowish orange to tan. | Hyphae are septate, highly irregular, and tend to become knobby and clubbed at ends (favic chandeliers) (Fig. 5.5). Chlamydoconidia are numerous. Microconidia and macroconidia are absent. Initial growth from clinical specimen may resemble yeast both macroscopically and microscopically. |
| T. violaceum | Grows slowly; matures in 14–21 days. In a typical primary culture it produces a conical colony with irregularly folded surface, very short velvety aerial hyphae and a deep violet colour. Subcultures are more downy, and they decrease in colour. Reverse is lavender to purple. | Irregularly branched hyphae with intercalary chlamydoconidia (Fig. 5.10). Microconidia and macroconidia are not usually seen on SDA, but a few may form on thiamine-enriched media. |
| T. verrucosum | Growth is slow. It matures in 14–21 days. Unlike other dermatophytes, this fungus grows best at 37°C. The colony is raised, irregularly folded and (on enriched media) covered with very short aerial hyphae. Usually white, but may be gray or yellow. Reverse varies from nonpigmented to yellow. | On SDA at 37°C it forms hyphae with many chlamydoconidia and some antler-like branches. On media, enriched with thiamine, it produces many small, delicate, single microconidia and occasional long, thin, irregular, macroconidia. |
| M. audouinii | M. audouinii grows slowly, producing a gray colony with short aerial hyphae and usually with a radially folded surface. On the reverse side the centre of the colony is reddish brown (pigment is best seen on potato dextrose agar). | Hyphae are septate with terminal chlamydoconidia that are often pointed on the end. Pectinate hyphae are commonly seen. It sporulates poorly on SDA, and the spindle-shaped macroconidia which characterize the genus may be lacking in many strains. Rate of growth and sporulation are increased by addition of yeast extract to the medium. |
| M. canis | Grows more rapidly, sporulates more freely and is more deeply pigmented than M. audouinii. The colony has abundant coarse, woolly aerial mycelium. The colour of the colony is white to bright yellow with bright yellow to orange-brown on reverse. | Hyphae are septate with abundant, thick-walled, rough, spindle-shaped, macroconidia which usually are 10–25 × 35–110 µm in size. The macroconidium may be divided into as many as 15 cells by septa. Microconidia are clavate, sessile borne laterally directly from the hyphae and are less numerous than macroconidia. |
| M. gypseum | It grows rapidly. The colony is fawn brown to buff or reddish brown. The reverse of the colony may be yellow, orange-tan, brownish red, or purplish red in spots. | Septate hyphae. Macroconidia (8–16 × 22–60 µm) are produced in greater numbers. They are broadly spindle-shaped with relatively thin walls and 4–6 septa. Club-shaped microconidia are usually present along the hyphae. |
| M. gallinae | Grows slowly and produces in two weeks a conical, folded and wrinkled colony with short aerial hyphae which may be white or pink. Reverse is yellow at first and later has a red pigment that diffuses into the medium. | Hyphae are septate. Macroconidia are 6–8 × 15–50 µm with 4–10 septa. Walls of macroconidia are relatively thin and usually smooth but sometimes slightly rough at the tip. Microconidia are clavate and are usually abundant. |

*(Contd.)*

## SECTION 2 : Superficial Cutaneous Mycoses

| Species | Colony character | Microscopic morphology |
|---|---|---|
| *M. vanbreuseghemii* | Growth moderately rapid; matures within 7 days. Surface is yellowish, cream or pink; powdery to downy. Reverse is colourless or yellow to orange-tan. | Hyphae are septate; macroconidia are long (10–12 × 58–62 µm); up to 12 septa, thick walls smooth to spiny; numerous microconidia. |
| *M. ferrugineum* | Grows slowly on SDA; matures in 12–20 days. Produces an irregularly folded, glabrous, reddish-yellow to orange-yellow colony with almost waxy surface. Reverse is usually brownish tan but may be colourless, yellow or red. | Hyphae are septate; some are long and straight with prominent cross-walls; these are called "bamboo" hyphae. Other hyphae are irregularly branched, clubbed, and fragmented, and may have intercalary chlamydoconidium-like cells. Macroconidia, rarely produced, resemble those of *M. canis* and *M. cookei*. |
| *M. cookei* | Growth moderately rapid; matures within 7 days. Surface yellowish, reddish or tan, powdery or granular; reverse deep purple-red. | Hyphae are septate and branched. Macroconidia are numerous, oval (10–15 × 30–50 µm), thick walled, and rough, with 5–8 cells. Club-shaped microconidia are usually abundant. |
| *M. nanum* | Growth moderately rapid; matures in 7 days. Surface cream to tan, powdery or downy; reverse reddish brown. | Septate hyphae; macroconidia (4–8 × 12–18 µm) are rough, fairly thin-walled and ovate or elliptical, having 1–3 cells (usually 2). Microconidia are clavate, 2–5 µm, and are rare to moderate. |
| *M. persicolor* | Flat powdery to cottony, buff to peach colony. Reverse is pink to reddish-brown. | Macroconidia are rare, clavate to fusiform and have minutely echinulate walls. Microconidia are clavate and abundant. |
| *E. floccosum* | Colonies grow rapidly; mature within 10 days. Surface of the colony is brownish-yellow to olive-gray or khaki. The centre of the colony is marked by irregular concentric and radial folds and furrows. After several weeks, fluffy white sterile mycelium covers the colony. Reverse is orange to brownish, sometimes with a thin yelllow border. | Septate hyphae; microconidia are never produced, therefore, if microconidia are observed in an unknown culture of a dermatophyte, *E. floccosum* can be excluded. Numerous macroconidia (7–12 × 20–40 µm), seen best in young cultures, are smooth, both thin and slightly thick-walled and club-shaped with round ends. They contain 2–6 septa and are found singly or in clusters. |

### Cellophane tape mount
See Appendix C.

### Hair perforation test
Hair perforation test is useful in differentiating *T. rubrum* from *T. mentagrophytes*. To observe hair perforation, short (5–10 mm) strands of human hair (ideally hair from a child under the age of 18 months) are placed in a petri dish with 20 ml of distilled water and autoclaved. Two to three drops of 10% sterilized yeast extract are added to the petri dish and hair strands are inoculated with small fragments of test fungus grown on SDA. It is incubated at 25–30°C and the hair strands are removed and microscopically examined in lactophenol cotton blue (LPCB) at weekly intervals for up to 1 month. **T. rubrum which may be morphologically similar to T. mentagrophytes, usually causes only surface erosion of hair shafts in this test, whereas T. mentagrophytes causes wedge-shaped perforation perpendicular to hair shaft** (Fig. 5.11). *M. canis* and *M. gypseum* also show wedge-shaped perforation perpendicular to hair shaft.

### Urease test
Urease test is useful for distinguishing isolate of

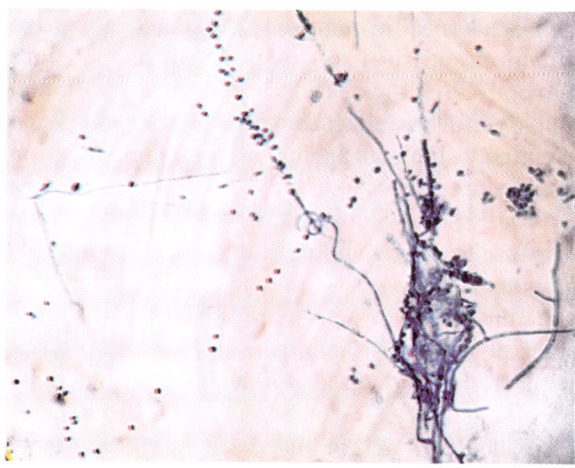

**Fig. 5.6.** Lactophenol cotton blue preparation of culture of *Trichophyton mentagrophytes* (×400).

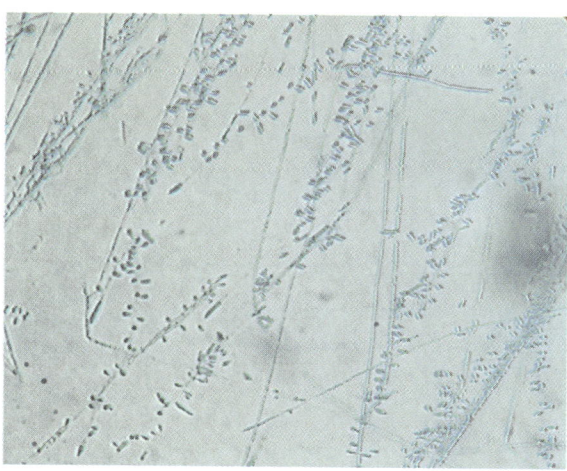

**Fig. 5.8.** Lactophenol cotton blue preparation of culture of *Trichophyton rubrum* (×400).

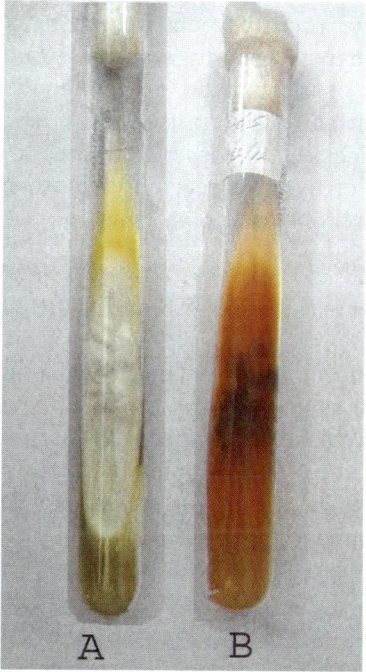

**Fig. 5.7.** Growth of *Trichophyton rubrum* on Sabouraud dextrose agar; surface (A) and reverse (B) view.

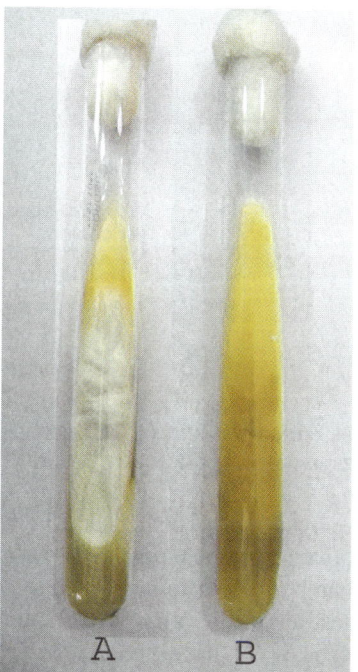

**Fig. 5.9.** Growth of *Trichophyton tonsurans* on Sabouraud dextrose agar; surface (A) and reverse (B) view.

*T. mentagrophytes* from that of *T. rubrum*. Urease splits urea in Christensen's medium, producing ammonia, which raises the pH and causes a colour shift of the phenol red indicator from amber to bright pink. For example, *T. mentagrophytes* produces a bright pink colour (positive), while *T. rubrum* produces no colour change (negative). A tube of Christensen's urea agar is very lightly inoculated with

## SECTION 2 : Superficial Cutaneous Mycoses

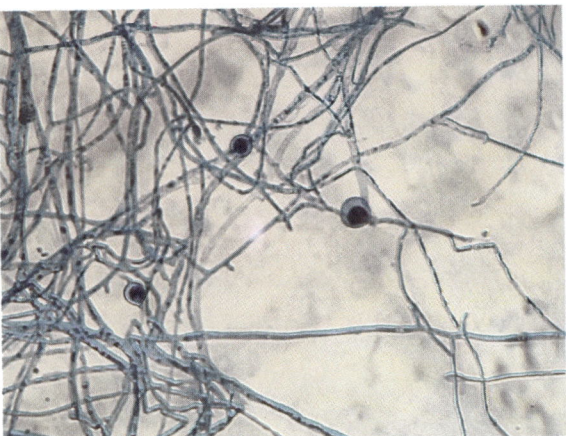

**Fig. 5.10.** Lactophenol cotton blue preparation of culture of *Trichophyton violaceum* showing intercalary chlamydoconidia (×400).

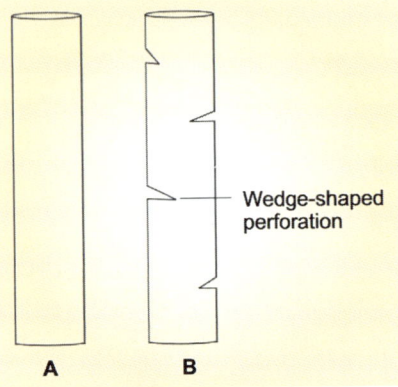

**Fig. 5.11.** Hair perforation test. (A) Normal hair. (B) Hair showing wedge-shaped perforation.

the dermatophyte and incubated at 25–30°C for 7 days. A positive reaction is indicated by a change of the original amber colour to bright pink.

Urease test also aids in the identification of the urease-positive *Cryptococcus*, *Rhodotorula*, *Malassezia* and *Trichosporon* from urease-negative *Candida*, *Saccharomyces*, *Geotrichum*, etc.

### Immunology

Dermatophyte colonization is characteristically limited to dead keratinized tissue of the stratum corneum and results in either a mild or intense inflammatory reaction. The cornified layers of the skin lack a specific immune system to recognize this infection and rid itself of it. Nevertheless, both humoral and cell-mediated reactions, and specific and non-specific host defence mechanisms respond and eventually eliminate the fungus, preventing invasion into the deeper viable tissue.

The host develops a variety of antibodies as a response to a dermatophyte infection, i.e., immunoglobulin M (IgM), IgG, IgA and IgE. However, they apparently do not help to eliminate the infection since high level of antibodies is found in patients with chronic infection. IgE mediates immediate hypersensitivity. Development of CMI, which is correlated with delayed hypersensitivity, is usually associated with clinical cure and with exclusion of the dermatophyte elements from the stratum corneum. Lack of CMI or defective CMI prevents an effective response, and predisposes the host to chronic or recurrent dermatophyte infection. Delayed hypersensitivity response to intradermal injections of trichophytin are commonly observed in the normal population. These responses are probably caused by earlier exposures to dermatophytosis, or by cross reactivity with one or more related environmental organisms.

### Treatment

Oral agents such as terbinafine, itraconazole, fluconazole, voriconazole and posaconazole are prescribed in various treatment regimens. Topical antifungal agents used in dermatophyte infections include Whitfield's ointment, tolnaftate (cream, powder, lotion), miconazole, clotrimazole, econazole, ketoconazole (cream, powder, lotion, spray, shampoo), amorolfine (cream, nail lacquer) and cyclopyroxolamine (cream).

### Important Questions

1. Name various genera and species of dermatophytes. Tabulate differences between various genera of dermatophytes.
2. Discuss laboratory diagnosis of dermatophytoses.
3. Write short notes on
   (a) Hair perforation test
   (b) Urease test.

## Multiple Choice Questions

1. Which of the following genera of fungi is **not** included under dermatophytes?
   (a) *Candida*.
   (b) *Trichophyton*.
   (c) *Microsporum*.
   (d) *Epidermophyton*.

2. Microconidia are not formed by which of the following dermatophytes?
   (a) *Trichophyton*.
   (b) *Microsporum*.
   (c) *Epidermophyton*.
   (d) All of the above.

3. Which of the following fungi is geophilic?
   (a) *Trichophyton rubrum*.
   (b) *Trichophyton audouinii*.
   (c) *Epidermophyton floccosum*.
   (d) *Microsporum gypseum*.

4. Which of the following fungi is anthropophilic?
   (a) *Trichophyton rubrum*.
   (b) *Trichophyton ajelloi*.
   (c) *Trichophyton verrucosum*.
   (d) *Microsporum canis*.

5. Favus is caused by
   (a) *Trichophyton rubrum*.
   (b) *Trichophyton schoenleinii*.
   (c) *Trichophyton mentagrophytes*.
   (d) *Trichophyton tonsurans*.

6. Which of the following dermatophytes causes hair perforation?
   (a) *Trichophyton rubrum*.
   (b) *Trichophyton tonsurans*.
   (c) *Trichophyton mentagrophytes*.
   (d) *Trichophyton violaceum*.

7. In which of the following genera of dermatophytes teleomorph state has **not** been described?
   (a) *Trichophyton*.
   (b) *Microsporum*.
   (c) *Epidermophyton*.
   (d) None of the above.

8. Id reaction is seen in patients suffering from:
   (a) dermatophytosis.
   (b) histoplasmosis.
   (c) blastomycosis.
   (d) Coccidioidomycosis.

9. The infection of the skin caused by non-dermatophytic fungi and the cutaneous manifestations of systemic mycoses are known as:
   (a) dermatophytosis.
   (b) dermatophytid.
   (c) dermatomycosis.
   (d) ectothrix.

10. Which of the following dermatophytes is urease-positive?
    (a) *Trichophyton mentagrophytes*.
    (b) *Trichophyton rubrum*.
    (c) *Trichophyton tonsurans*.
    (d) *Trichophyton schoenleinii*.

11. Which of the following statements is **true** about cultivation of dermatophytes on Sabouraud dextrose agar?
    (a) Cultures are incubated at 37°C to inhibit saprophytic fungi.
    (b) Cultures should not be considered negative before 4 weeks of incubation.
    (c) Dermatophytes cannot be isolated from nail specimens.
    (d) Medium containing cycloheximide is inhibitory.

12. Which of the following mycoses is contagious, directly host-to-host transmissible disease of humans and animals?
    (a) Blastomycosis.
    (b) Histoplasmosis.
    (c) Dermatophytoses.
    (d) Sporotrichosis.

### ANSWERS TO MCQs

1. (a), 2. (c), 3. (d), 4. (a), 5. (b), 6. (c), 7. (c), 8. (a), 9. (c), 10. (a), 11. (b), 12. (c).

### Further Reading

1. Almeida SR. Immunology of dermatophytosis. *Mycopathologia* 2008.
2. Caddell JR. Differentiating the dermatophytes. *Clin Lab Sci* 2002; 15: 13–5.
3. Duek L, Kaufman G, et al. The pathogenesis of dermatophyte infections in human skin sections. *J Infect* 2004; 48: 175–80.

4. Fuller LC, Child FJ, et al. Diagnosis and management of scalp ringworm. *BMJ* 2003; 326: 539–41.
5. Galhardo MC, Wanke B, et al. Disseminated dermatophytosis caused by *Microsporum gypseum* in an AIDS patient: response to terbinafine and amorolfine. *Mycoses* 2004; 47: 238–41.
6. Gupta AK, Tu LQ. Dermatophytes: diagnosis and treatment. *J Am Acad Dermatol* 2006; 54: 1050–55.
7. Liu D, Pearce L, et al. PCR identification of dermatophyte fungi *Trichophyton rubrum*, *T. soudanense* and *T. gourvillii*. *J Med Microbiol* 2002; 51: 117–22.
8. Malik AK, Arora DR, et al. Animal dermatophytosis in North India. *Indian Vet Med J* 1984; 8: 93–96.
9. Rodwell GE, Bayles CL, et al. The prevalence of dermatophyte infection in patients infected with human immunodeficiency virus. *Int J Dermatol* 2008; 47: 339–43.

# SECTION 3

## SUBCUTANEOUS MYCOSES

**Chapter 6**   Mycetoma
**Chapter 7**   Sporotrichosis
**Chapter 8**   Chromoblastomycosis
**Chapter 9**   Phaeohyphomycosis
**Chapter 10**  Lobomycosis

# CHAPTER 6

# Mycetoma

Mycetoma is a localized swollen lesion, usually on foot (Fig. 6.1) or hand (Fig. 6.2), less often on shoulders, buttocks, head, or any site which is subject to trauma. Location of extrapedal lesions depends upon what part of the body is subject to traumatic inoculation with the etiologic agent. The lesion begins at the site of trauma and continues to spread locally over the ensuing months and years. It involves skin, subcutaneous tissue, fascia and bone. The lesion contains **granulomas** and **abscesses** which suppurate and drain through **sinus tracks**. The pus contains **grains** or **granules**, which are macrocolonies of the etiologic agent that are extruded through the sinuses. They vary from microscopic in size to more than 2 mm in diameter. The size, colour, shape and texture of grains as well as the dimensions of the fungal hyphae within the grains, vary with the species of fungus. Grains are white, yellow, pink, red or black depending upon the species of etiologic agent. Microscopic examination of the grains even without culture permits the experienced mycologist to identify the species of fungus.

Mycetoma is popularly known as **"Madura foot"** or **"maduromycosis"**. The disease was first recognized in India by Gill (1842) and Colebrook (1846) who worked in medical dispensary at Madurai, Tamil Nadu in southern India. The name

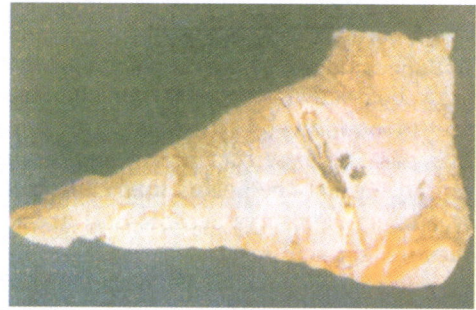

Fig. 6.1. Mycetoma foot showing black granules.

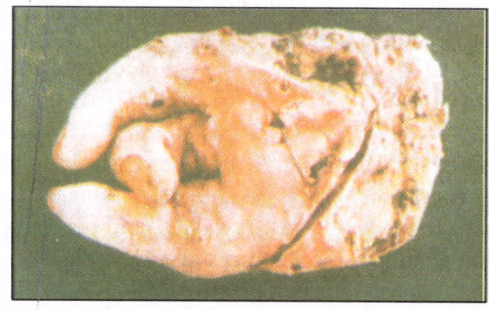

Fig. 6.2. Mycetoma hand showing black granules.

"Madura foot" though of ancient standing is a misnomer even for mycetoma localized in the feet. For generations it has created confusion by identifying the island of Madura, northeast of Java

(Indonesia) rather than the town of Madurai in South India. Therefore, it is proposed that "Madurai foot" henceforth should replace the incorrect designation of Colebrook hitherto used.

## Differential diagnosis

1. Mycetoma should be differentiated from **actinomycosis**, which is an endogenous suppurative infection caused by *Actinomyces israelii* or other species of *Actinomyces* or related bacteria, affecting the sites that would be unusual for mycetoma, such as cervicofacial, thoracic, and pelvic sites (the latter is usually associated with the use of intrauterine devices). The branching bacteria that cause actinomycosis are non-acid-fast, anaerobic or microaerophilic none of which causes mycetoma. There is no history of penetrating external trauma. Draining sinuses originate in the viscera, not in subcutaneous tissue. The two diseases can resemble each other on biopsy, both showing grains in pyogenic foci that are surrounded by fibrosis and chronic inflammation. These bacteria are smaller than 1 µm in diameter. **The agents that cause actinomycetoma are always aerobic and are sometimes weakly acid-fast.**
2. Early lesions of mycetoma, without draining sinus, may be mistaken for a pyogenic granuloma.
3. **Mycotic granulomas** containing diffusely growing fungal elements are not classified as mycetomas.
4. Mycetoma should be differentiated from **fungus ball**. The latter develops in pre-existing pulmonary cavities such as tuberculosis or cystic disease. The inhaled conidia enter a cavity, germinate and produce abundant hyphae. It may also develop in maxillary sinus, and occasionally in the ethmoid, sphenoid and frontal sinuses. It is only saprophytic colonization without invasion of lung or sinus mucosa.
5. **Abscesses** containing colonies of staphylococci are not included under botryomycosis unless the colonies have an eosinophilic coating and the microscopic appearance of grains.
6. Mycetoma must be differentiated from **elephantiasis** of the foot, in which no sinus tracts are formed.

## Etiology and pathogenesis

An increasing number of different types of fungi, aerobic actinomycetes which occur as saprophytes in soil or on plants, and other bacteria have been named as causative agents of **eumycetoma**, **actinomycetoma** and **botryomycosis**, respectively (Table 6.1). Infection follows traumatic inoculation of the organism into the subcutaneous tissue from soil or vegetable source, e.g., thorns or splinters and results in **tumefactions, deformities**, and **draining sinuses discharging fungal colonies called grains or granules** (triad of symptoms).

Eumycetoma is endemic in the tropics and subtropics. The major endemic area is in Sudan; other areas are Mexico, Central and South America, India,

**Table 6.1.** Causative agents and colour of the grains of various types of mycetoma

| Causative agent | Colour of grains |
|---|---|
| **A. Eumycetoma** | |
| *Madurella mycetomatis* | Black |
| *M. grisea* | Black |
| *Exophiala jeanselmei* | Black |
| *Curvularia geniculata* | Black |
| *Leptosphaeria senegalensis* | Black |
| *Pyrenochaeta romeroi* | Black |
| *Acremonium* spp. | White |
| *Aspergillus nodulans* | White |
| *A. flavus* | White |
| *Fusarium moniliforme* | White |
| *Cylindrocarpon cyanescens* | White |
| *Neotestudina rosati* | White |
| *Scedosporium apiospermum* | White |
| **B. Actinomycetoma** | |
| *Actinomadura madurae* | White to yellow |
| *A. pelletieri* | Red to pink |
| *Nocardia brasiliensis* | White to yellow |
| *N. caviae* | White to yellow |
| *N. asteroides* | White to yellow |
| *N. otitidiscaviarum* | White to yellow |
| *Nocardiopsis dassonvillei* | Cream |
| *Streptomyces somaliensis* | Yellow |
| **C. Botryomycosis** | |
| *Staphylococcus aureus* | White |
| *Escherichia coli* | White |
| *Proteus* spp. | White |
| *Pseudomonas aeruginosa* | White |
| *Actinobacillus lignieresii* | Yellow |

Pakistan, Indonesia, other African countries, the Middle East, and occasionally in temperate zones including the United States. Actinomycetomas caused by *Nocardia* spp. are most common in Central America and Mexico. The actinomycete, *Streptomyces somaliensis*, is most often isolated from patients originating from Sudan, the Middle East and India. The causative organisms have been isolated from either soil or plant material including thorns from *Acacia* bushes in endemic areas. Mycetoma usually occurs in agriculture workers. Adult males are, therefore, most often infected.

After the fungi or bacteria enter the tissues, a period of growth and multiplication results in the production of colonies of etiologic agents. Between the colonies and the surrounding tissues of the host there is a suppurative inflammatory reaction which may be accompanied by an outer epithelioid and giant-cell granulomatous reaction. The outer surface of the colonies may be surrounded by an eosinophilic homogenous material (Splendore-Hoeppli material), sometimes with radiating or knobby extensions.

Mycetoma usually remains localized, although it spreads slowly to contiguous tissues. Extension to underlying bones and joints gives rise to periostitis, osteomyelitis and arthritis. X-ray study of mycetoma lesions is helpful for determining the extent of bone destruction (Fig. 6.3). In general the eumycetomas rarely metastasize, but actinomycetomas may disseminate via the lymphatics or blood vessels.

As seen in tissue sections, the causative agents are grains rather than individual elements of fungi or bacteria. If no grains have formed, the lesion cannot be classified as a mycetoma. Sometimes numerous sections must be examined microscopically to find a single grain. **No grain no mycetoma.** While there may be difficulty in differentiating some grains from colonies, the former are **more compact** and characteristically have a **cement-like matrix** and **outer shell or club-like arrangement of eosinophilic material**.

Chronic bacterial infections sometimes have clumps of etiologic agent encased in proteinaceous debris, forming a soft grain. This entity is known as botryomycosis. *Staphylococcus aureus* is the usual bacterial pathogen, but Gram-negative bacteria also can be responsible. The grains of botryomycosis are small, nonpigmented, with a prominent eosinophilic shell. Gram staining of a crushed grain readily distinguishes the grain of botryomycosis from those of mycetoma.

### Laboratory diagnosis

The diagnosis of mycetoma rests on the microscopic demonstration of the grains and the appropriate tissue reaction. There is a central zone of suppuration and a surrounding chronic inflammatory reaction which may include epithelioid and multinucleated giant cells. The grain is found surrounded by pus in the centre of the lesion. In old lesions fibrosis becomes prominent in areas between abscesses. Sometimes a foreign body, such as a thorn, is present in association with the mycotic grains providing a clue to penetrating injury. The methods of laboratory diagnosis of mycetoma include direct microscopy, histopathology and culture.

### Direct microscopy

An unruptured pustule is identified, cleaned with an alcohol swab and gently pierced with a sterile needle. The edges of the pustule are squeezed, and a small drop of pus and blood is extruded. This is then spread on a glass slide where it is possible to identify small (200 μm to more than 2 mm) granules that are white, yellow, pink, red or black. Grains of eumycetoma are white or yellow when the agents are hyaline molds or black when due to melanized fungi.

Granules are placed in a drop of 10% potassium hydroxide and crushed under a cover slip in order to

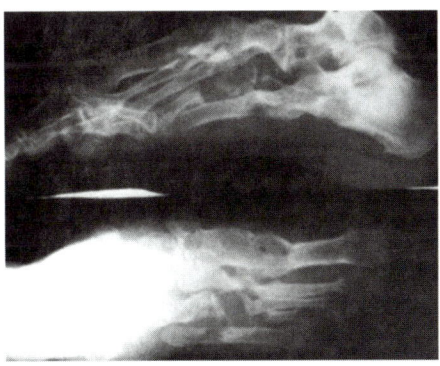

**Fig. 6.3.** Erosive X-ray changes in a mycetoma.

observe hyphal dimensions, septation, morphology, pigment formation in hyphal walls, interhyphal cementing material and consistency of grain. **Eumycotic grains** can be seen with 2–6 μm wide hyphae that often have large, globose swollen cells (chlamydoconidia), up to 15 μm or more at the margin.

**Actinomycotic grains** have filaments, with a diameter of 0.5–1 μm, as well as coccoid to bacillary elements. For a stained film the granule should be crushed in the pus in which it is found. The hyphae of the actinomycetes are Gram-positive, narrow filaments in a background of Gram-negative cementing material. Although, some eumycotic grains are Gram-positive, Gram stain, in general, is of limited value in demonstrating the presence of eumycetes.

*Culture and histopathology*

The fungi of mycetoma grow readily in culture. It is best to use conventional media such as Sabouraud dextrose agar (SDA) for primary isolation, using plates or tubes with and without antibiotics such as chloramphenicol and gentamicin. For culture a biopsy of deep tissues is best. Superficial tissues are usually contaminated with either bacteria or fungi. Wash the grains in sterile normal saline if contamination is suspected, crush them and spread the fragments as inoculum on agar slants.

Since the optimum temperature for growth differs, in the diagnosis of mycetoma of unknown etiology, some cultures should be incubated at room temperature and others at 35–37°C. The rate of growth is highly variable and therefore cultures should be kept for at least 3 weeks before they are discarded as negative. The isolate is identified by colonial morphology, patterns of sporulation, pigmentation, and growth rates.

When actinomycetoma is suspected by observation of Gram-positive filaments of crushed grains then these are washed several times with sterile normal saline and then inoculated on SDA without antibiotics, blood agar and brain-heart-infusion agar.

The infected tissue should be sectioned and stained with haematoxylin and eosin, Gomori methamine silver, periodic acid-Schiff and Brown and Brenn stain (tissue Gram stain). The stains are not necessary to visualize the grains, but are helpful in demonstrating the large hyphae and chlamydoconidia within, and to differentiate the grains of fungi from those of actinomycetes. Brief description of histological appearance and cultural characteristics of both fungal and bacterial agents causing mycetoma is given below:

### Madurella mycetomatis

Grains of *M. mycetomatis* are black, firm, and brittle; and the shape is globose, oval, or lobulated. They are usually 0.5–4 mm in size. Grains are composed of interlacing hyphae 2–5 μm in diameter. Terminal hyphal cells at the periphery of the grain may be 12–15 μm in diameter sometimes with exceptionally large (30 μm) swollen cells. **There is relatively little pigment in the walls of many hyphae, but the hyphal cells contain brown pigment particles.** The hyphae are embedded in brown cement substance. The cement substance is uniformly distributed in the whole grain (Figs. 6.4–6.6), thus differentiating it from the grain of *M. grisea*. The latter has a hollow appearance due to the peripheral distribution of cement substance.

*Colony morphology*

In culture, *M. mycetomatis* is extremely variable. Optimum temperature of growth is 37°C. The colony

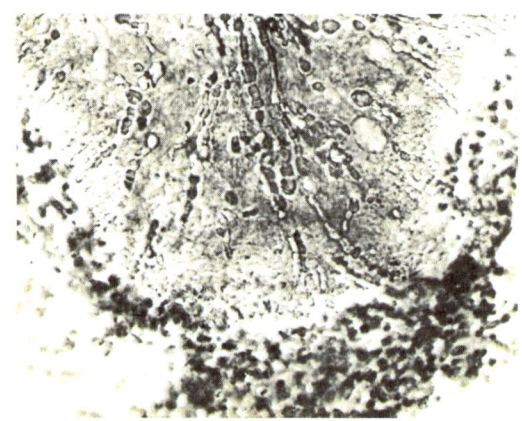

**Fig. 6.4.** Grain of *Madurella mycetomatis* with a ring of inflammatory cells. Radial arrangement of segmented hyphae at the periphery along with large variable sized spores is clearly visible. The cement substance is uniformly distributed in the whole grain (H&E stain, ×400).

# Mycetoma

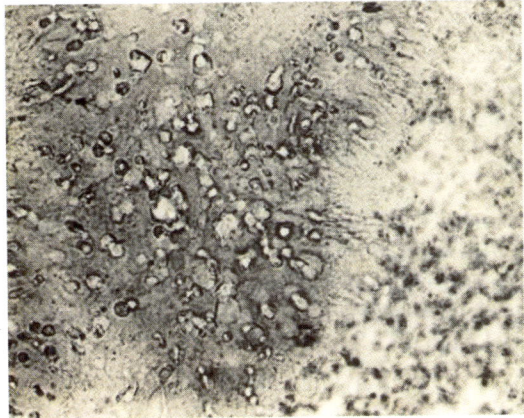

**Fig. 6.5.** Grain of *Madurella mycetomatis* with terminal hyphal cells outnumbering the hyphae (H&E stain, ×400).

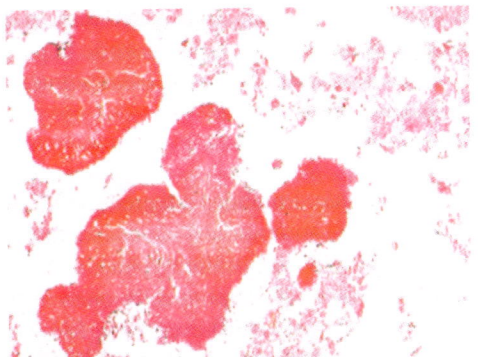

**Fig. 6.6.** Granulomatous reaction and the grain of *Madurella mycetomatis* in a patient with mycetoma foot (H&E stain, ×400).

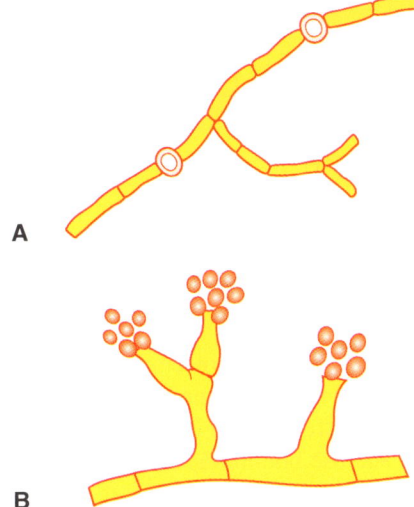

**Fig. 6.7.** Microscopic appearance of *Madurella mycetomatis* on Sabouraud dextrose agar (A) and on corn meal agar (B).

develops within 10 days. It grows much more slowly at 25°C. The colony may be smooth or folded and glabrous or powdery and ranges in colour from white to yellowish brown. There is usually a brown diffusible pigment in the agar. Reverse is dark brown.

### Microscopic morphology

On SDA, it forms only septate hyphae (1–6 μm in diameter) with numerous chlamydoconidium-like enlarged cells (Fig. 6.7A). On corn meal agar, some strains produce phialides that bear round or oval conidia at their tips (Fig. 6.7B). It may form large, black masses of modified hyphae (sclerotia) in old cultures. *M. mycetomatis* differs biochemically from *M. grisea* in assimilating lactose but not sucrose.

## Madurella grisea

The grains of *M. grisea* are black, 0.3–0.6 mm in diameter. They are soft when young, become firm in larger grains and become brittle upon drying. In the sections, grains of *M. grisea* show unpigmented or pale central areas with an outer brown fungus hyphae and brown interstitial cement substances. **The peripheral hyphae have pigmented walls but lack the brown granules of intracellular pigment characteristic of *M. mycetomatis*.**

### Colony morphology

*M. grisea* grows well at 25–30°C in 12 days than at 37°C. The surface is somewhat folded in the centre with radial grooves towards the periphery. Very short, tan or gray aerial hyphae cover a dark gray or olive-brown mycelial mat. Reverse is dark. May form diffusible pigment, but not as commonly as does *M. mycetomatis*.

### Microscopic morphology

Hyphae are septate, branched, dark and mostly wide (3–5 μm in diameter). These hyphae sometimes appear to be made up of chains of rounded cells, suggesting a budding process (Fig. 6.8). Thinner (1–3 μm in diameter), cylindrical, branched hyphae are

## SECTION 3 : Subcutaneous Mycoses

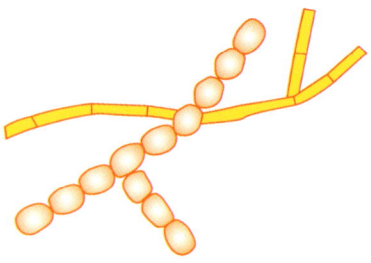

**Fig. 6.8.** Microscopic appearance of culture of *Madurella grisea*.

also present. Conidia are not commonly formed. Chlamydoconidia are occasionally produced.

*M. grisea* differs from *M. mycetomatis* in assimilating sucrose but not lactose.

### Pyrenochaeta romeroi

*P. romeroi* produces soft, black, spherical or tubular grains which are 0.5–1.5 mm in diameter.

*Colony morphology*

It produces a dark downy colony with a black under-surface. Most strains grow slowly at 37°C, but optimum temperature is 30°C. The colony, expands rapidly and produces pycnidia. These have thick outer walls.

*Microscopic morphology*

The fungus produces brownish-black ostiolate pycnidia 50–150 × 100–300 μm in size. These contain elliptical and yellowish pycnidiospores which are about 1 μm in diameter. These are produced by phialides in chains.

### Scedosporium apiospermum

*S. apiospermum* produces white, soft to firm, sub-spherical and lobulated grains measuring 0.5–1.0 mm in diameter. The hyphae which constitute the grain are hyaline, 2–5 μm in diameter but much wider (15–20 μm) at the periphery. Border is eosinophilic.

*Colony morphology*

Colonies are rapidly growing. Surface has a spreading, white, cottony, aerial mycelium which later turns gray or brown. Reverse is at first white but usually becomes gray or black.

*Microscopic morphology*

Hyphae are septate (2–4 μm in diameter) with simple long or short conidiophores bearing conidia singly or in small groups. Conidia are 4–7 × 5–12 μm in size.

### Acremonium spp.

The main species implicated in mycetoma are *A. kiliense*, *A. falciforme* and *A. recifei*. The grains produced by *Acremonium* spp. are white to pale yellow, soft, 0.5–1.0 mm in diameter and variable in shape. They are composed of dense mass of slender, septate, hyaline hyphae with occasional vesicles or swollen hyphae.

*Colony morphology*

Colonies of all the three species are slow growing at first compact, glabrous; later become feltlike, powdery, or cottony. The colour is white to pink. On the undersurface there is usually a clear pigmentation that is pink to rose in colour.

*Microscopic morphology*

Hyphae are septate. Phialides are erect, unbranched, tapering and most (but not all) have a septum at the base delimiting them from the hyphae. Conidia are oblong (2–3 × 4–8 μm) and usually one-celled but occasionally two-celled. The conidia form easily disrupted clusters at the tips of the phialides (Fig. 6.9).

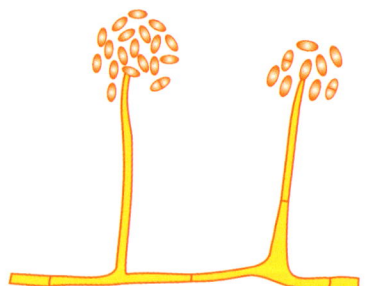

**Fig. 6.9.** Microscopic appearance of culture of *Acremonium* spp.

### Curvularia geniculata

*C. geniculata* grains are black to dark brown, firm, and 0.5–1.0 mm or more in size. In tissue sections, grains are spherical, ovoid, or irregularly shaped and are often surrounded by a zone of epitheloid cells.

# Mycetoma

The periphery of the grain is a dense, interwoven mass of dematiaceous mycelium and thick-walled, chlamydoconidia-like cells embedded in a cement-like substance. The interior of the grain is vacuolar and consists of a loose network of septate hyphal filaments.

### Colony morphology
In culture, *C. geniculata* develops a rapidly growing, floccose to downy, olive gray to black colony.

### Microscopic morphology
Microscopically, the melanized, septate hyphae bear solitary conidiogenous cells. They are smooth walled, predominantly five-celled, curved, with the swollen median cells pale to dark brown, in contrast to the lighter end cells.

## Exophiala jeanselmei
Grains of mycetoma produced by *E. jeanselmei* are black, 0.5–2.0 mm in diameter and irregular in shape.

In tissue sections, grains appear as hollow structures or as sinuous bands that are vermiform. The external surface is composed of brown thick-walled hyphae and thick-walled chlamydoconidia-like cells. The grains are cement-free. Within the hollow grains, smaller, degenerated hyphal fragments with leucocytes and giant cells may be seen.

### Colony morphology
It forms a distinct colony that changes with time from a predominance of yeast-like cells, which form a glabrous mucoid colony with dark pigmentation, to a downy colony containing a lot of mycelium with aerial hyphae. Reverse is black.

### Microscopic morphology
Young culture consists of many yeast-like budding cells. Eventually, septate hyphae form with numerous conidiogenous cells that are slender, tubular, sometimes branched, and characteristically tapered to a narrow, elongated tip. The conidia are oval 1–3 × 2–6 µm in size and gather in clusters at the end and sides of the conidiophore and at points along the hyphae (Fig. 6.10). Conidium formation is often best exhibited on cornmeal agar or potato dextrose agar. Chlamydoconidia may be present.

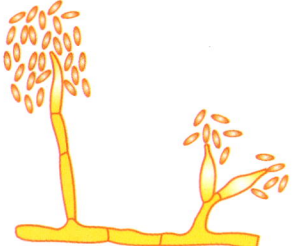

**Fig. 6.10.** Microscopic appearance of culture of *Exophiala jeanselmei*.

## Leptosphaeria senegalensis
It produces hard, black grains which are 0.5–4.0 mm in diameter. In tissue sections, the grains are round to polylobulated, with large vesicles. At the periphery, the mycelium is embedded in a black cement-like substance. The central portion of the grain consists of a loose network of hyphae.

### Colony morphology
It grows rapidly to produce a downy colony with a gray to black reverse pigmentation.

### Microscopic morphology
Asci are produced in older colonies and these contain eight oval ascospores that are long, measuring up to 30 µm in length.

## Actinomadura madurae
The grains of *A. madurae* are white, 1–5 mm in diameter, irregular and serpiginous in shape due to an irregular, relatively unstained and empty centre and a broad zone of deep blue (haematoxylinophilic) stained margin (Fig. 6.11). Mycelial filaments are delicate 0.5–1 µm in diameter and branching. The hyphae and the grains are surrounded by eosinophilic material.

### Colony morphology
In primary culture, growth develops slowly and is more reliable and rapid on Lowenstein-Jensen medium, than on SDA. Colonies are waxy, cerebriform at the centre with a flat peripheral zone, so membranous and tough that attempts to remove a portion may result in tearing out a triangular sector, and the colour varies from white to yellow, pink or red.

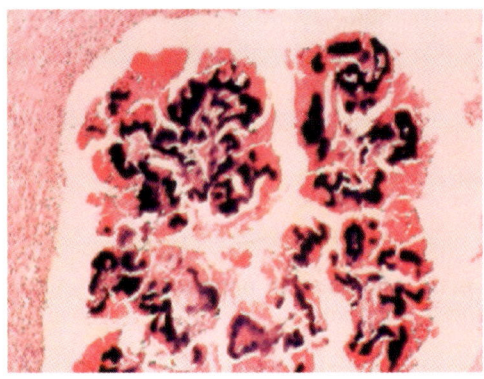

**Fig. 6.11.** Grain of *Actinomadura madurae* (H&E stain, ×400).

*Microscopic morphology*

Hyphae are 0.5–1 μm in diameter, Gram-positive and non-acid-fast.

### Actinomadura pelletieri

The grains of *A. pelletieri* are red, hard, spherical or oval 300–500 μm in diameter. In haematoxylin and eosin stained sections, the entire grain stains intensely with haematoxylin and its border is sharply delimited without the fringe of hyphal tips which characterize the granule of *A. madurae*, but many granules are bordered by a narrow eosinophilic zone. Hyphae are 0.5–1 μm in diameter, Gram-positive and non-acid-fast.

*Colony morphology*

In culture, colonies of *A. pelletieri* are small. The colour is red and surface is waxy on SDA and often covered with short white aerial hyphae on Lowenstein-Jensen medium.

### Nocardia brasiliensis

Grains of *N. brasiliensis* are white to yellow, soft, irregularly spherical, often lobulated less than 1 mm in diameter. The hyphae in the grain are Gram-positive and acid-fast.

*Colony morphology*

In culture, it produces a small, heaped, wrinkled or folded colony, yellow to orange in colour. It coagulates milk, liquefies gelatin and casein and does not utilize paraffin.

*Microscopic morphology*

The smear shows Gram-positive, acid-fast, branched filaments that fragment into bacillary forms. Acid-fast and aerobic nature of the organism serves to differentiate a nocardial mycetoma from actinomycosis.

### Nocardia caviae

The grains of *N. caviae* are similar to those of *N. brasiliensis*. The colonies on SDA are yellow to orange, with sparse, and short aerial hyphae and a close resemblance to *N. asteroides*. It differs from the latter by its ability to decompose xanthine and hypoxanthine and by formation of acid from inositol and mannitol. It differs from *N. brasiliensis* by its ability to decompose xanthine and by its inability to hydrolyze casein and tyrosine.

### Nocardia asteroides

The grains of *N. asteroides* are white, soft, irregular, and small in size measuring less than 0.5 mm.

*Colony morphology*

The colonies are glabrous, chalky, folded or wrinkled, white to orange pink in colour and have aerial hyphae.

*Microscopic morphology*

Microscopically it resembles *N. brasiliensis*.

### Streptomyces somaliensis

Grains produced by *S. somaliensis* are spherical or lobate, 0.5–2 mm in diameter, yellow to brown, smooth, hard and brittle. When the grains are pressed between two glass slides, they tend to break into angular fragments. In haematoxylin and eosin-stained sections, the centre of the grain is basophilic and often cracked owing to the brittleness of the grains. The peripheral part is smooth, narrow and eosinophilic (Fig. 6.12). Gram-stained smears show delicate Gram-positive branching filaments 0.5–1 μm in diameter and they are non-acid-fast.

*Colony morphology*

In culture, *S. pelletieri* grows rapidly. Growth is better on Lowenstein-Jensen medium than on SDA. Colonies are folded or cerebriform.

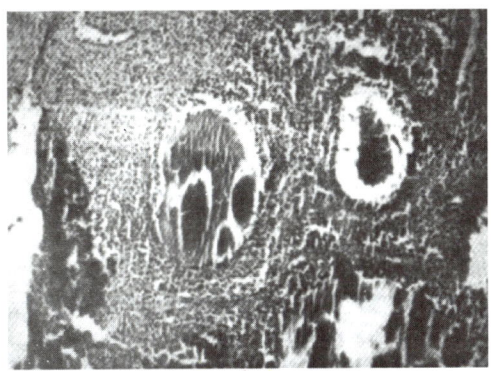

**Fig. 6.12.** Grains of *Streptomyces somaliensis* with abundant inflammatory exudate (H&E stain, ×400).

Diagnostic characteristics of grains of important eumycetomas and actinomycetomas are given in Table 6.2.

## Epidemiology of mycetoma in India

Mycetoma is prevalent in almost all parts of India. Actinomycetoma is more commonly encountered than eumycetoma. In India, *A. madurae* is a major cause of actinomycetoma responsible for 31% of recorded cases and is the predominant pathogen in the northern and southern regions. *A. pelletieri* is rarely seen in northern India, and most of the cases reported from South are from Tamil Nadu. Though once considered to be rare in Asia, *Nocardia* has been found in considerable number of cases. This has been reported as the most common causative agent in Kolkata, Mumbai and Pondicherry, and it is second largest group of actinomycetes causing mycetoma in South India. *S. somaliensis* is said to cause 3–10% of mycetoma cases. It is more common in southern region. However, it is dominant pathogen in Rajasthan.

The commonest causal agent of eumycetoma is *M. mycetomatis*. It is the major cause of black grain mycetoma in the dry, arid regions of the North. In the East, black grain mycetoma is caused by *M. grisea*. In the South, *M. mycetomatis* is either the dominant pathogen or the second largest group.

Chugh, Arora (first author), et al., in 1975 reported 43 cases of mycetoma from Haryana. Eumycetoma and actinomycetoma were seen in 33 and 10 cases respectively. *Madurella mycetomatis* was the commonest causative agent, being present in 33 of them. *Actinomadura madurae* was seen in six, *Streptomyces somaliensis* in three and *Nocardia* species was seen in one case. Of the 43 cases, foot was involved in 33 cases. In two cases each, hand and perineum were involved. In one case each, leg, patella, inguinal region, chest wall, scalp and mastoid were involved.

Most of the causal agents of mycetoma have been isolated from either soil or plants. These include *N. asteroides*, *N. brasiliensis*, *N. caviae*, and *M. mycetomatis*.

## Treatment

Localized lesions can be excised. In other cases, medical treatment should first be attempted, although chemotherapy of eumycetomas has, so far, been found to be quite unsatisfactory in most cases. However, certain fungi have been found to be relatively sensitive *in vitro* to therapeutic agents such as amphotericin B. *M. mycetomatis* is sensitive to ketoconazole in about 60% of the cases. Griseofulvin, terbinafine and itraconazole may be used in eumycetomas caused by other fungi. Actinomycetomas may be susceptible to chemotherapeutic agents. Combination of dapsone with streptomycin has been reported to give good results. Rifampicin and amikacin may also be used. Radical surgery, usually amputation, should be considered carefully.

## BOTRYOMYCOSIS (SCHIZOMYCETOMA)

Botryomycosis is chronic, purulent, "sulphur" grain-producing pyogranulomatous lesion of cutaneous or subcutaneous tissue and is caused by bacteria. Botryomycosis resembles actinomycosis and mycetoma in both clinical and histologic features. It is caused by *Staphylococcus aureus*, *Escherichia coli*, *Proteus* spp., *Pseudomonas aeruginosa*, and *Actinobacillus lignieresii* (Table 6.1).

Histologic sections from diseased tissues reveal neutrophils, lymphocytes, eosinophils, plasma cells, and fibroblasts, as well as histiocytes and scattered foreign body giant cells. The "sulphur" grains are found in the centre of the granulomas and are covered by neutrophils. The grains are soft and composed of the causative organisms measuring up to 1 mm in diameter. The eosinophilic shell around the grains is PAS-positive.

## SECTION 3 : Subcutaneous Mycoses

**Table 6.2.** Diagnostic characteristics of grains of important eumycetomas and actinomycetomas

| Classification | Species | Colour | Size | Texture | Properties |
|---|---|---|---|---|---|
| Actino-mycetoma grains | Actinomadura madurae | White to yellow | 1–5 mm | Soft to hard | Non-acid-fast periphery stained by H&E. |
| | Actinomadura pelletieri | Red to pink | 0.3–0.5 mm | Soft to hard | Non-acid-fast, variable H&E staining. |
| | Nocardia brasiliensis | White to yellow | < 1 mm | Soft | Acid-fast, variable H&E staining. |
| | Streptomyces somaliensis | Yellow to brown | 0.5–2 mm | Hard | Non-acid-fast, with H&E staining grain shows cracks owing to the brittleness of grains. |
| Eumycetoma grains | Madurella mycetomatis | Black | 0.5–4 mm | Firm and brittle | Hyphae 2–5 µm in diameter, terminal hyphal cells at the periphery are 12–15 µm in diameter. Brown cement substance is uniformly distributed in the whole grain. |
| | Madurella grisea | Black | 0.3–0.6 mm | Hard | Unpigmented or pale central areas with an outer brown fungal hyphae and brown interstitial cement substance. The peripheral hyphae have pigmented walls. |
| | Exophiala jeanselmei | Black | 0.5–2 mm | Brittle | Brown thick-walled hyphae and thick-walled chlamydoconidia-like cells. |
| | Leptosphaeria senegalensis | Black | 0.5–4 mm | Hard | Lobulated, dark periphery with loose network of hyphae and chlamydoconidia in cemented periphery. |
| | Acremonium spp. | White to pale yellow | 0.5–1 mm | Soft | Round to polylobulated, with large vesicles. At the periphery, the mycelium is embedded in a black cement substance. The central portion of the grain consists of a loose network of hyphae. |
| | Scedosporium apiospermum | White | 0.5–1 mm | Soft | Hyphae which constitute the grain are hyaline, 2–5 µm in diameter but much wider (15–20 µm) at the periphery. Border is eosinophilic. |

 **Important Questions**

1. Discuss etiology, pathogenesis and laboratory diagnosis of mycetoma.
2. Write short notes on
   (a) Differential diagnosis of mycetoma
   (b) Epidemiology of mycetoma in India.

**Multiple Choice Questions**

1. Which of the following causative agents of mycetoma **does not** form black grains?
   (a) *Madurella mycetomatis.*
   (b) *Actinomadura madurae.*
   (c) *Exophiala jeanselmei.*
   (d) *Pyrenochaeta romeroi.*

2. Which of the following causative agents of mycetoma forms black grains?
   (a) *Madurella grisea*.
   (b) *Actinomadura pelletieri*.
   (c) *Nocardia asteroides*.
   (d) *Actinomadura madurae*.

3. Mycetoma follows traumatic inoculation of the organism into the subcutaneous tissue from soil or vegetable source, e.g., thorns or splinters and results in:
   (a) tumefactions.
   (b) deformities.
   (c) draining sinuses discharging grains.
   (d) All of the above.

4. Which of the following fungi produces asci containing eight oval ascospores?
   (a) *Leptosphaeria senegalensis*.
   (b) *Madurella mycetomatis*.
   (c) *Pyrenochaeta romeroi*.
   (d) *Scedosporium apiospermum*.

5. Which of the following actinomycetes possesses acid-fast filaments?
   (a) *Actinomadura madurae*.
   (b) *Actinomadura pelletieri*.
   (c) *Nocardia brasiliensis*.
   (d) *Streptomyces somaliensis*.

6. Which of the following actinomycetes produces red to pink grain mycetoma?
   (a) *Actinomadura madurae*.
   (b) *Actinomadura pelletieri*.
   (c) *Nocardia brasiliensis*.
   (d) *Streptomyces somaliensis*.

7. Which of the following is classified as mycetoma?
   (a) Actinomycosis.
   (b) Mycotic granuloma.
   (c) Fungus ball.
   (d) None of the above.

8. White grain mycetoma is caused by
   (a) *Acremonium* spp.
   (b) *Curvularia geniculata*.
   (c) *Exophiala jeanselmei*.
   (d) *Pyrenochaeta romeroi*.

9. *Madurella mycetomatis* assimilates:
   (a) sucrose.
   (b) lactose.
   (c) Both of the above.
   (d) None of the above.

10. The signs of mycetoma are:
    (a) chains of subcutaneous nodules along the lymphatic vessels.
    (b) circular lesion with active borders.
    (c) subcutaneous infection of foot or leg with swelling, draining sinus tracts and discharging grains.
    (d) verrucous, crusted and ulcerated lesions.

11. Which of the following specimens should be collected for the diagnosis of mycetoma?
    (a) Sputum.
    (b) Blood.
    (c) Grain.
    (d) Scrapings.

12. Which of the following characteristics of a grain are used to aid in identifying the causative agent of mycetoma?
    (a) Colour.
    (b) Texture.
    (c) Microscopic morphology.
    (d) All of the above.

### ANSWERS TO MCQs

1. (b), 2. (a), 3. (d), 4. (a), 5. (c), 6. (b), 7. (d), 8. (a), 9. (b), 10. (c), 11. (c), 12. (d).

### Further Reading

1. Ahmed AO, van Leeuwen, et al. Mycetoma caused by *Madurella mycetomatis*: a neglected infectious burden. *Lancet Infect Dis* 2004; 4: 566–74.
2. Anandi V, Jeya M, et al. Actinomycotic mycetoma of thumb. *Indian J Med Microbiol* 1997; 15: 43–4.
3. Arif M, Khan ZR, Moolla I. Madura foot. *J Afr Med J* 2007; 97: 834–5.
4. Arora B, Arora DR, Yadav SPS. Maduromycosis of maxillary antrum. *Indian J Otolaryng* 1989; 41: 111–2.
5. Arora B, Gupta S, Arora DR. Primary mycetoma of patella – a case report. *Indian J Orth* 1979; 13: 84–6.

6. Arora DR, Chugh TD. Histological and histochemical study of grain of *Madurella mycetomatis*. *J Indian Med Assoc* 1974; 65: 10–3.
7. Chugh TD, Arora DR. Mycetoma caused by *Streptomyces somaliensis*. *Indian J Pathol Bacteriol* 1975; 18: 49–53.
8. Chugh TD, Arora DR, et al. Mycetoma. *Indian J Med Res* 1975; 63: 1408–12.
9. Chhabra HL, Chugh TD, Keswani RK, Arora DR, et al. Mycetoma in the perineum. *Indian J Pathol Microbiol* 1976; 19: 71–74.
10. Fahl AH. Mycetoma: a thorn in flesh. *Trans R Soc Trop Med Hyg* 2004; 98: 3–11.
11. Kemper CA. Eumycetoma. *Curr Treat Option Infect Dis* 2000; 2: 533–8.
12. Lichon V, Khachemoune A. Mycetoma: a review. *Am J Clin Dermatol* 2006; 7: 315–21.

# CHAPTER 7

# Sporotrichosis

Sporotrichosis is a chronic pyogranulomatous infection of the skin and subcutaneous tissue, although it may become disseminated by lymphatic spread involving bones, joints, lungs and central nervous system. It is caused by *Sporothrix schenckii* which has a worldwide distribution with some highly endemic areas – Brazil, India, Mexico, Japan, Peru, Uruguay, and South Africa. The regional distribution of cases of sporotrichosis reported from India from 1932 to 2002 indicates that the disease is endemic in Assam, West Bengal, Himachal Pradesh and probably in Uttar Pradesh as well as other northern states. Of the 205 cases reported, 91 (44.4%) originated from West Bengal, 56 (27.3%) from Himachal Pradesh, and 45 (22.0%) from Assam. The remaining 13 (6.3%) cases occurred sporadically and were reported from Punjab, Chandigarh, Uttar Pradesh, Bihar, Tripura, Meghalaya and Karnataka.

The first case of sporotrichosis was reported by Schenck, from the Johns Hopkins Hospital in Baltimore in 1898. In 1908 in Brazil, Splendore described the asteroid bodies seen around *S. schenckii* that became very useful in the histologic diagnosis of sporotrichosis.

## Morphology and cultural characteristics

*S. schenckii* is a **dimorphic fungus**. In tissues and

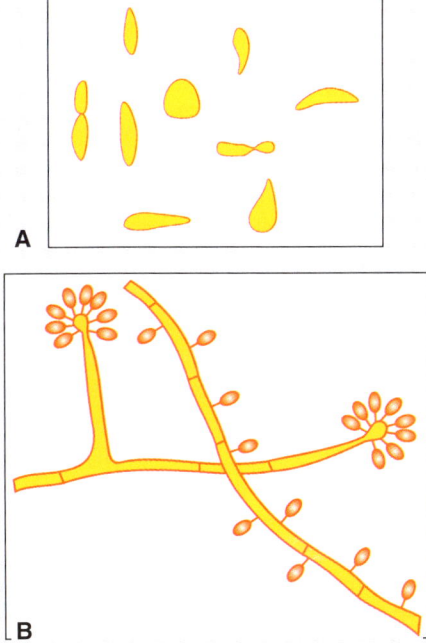

**Fig. 7.1.** *Sporothrix schenckii*: (A) yeast phase; and (B) mycelial phase.

in supplemented agar, such as brain-heart-infusion agar at 35–37°C, it is yeast-like and appears in the form of spherical, oval, or elongated ("cigar-shaped") cells 2–6 μm in diameter with single or rarely multiple buds. Budding is on a narrow base. In this form, the colonies are off-white with a cream texture and the organism reproduces by budding (Fig. 7.1A).

In culture on Sabouraud dextrose agar at 25–30°C, the fungus grows as a mold. Colonies appear within 3–5 days. These are cream-coloured initially, smooth and moist, gradually becoming dark brown or black and filamentous in texture. Some isolates are black from the beginning. Microscopic examination reveals thin (1–2 µm in diameter), septate and branching hyphae. Tapering conidiophores arise at right angles from the hyphae. The apex of the conidiophore is often slightly swollen and bears many small tear-shaped or round conidia (2–3 × 2–6 µm) on delicate threadlike denticles forming a "rosette-like" cluster in young cultures. Dark-walled conidia are also produced along the sides of the hyphae and may be more readily viewable than the rosette in mature cultures (Fig. 7.1B).

## Pathogenesis

The fungus is found in soil, decaying wood, thorns and on infected animals, including horses, cats, rats and dogs. Infection with *S. schenckii* typically occurs by direct skin inoculation from contaminated soil or thorny plants. **Sporotrichosis is a recognized occupational hazard of gardeners and farmers.** Also at risk are manual labourers who wear little protective clothing or footwear, and thus have increased potential for exposure to the fungus. Sporotrichosis is not contagious, although transmission has been recorded in a family from a cat.

The commonest type of sporotrichosis follows the subcutaneous implantation of conidia in a penetrating wound caused by a thorn or splinter. After an incubation period of 1–10 weeks or longer, reddish-purple, necrotic, nodular cutaneous lesion appears that commonly ulcerates. Satellite lesions sometimes arise. In most cases, yeast cells from the initial lesion are phagocytosed and carried into the lymphatic system where a line of cutaneous ulcerative lesions then develop in an ascending fashion along lymph channels. Extracutaneous sporotrichosis can also occur in organ transplant recipients who are receiving immunosuppressive therapy for the prevention of organ rejection.

Sporotrichosis is one of the **opportunistic infections encountered in AIDS patients**. In these patients it becomes disseminated and the prognosis is grave. Disseminated infections may involve one or more joints or organ systems, including central nervous system. *S. schenckii* may also cause eye infections, sinusitis, infection of the vocal cords, pyelonephritis and pulmonary infections.

## Oral manifestations

Nonspecific ulceration of the oral, nasal and pharyngeal mucosa also occurs in this disease, usually associated with regional lymphadenopathy. Lesions heal by soft, pliable scars even though the organisms may still be present in the tissues.

## Laboratory diagnosis

Although the yeast form may be seen occasionally in a Gram-stained smear, a wet mount from pus, or a biopsy specimen, direct examination of such material is often not helpful because of the paucity of fungal cells. Histopathological examination of lesions reveals a central necrotic region with associated infiltration of neutrophils, macrophages, and giant cells. *S. schenckii* appears in the form of spherical budding cells 2–6 µm in diameter and is often cigar-shaped. With ordinary stains, they are difficult to find, but can be detected through examination of serially sectioned tissue that has been stained with special fungal stains, e.g., periodic acid Schiff (PAS) or Gomori methenamine silver stain (GMS). Fluorescent antibody technique also facilitates detection of these organisms.

**Asteroid body** is often cited as a characteristic microscopic feature in cases of sporotrichosis. With H&E staining it shows central budding yeast cell with eosinophilic material radiating from it (Fig. 7.2). The eosinophilic material is formed by antibodies or antigen-antibody complexes (Splendore-Hoeppli material). It protects the yeast form from further attack by the immune system. Yeast cell in the centre of the asteroid body remains viable and can germinate *in vitro*, producing conidia after incubation at 25–30°C.

*S. schenckii* and *Histoplasma capsulatum* var. *capsulatum* may both appear as small, round or oval

# Sporotrichosis

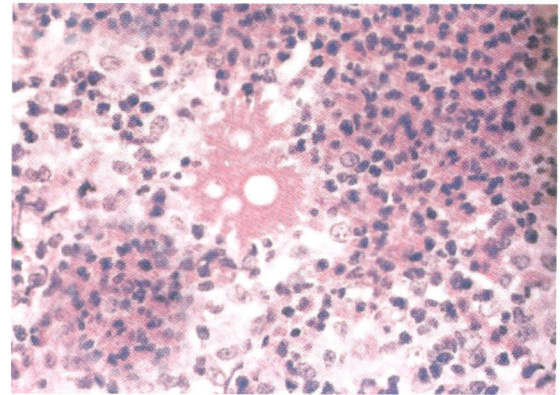

**Fig. 7.2.** Asteroid body in sporotrichosis. Yeast-like cells are surrounded by eosinophilic Splendore-Hoeppli material (haematoxylin and eosin stain, ×400).

cells, but the neutrophilic inflammatory reaction of sporotrichosis is not characteristic of histoplasmosis. *Candida glabrata*, which appears as small, oval yeast cells, produces a suppurative tissue reaction but does not usually generate granulomas. This fact assists in differentiating it from *Sporothrix*.

In most human lesions very few yeast-like organisms can be increased by inoculating pus from human sporotrichosis into an experimental animal such as mouse or rat. Intraperitoneal injection of the fungus in a male mouse causes orchitis within a week or 10 days. The cigar-shaped cells and large spherical bodies up to 8 μm in diameter are found in abundance in the testes of the mice.

The diagnosis is confirmed by **isolation of the causative organism** from the site of infection. Sputum, synovial fluid, CSF, biopsy specimens, exudates and, rarely blood have been reported to yield *S. schenckii* when cultured. Growth of the organism occurs within 3–5 days. Culture is superior to histopathologic methods in terms of diagnostic yield, because the organism is not abundant in tissues and is visualized poorly with haematoxylin and eosin and PAS stains.

**To induce mycelial to yeast conversion**, the fungus is inoculated on blood agar or brain-heart-infusion agar tubes and incubated at 35–37°C. The formation of yeast colonies may require several subcultures. Complete conversion seldom occurs, but a portion of the colony will develop cigar-shaped yeast-like cells.

A **latex agglutination test** for detection of antibodies against *S. schenckii* is available for the diagnosis of the extracutaneous forms of sporotrichosis.

A **skin test** with sporotrichin antigen is positive in all patients with cutaneous sporotrichosis.

## Treatment

Potassium iodide, five drops initially, increasing to 4–6 ml of saturated potassium iodide three times daily is effective in localized types, and should be continued for 3–4 weeks after clinical cure. The alternatives are itraconazole 100–200 mg/day or terbinafine 250 mg/day. Intravenous amphotericin B or miconazole may also be helpful.

 **Important Questions**

1. Discuss morphology, cultural characteristics, pathogenesis and laboratory diagnosis of sporotrichosis.
2. Write short notes on:
   (a) Asteroid body
   (b) Epidemiology of spirotrichosis in India.

## Multiple Choice Questions

1. Which of the following is **not** a dimorphic fungus?
   (a) *Sporothrix schenckii*.
   (b) *Histoplasma capsulatum*.
   (c) *Aspergillus fumigatus*.
   (d) *Blastomyces dermatitidis*.
2. Asteroid body is often cited as a characteristic microscopic feature in cases of:
   (a) sporotrichosis.
   (b) chromoblastomycosis.
   (c) histoplasmosis.
   (d) coccidioidomycosis.
3. *Sporothrix schenckii* is found in:
   (a) soil, decaying wood and thorns.
   (b) in bird droppings.
   (c) in bat droppings.
   (d) All of the above.
4. Which of the following laboratory approaches is most likely to lead to a diagnosis of sporotrichosis?

(a) Direct examination of pus from skin lesions.
(b) Culture of pus from skin lesion.
(c) Serology.
(d) Histopathology of biopsied skin lesion.

5. Colonies of *Sporothrix schenckii* begin as moist, yeast-like white or cream-coloured, later becoming dark brown to black within 1–2 weeks. What causes the dark brown to black colour to develop?
    (a) *Sporothrix schenckii* is a dematiaceous fungus.
    (b) Black conidia are formed on small denticles in a rosette-like clusters on apically swollen denticles.
    (c) Dark-walled conidia are produced along the sides of the hyphae.
    (d) None of the above.

6. Splendore-Hoeppli material is found surrounding:
    (a) yeast cells of *Sporothrix schenckii*.
    (b) grains of actinomycetoma, botryomycosis and actinomycosis.
    (c) hyphae of Entomophthorales.
    (d) All of the above.

## ANSWERS TO MCQs

1. (c), 2. (a), 3. (a), 4. (b), 5. (c), 6. (d).

### Further Reading

1. Agarwal S, Gopal K, et al. Sporotrichosis in Uttarakhand (India): a report of nine cases. *Int J Dermatol* 2008; 47: 367–71.
2. Alves SH, Aurelio PL, et al. Subcutaneous bilateral sporotrichosis: a rare presentation. *Mycopathologia* 2004; 158: 285–7.
3. Barros MB, Schubach AO, et al. An epidemic of sporotrichosis in Rio de Janeiro, Brazil: epidemiological aspects of a series of cases. *Epidemiol Infect* 2008; 136: 1192–6.
4. Bernardes-Engemann AR, Costa RC, et al. Development of an enzyme-linked immunosorbent assay for the serodiagnosis of several clinical forms of sporotrichosis. *Med Mycol* 2005; 43: 487–93.
5. Bustamante B, Campos PE. Endemic sporotrichosis. *Curr Opin Infect Dis* 2001; 14: 145–9.
6. Callens SF, Kitetele F, et al. Pulmonary *Sporothrix schenckii* infection in an HIV-positive child. *J Trop Pediatr* 2006; 52: 144–6.
7. de Lima Prearo CA, Daniguchi DP, et al. Bilateral sporotrichosis. *Mycoses* 2002; 45: 415–7.
8. Fontes PC, Kitakawa D, et al. Sporotrichosis in an HIV-positive man with oral lesion: a case report. *Acta Cytol* 2007; 51: 648–50.
9. Gori S, Lupetti A, et al. Pulmonary sporotrichosis with hyphae in a human immunodeficiency virus infected patient: a case report. *Acta Cytol* 1997; 41: 519–21.

# CHAPTER 8

# Chromoblastomycosis

Chromoblastomycosis is a chronic, localized fungal infection of skin and subcutaneous tissue. It is caused by several darkly pigmented, soil inhabiting phaeoid (dematiaceous) fungi. Five principal agents of chromoblastomycosis have been recognized since 1915 – *Phialophora verrucosa*, *Fonsecaea pedrosoi*, *F. compacta*, *Cladophialophora carrionii*, and *Rhinocladiella aquaspersa*.

Chromoblastomycosis has been reported from Central, South and North America, Cuba, Jamaica, Martinique, and also from many other countries including India, South Africa, Madagascar, Australia and northern Europe. The causative organisms have been isolated from soil and decaying vegetation in high-prevalence areas. It more often involves males more than 30 years old and those who work outdoor without footwear. The term **chromomycosis** includes chromoblastomycosis and a variety of other unrelated diseases caused by dematiaceous fungi, such as **phaeohyphomycosis**.

## Pathogenesis

Infection occurs following a wound or slight abrasion of the skin which is contaminated with soil or vegetable matter containing the causative fungi. In rare instances, splinters that presumably harboured the fungus and initiated the infection are found within infected tissue. Some patients are able to recount specific trauma to the affected site as a possible initiating event, but more commonly a traumatic event is not recalled, and it is thought that infection in these cases occurs through minor breaks in skin integrity. Person-to-person spread of chromoblastomycosis has not been documented.

Lesions develop most commonly on the distal lower extremities, a location compatible with exposure of damaged skin to soil. These may also involve arms, face and neck. Five types of chromoblastomycotic lesions occur:

1. The primary skin lesion is a **small papule** that gradually enlarges over weeks to months to form a **superficial nodule** with an irregular, friable surface. Lesions continue to evolve, often over many years.
2. **The verrucous lesions** are warty and hyperkeratotic.
3. **Tumorous lesions** are larger than **nodular lesions**, with raised surface projections that may be covered by crusting and epidermal debris. These lesions can become very large, and their surface texture has been compared with that of cauliflower.
4. **Plaque lesions**, the least common type, are flat, reddish and scaly.

5. **Cicatricial (scarring) lesions** have irregular borders and expand at their periphery with central healing and scarring.

"**Black dots**" may be observed on the surface of lesions. Samples of material from these areas are particularly useful for microscopic examination.

The lesions are usually painless unless the presence of secondary infection causes itching and pain. Satellite lesions are produced by scratching, and there may be lymphatic spread to adjacent areas. Haematogenous spread has occurred but is rare, and brain abscesses have been described. Secondary infection may eventually lead, after several years, to lymphatic stasis with the production of elephantiasis. *Squamous carcinomas may develop in chronic lesions.*

Tissue reaction in skin shows a characteristic pseudoepitheliomatous hyperplasia with hyperkeratosis and parakeratosis. Inflammation is generally granulomatous. It is often accompanied by a suppurative reaction, possibly from a secondary infection, causing satellite microabscesses.

## Laboratory diagnosis

1. Superficial crusts scraped from the lesions, preferably from an area containing "black dots", may contain brown-pigmented, branched, distorted, septate hyphae (3–5 μm in diameter) which are easily seen upon microscopic examination after digestion in potassium hydroxide.
2. In pus, granulation tissue obtained by curettage, or in biopsy specimens of epidermis and subcutaneous tissue, the fungus is present in the form of rounded, thick-walled, brown cells with a diameter of 5–12 μm. They have horizontal and/or vertical septations. They reproduce by equatorial splitting and not by budding. They are known as **sclerotic bodies** (Fig. 8.1). These structures were at one time thought to be budding yeast cells, resulting in the name chromoblastomycosis (*chromo*: coloured, *blasto*: budding, *mycosis*: fungal infection). Sclerotic bodies are seen within giant cells, rarely in macrophages or extracellularly in microabscesses. **The fungi typically migrate to the surface of the skin and are seen as "black dots" in the keratin scales.**

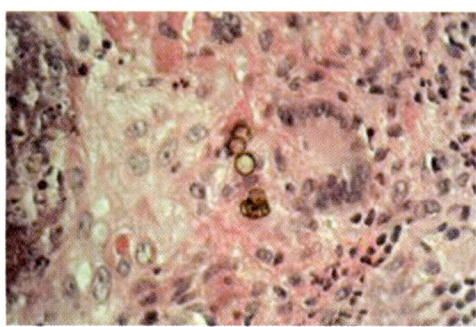

**Fig. 8.1.** Chromoblastomycosis showing sclerotic bodies (H&E stain, ×400).

3. Because the causative agents cannot be distinguished on the basis of histologic features, culture of lesion material is necessary. Crusts, pus, and biopsy material are inoculated on culture media both with and without antibiotics because of the possibility of bacterial contamination, and inoculated plates should be incubated at 25–30°C. In most cases colonies are formed within 2 weeks; but cultures should be held for 4 weeks before being reported as negative.

## Mycology

### *Phialophora verrucosa*

*Colony morphology*

On Sabouraud dextrose agar (SDA) growth appears in 7–12 days. The colony is dark greenish brown to black with a close matlike olive to gray mycelium. Some strains are heaped and granular; others are flat. Colonies become embedded in the medium. Reverse is black.

*Microscopic morphology*

Hyphae are brown, branched and septate. Conidiogenous cells are phialides, vase-like in shape, with a prominent collarettes (Fig. 8.2) Conidia measure 1–3 × 2–4 μm, are one-celled, ellipsoidal and accumulate at the apex of the phialide, giving the appearance of a vase of flowers.

### *Fonsecaea pedrosoi*

*Colony morphology*

Colonies are dark green, gray or black, covered with silvery, velvety mycelium. Colonies are usually flat

# Chromoblastomycosis

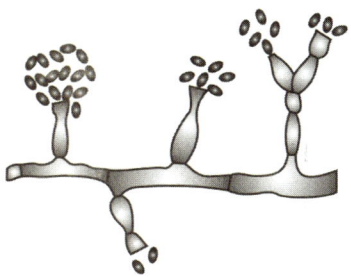

**Fig. 8.2.** *Phialophora verrucosa* sequentially forms conidia at the orifice of phialides which bear distinctive cuplike collarettes.

and then develop a convex cone-shaped protrusion in the centre. Colonies become slightly embedded in the medium. Reverse is black.

### Microscopic morphology

Hyphae are septate, branched and brown. Conidia are dark, 1.5–3.0 × 2.5–6.0 μm. Conidiation is enhanced on cornmeal agar or potato dextrose agar. Four types of conidial formation may be seen (Fig. 8.3):

1. **Fonsecaea-type:** Conidiophores are septate and erect. Distal end of the conidiophore develops swollen projections (denticles) that bear primary single-celled ovoid conidia. Denticles on the primary conidia support secondary single-celled conidia that may produce tertiary conidia.
2. **Rhinocladiella-type:** Conidiophores are septate and erect. Swollen denticles bear ovoid conidia at the tip and along the side of the conidiophore. Usually only primary conidia develop; secondary conidia are rare.
3. **Phialophora-type:** Phialides are vase-shaped with terminal cuplike collarettes. Round to oval conidia accumulate at the apex at the philide, giving appearance of 'flowers in vase'.
4. **Cladosporium-type:** Conidiophores are erect and give rise to large primary shield-shaped conidia. The latter, in turn, produce short, branching chains of oval conidia. This type of conidia formation predominates in *Fonsecaea pedrosoi*.

## Fonsecaea compacta

### Colony morphology

*F. compacta* grows slowly on SDA. Surface is dark-

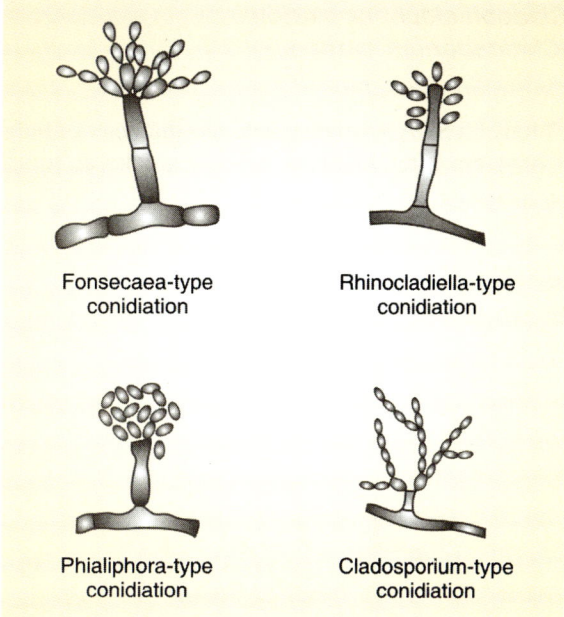

**Fig. 8.3.** Types of conidial formation in *Fonsecaea pedrosoi*.

green to black, heaped, and brittle, with irregular indented border. After 2–3 weeks tufts of brownish hyphae appear over the surface. Reverse is black.

### Microscopic morphology

Microscopically, hyphae are septate, brown, and branched and bear predominantly fonsecaea-type conidiophores that produce short chains and masses of rounded conidia (1.5–3 μm in diameter). The conidia are cask-shaped and separated from each other by septa of wide diameters. This results in compact head, the conidia of which are not easily dissociated (Fig. 8.4). Rhinocladiella-, cladosporium- and phialophora-type conidiation may also be seen.

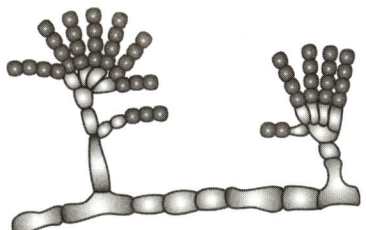

**Fig. 8.4.** *Fonsecaea compacta*.

## Cladophialophora carrionii (Cladosporium carrionii)

### Colony morphology

Colony on SDA is small, reaching a diameter of only 3 or 4 cm after incubation for 4 weeks at room temperature. It is olivaceous-black and velvety in texture.

### Microscopic morphology

Brown septate hyphae with elongate conidiophores bearing outwardly spreading, sparsely branching, long chains of ellipsoidal, symmetrical, one-celled conidia that measure 2.2–2.6 × 4.5–6.0 μm (Fig. 8.5).

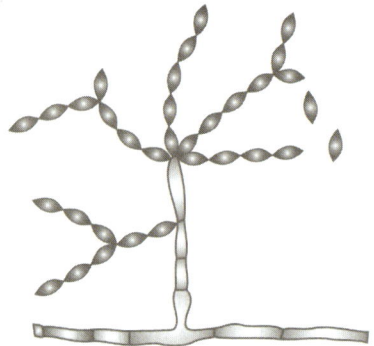

**Fig. 8.5.** *Cladophialophora carrionii.*

## Rhinocladiella aquaspersa

### Colony morphology

Colonies of *Rhinocladiella aquaspersa* are moderately rapid growing, floccose olivaceous-black, reverse is dark olivaceous.

### Microscopic morphology

Hyphae are smooth or slightly rough walled. The conidiophores are straight, unbranched, thick-walled and dark brown. Conidia are smooth, thin-walled, ellipsoidal or clavate 2 × 5 μm in size. They are arranged like bottle brush (Fig. 8.6).

### Treatment

Surgical excision is the best treatment for small or early lesions, and antifungal medications for more extensive disease. Itraconazole with or without flucytosine is often successful. If the causative organism is *C. carrionii* then response to itraconazole

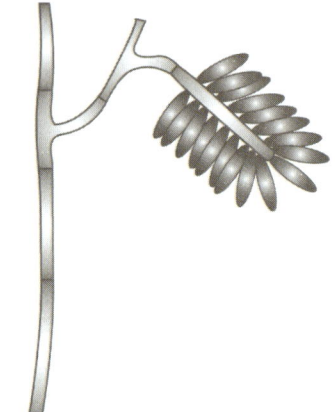

**Fig. 8.6.** *Rhinocladiella aquaspersa.*

alone is thought to be better. Terbinafine 250 mg/day may also be effective.

### Important Questions

1. Discuss morphology, pathogenesis and laboratory diagnosis of chromoblastomycosis.
2. Write short notes on:
   (a) Sclerotic bodies
   (b) Cultural characteristics of fungi causing chromoblastomycosis.

### Multiple Choice Questions

1. Sclerotic bodies are seen in:
   (a) mycetoma.
   (b) actinomycosis.
   (c) chromoblastomycosis.
   (d) phaeohyphomycosis.
2. Which of the following fungi **does not** cause chromoblastomycosis?
   (a) *Aspergillus fumigatus*.
   (b) *Phialophora verrucosa*.
   (c) *Fonsecaea pedrosoi*.
   (d) *Cladophialophora carrinii*.
3. Which of the following fungi shows fonsecaea-type, rhinocladiella-type, phialophora-type and cladosporium-type conidiation?
   (a) *Phialophora verrucosa*.
   (b) *Fonsecaea pedrosoi*.
   (c) *Fonsecaea compacta*.
   (d) *Cladophilophora carrinii*.

4. In which of the following fungi conidia are arranged like bottle brush?
   (a) *Rhinocladiella aquaspersa*.
   (b) *Cladophialophora carrionii*.
   (c) *Fonsecaea compacta*.
   (d) *Phialophora verrucosa*.

5. Squamous carcinomas may develop in chronic lesions of:
   (a) histoplasmosis.
   (b) chromoblastomycosis.
   (c) coccidioidomycosis.
   (d) aspergillosis.

## ANSWERS TO MCQs

1. (c), 2. (a), 3. (b), 4. (a), 5. (b).

### Further Reading

1. Attapattu MC. Chromoblastomycosis: a clinical and mycological study of 71 cases from Sri Lanka. *Mycopathologia* 1997; 137: 145–51.
2. Dixon DM, Polak-Wyss A. The medically important dematiaceous fungi and their identification. *Mycoses* 1991; 34: 1–18.
3. Fader RC, McGinnis MR. Infections caused by dematiaceous fungi: chromoblastomycosis and phaeohyphomycosis. *Infect Dis Clin N Am* 1988; 2: 925–38.
4. Kumar B. Chromoblastomycosis in India: two more cases. *Int J Dermatol* 2000; 39: 800.
5. Kutty MK, Majumdar M. Chromoblastomycosis. *Southeast Asian J Trop Med Public Health* 1971; 2: 86–7.
6. Lopez Martinez R, Mendez Tovar LJ. Chromoblastomycosis. *Clin Dermatol* 2007; 25: 188–94.
7. Perez-Blanco M, Hernandez Valles R, et al. Chromoblastomycosis in children and adolescents in the endemic area of the Falcon State, Venezuela. *Med Mycol* 2006; 44: 467–71.
8. Salgado CG, da Salva JP, et al. Cutaneous diffuse chromoblastomycosis. *Lancet Infect Dis* 2005; 5: 528.

# CHAPTER 9

# Phaeohyphomycosis

Phaeohyphomycosis is **a mycotic infection caused by phaeoid (dematiaceous, brown-pigmented) fungi where the tissue morphology of the causative organism is mycelial**. This separates it from other clinical types of disease involving brown-pigmented fungi where the tissue morphology of the organism is a grain (eumycotic mycetoma) or sclerotic body (chromoblastomycosis).

Phaeoid fungi are worldwide in soil, thorns, splinters, and decaying plant material. Infection is acquired by penetrating injury with conidia-containing soil or plant material. The respiratory route is suspected in cerebral abscess disease. Phaeohyphomycosis may be divided into superficial, cutaneous, subcutaneous, corneal, sinus and systemic.

## SUPERFICIAL PHAEOHYPHOMYCOSIS

This includes **tinea nigra** and **black piedra** (see Chapter 4).

## CUTANEOUS PHAEOHYPHOMYCOSIS

***Dermatomycosis and onychomycosis:*** Some fungi causing phaeohyphomycosis are capable of causing dermatomycosis and onychomycosis similar to those caused by dermatophytes. They involve only keratinized tissue. It leads to dark pigmentation of the nail and an associated paronychia. Clinically, this condition may be indistinguishable from that of dermatophytosis. *Exophiala jeanselmei* causes onychomycosis, and *Nattrassia mangiferae* and *Alternaria* spp. may cause both types of infection.

Dematiaceous hyphae may be seen in nail scrapings examined in 30% KOH containing 40% dimethyl sulfoxide, but the presence of hyaline-appearing hyphae does not rule out these organisms.

## SUBCUTANEOUS PHAEOHYPHOMYCOSIS

Subcutaneous phaeohyphomycosis occurs worldwide, usually following the traumatic implantation of fungal elements from contaminated soil, thorns or wood splinters. It is more common in warm climates, and immunocompromised individuals are at increased risk. Person-to-person spread does not occur.

At the site of prior trauma patient develops a single, well-developed subcutaneous mass or nodule measuring 1–7 cm in diameter. Initially the lesion is firm, but the centre of the nodule may later become necrotic and liquefy, resulting in fluctuance. Such lesion may be aspirated for diagnostic purposes. KOH preparation reveals the presence of septate, irregularly swollen hyphae that may or may not be branched. Dark yeast-like elements may also be seen either singly or in chains. Some of the resected cysts may contain the original wood splinter that introduced fungus into tissues.

Culture of the material from aspirated or excised lesions is inoculated on media both with and without cycloheximide and chloramphenicol, and incubated at 25–30°C. Growth appears in 2 weeks, but plates should be kept for at least 4 weeks before being discarded as negative. The organisms most commonly isolated from these cases include *Exophiala*, *Phialophora*, and *Bipolaris* species.

## CORNEAL PHAEOHYPHOMYCOSIS (KERATITIS)

Over 20 dematiaceous species from 11 genera have been reported to cause mycotic keratitis or keratomycosis (see Chapter 22).

## FUNGAL SINUSITIS

Fungal sinus infections with dematiaceous fungi can present in three main categories – allergic fungal sinusitis, fungus ball, and invasive fungal sinusitis. Invasive fungal sinusitis can be further subdivided into three categories – acute necrotizing, chronic, and granulomatous.

- **Allergic fungal sinusitis** is characterized by the presence of "allergic mucin" (a mixture of layers of basophilic mucus and sheets of eosinophils with Charcot Leyden crystals and sparse fungal hyphae). Dematiaceous fungi have been grown in more than 80% cases, with the most commonly implicated dematiaceous fungi being *Bipolaris*, *Curvularia*, *Exserohilum*, *Alternaria* and *Cladosporium* spp. Nasal obstruction and discharge with headache are the most common presenting complaints. Patient may also develop periorbital swelling, proptosis, and visual disturbances.
- **Fungus ball** produces disease primarily by obstruction. There is no fungal invasion into local soft tissue or bone in allergic fungal sinusitis and fungus ball.
- **Invasive fungal sinusitis** manifests by extension of the infection into host tissue such as bone and even the brain.

## SYSTEMIC PHAEOHYPHOMYCOSIS

Disseminated phaeohyphomycosis results by the spread of the dematiaceous pathogen from a previously colonized or infected body site. Dissemination can originate from the lungs or infected sinus tissue following inhalation of fungal cells or conidia. Direct extension from the sinus or haematogenous spread of the fungus to one or more distant sites of the body can result in visceral infections of the heart and heart valves, brain, joints, bone, kidney, liver, lymphatics, pancreas, and other organs. Affected individuals are frequently immunocompromised, but both disseminated and localized infections have been seen in seemingly immunocompetent individuals.

**Cerebral phaeohyphomycosis:** Cerebral infections caused by dematiaceous fungi have a worldwide distribution. Most of the commonly encountered dematiaceous fungi causing cerebral phaeohyphomycosis produce mainly brain abscess. These fungi include *Cladophialophora bantiana*, *Ochroconis gallopavum*, *Exophiala* (*Wangiella*) *dermatitidis*, *Curvularia pallescens*, *Fonsecaea pedrosoi*, and *Bipolaris spicifera*.

Most patients with cerebral phaeohyphomycosis present with symptoms and physical signs of an intracerebral mass lesion. Patient complains of headache, seizures, altered mental status and fever.

### Laboratory diagnosis

The diagnosis of phaeohyphomycosis is established in the laboratory by KOH mount, histopathology and culture. There are no available serologic tests to diagnose infection with these fungi.

### KOH mount

The aspirates from cysts and curettings from the cutaneous and corneal lesions, and biopsy material are examined in KOH wet mount. In case of phaeohyphomycosis, the fungus is present in the form of brown-pigmented septate hyphae 2–6 μm in diameter.

### Histopathology

The pathological features are similar regardless of the etiologic agent. In systemic phaeohyphomycosis lesions of a given organ may occur as single or multiple abscesses. The abscesses are usually circumscribed and encapsulated granulomas, the walls of which comprise epithelial histiocytes and giant cells surrounded by connective tissue. The centre of the granulomas contain necrotic debris, fibrin, and degenerated polymorphonuclear cells.

Within the necrotic debris and inflammatory infiltrates, as well as in the giant cells, fungal elements can be observed. The fungus in the tissue is present in the form of brown-pigmented, septate hyphae (2–6 µm in diameter) (Fig. 9.1). They occur singly or in small aggregates. They often have closely spaced, constricted septations producing a moniliform ("string of beads") appearance. Large, bizarre, thick-walled vesicular swellings (≥ 25 µm in diameter), resembling chlamydoconidia may be seen along, or at the end of the hyphae. Yeast-like cells producing buds singly or in chains are also commonly present. **Special fungal stains such as Gomori methenamine silver and periodic acid-Schiff mask the natural colour of the hyphae, but in haematoxylin and eosin sections the brown colour may be obvious.** In some cases, however, the hyphae appear unpigmented and a specific stain for melanin, Masson Fontana stain, must be used to reveal the presence of the fungal pigment.

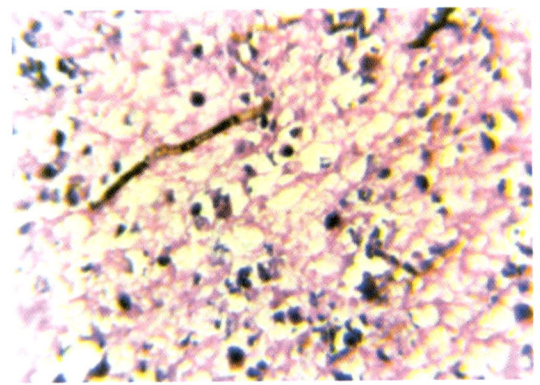

**Fig. 9.1.** Phaeohyphomycosis showing brown septate fungal hypha (H&E stain, ×400).

## Mycology

### Cladophialophora bantiana

*Cladophialophora bantiana* (formerly *Phialophora bantianum*) has a predilection for the central nervous system. It is the most commonly isolated causative agent of **cerebral phaeohyphomycosis**. This organism appears to be acquired through the respiratory tract, therefore, *a biological safety cabinet must be used when handling this organism*. It is only rarely involved in cutaneous and subcutaneous infection.

### Colony morphology

Colonies are olive-gray to brown or black, slightly folded, with moderate growth rate. Growth matures within 15 days.

### Microscopic morphology

Microscopic examination of lactophenol cotton blue preparation reveals brown septate hyphae with conidiophores that are similar to the vegetative hyphae. Conidiophores bear long sparsely branched, wavy chains of spindle-shaped conidia (2.5–5 × 6–11 µm). The conidia do not display conspicuous scars of attachment (Fig. 9.2).

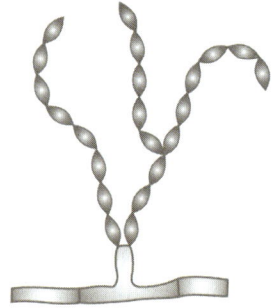

**Fig. 9.2.** *Cladophialophora bantiana*.

### Ochroconis gallopava

This fungus has predilection for the central nervous system. It displays good growth up to 45°C and fails to grow on media containing cycloheximide.

### Colony morphology

On SDA colonies are woolly and dark olive-gray, reddish brown, or gray-black. Reverse is dark. A red to brown pigment usually diffuses into the medium.

### Microscopic morphology

Hyphae are septate, with conidiophores that are hyaline, erect, and sometimes knobby or bent at the point of conidial formation. Hyaline to pale brown, clavate, two-celled conidia measuring 11–18 × 2.5–4.5 µm and constricted at the septum are borne at the tip of denticles. However, young conidia may be round and single-celled (Fig. 9.3)

## Phaeohyphomycosis

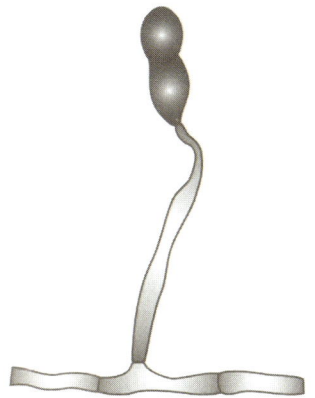

Fig. 9.3. *Ochroconis gallopava*.

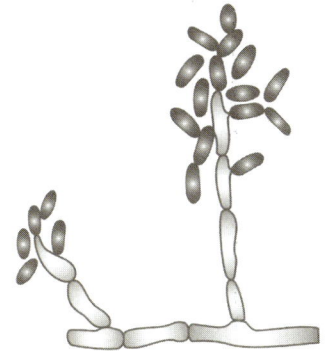

Fig. 9.4. *Exophiala dermatitidis*.

### Exophiala (Wangiella) dermatitidis

*E. dermatitidis* causes subcutaneous, ocular, systemic and cerebral forms of phaeohyphomycosis. Predilection for the central nervous system is associated with high mortality. Respiratory tract colonization is common in cystic fibrosis.

#### Colony morphology

Growth appears slowly. At first the colony is black, moist, shiny, and yeast-like. After 3–4 weeks or upon repeated subculture, olive-gray aerial hyphae develop at the periphery and sometimes near the centre of the colony. Reverse is dark.

#### Microscopic morphology

Microscopically, young cultures are composed of dark oval to round, budding, yeast-like cells. These eventually produce septate, pigmented hyphae. Single-celled conidia (2–3 × 3–6 µm) are subglobose to elliptical and accumulate at the apices of conidiogenous cells (Fig. 9.4).

### Curvularia spp.

*Curvularia* spp., common inhabitants of dead plant material may cause fungal keratitis, sinusitis, mycetoma and phaeohyphomycosis at various sites, including nails, subcutaneous tissue, and systemic organs. Occasionally, dissemination to brain may occur. They are also encountered as contaminants.

#### Colony morphology

Colonies display rapid growth. These are dark, olive-green to brown or black with a pinkish gray, woolly surface. Reverse is dark.

#### Microscopic morphology

Hyphae are septate and dark. Conidiophores are simple or branched and bent or knobby at points of conidium formation. Conidia are large 8–14 × 21–35 µm in size. They usually contain 4 cells. Due to swelling of a central cell they appear curved (Fig. 9.5). Conidia differ from those of *Bipolaris* spp. by having a central cell that is darker than end cells, a thinner cell wall, narrower septations between cells, and a distinct curve that develops with age.

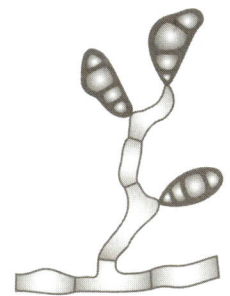

Fig. 9.5 *Curvularia* spp.

### Bipolaris spp.

*Bipolaris* spp. cause subcutaneous lesions, keratitis, peritoneal dialysis-associated peritonitis, and central nervous system phaeohyphomycosis. They may also be present as contaminants in clinical specimens.

#### Colony morphology

Colonies are moderately fast growing, gray to

blackish brown with a matted centre and raised grayish periphery. The reverse is dark brown to black.

### Microscopic morphology

Microscopic morphology shows dark septate hyphae. Conidiophores bend at the point where elliptical to oval, thick-walled conidia are formed thus producing a knobby zigzag appearance. The conidia are brown, oblong to cylindrical (6–13 × 14–39 µm) appear thick-walled, and have 3–5 septations and a slightly protruding hilum (Fig. 9.6).

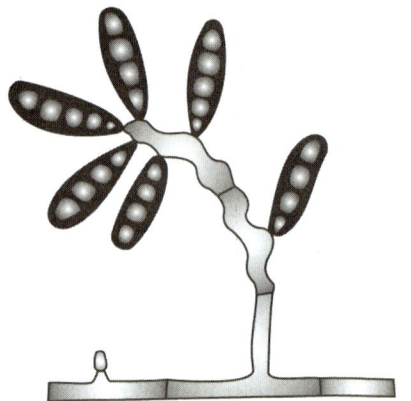

**Fig. 9.6.** *Bipolaris* spp.

## Exophiala jeanselmei

It causes mycetoma and phaeohyphomycosis.

### Colony morphology

Rate of growth is slow. When incubated at 25–30°C, growth matures within 14 days. At 37°C, it grows more slowly or not at all. Colonies on SDA are brownish-black or greenish-black. They then become covered with short, velvet grayish hyphae. Reverse is black.

### Microscopic morphology

Young culture consists of many yeast-like budding cells. Eventually septate hyphae form with numerous conidiogenous cells that are slender, tubular, sometimes branched and characteristically tapered to a narrow, elongated tip. The conidia are oval, measure 1–3 × 2–5 µm in size. They gather in clusters at the end and sides of conidiophore and at points along the hyphae (Fig. 9.7).

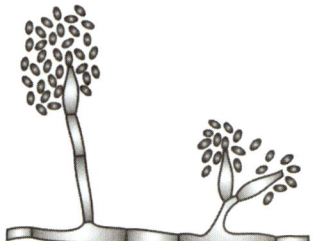

**Fig. 9.7.** *Exophiala jeanselmei.*

## Neoscytalidium dimidiatum (Scytalidium dimidiatum)

It is a common agent of dermatomycosis and onychomycosis in patients living in or immigrating from tropical areas. Invasive disease may occur in immunocompromised hosts.

### Colony morphology

Growth is rapid. It matures in 3 days. Colonies are usually woolly. The surface is gray to brown with a dark reverse or may be white to cream or gray with a buff to yellowish reverse in melanin-deficient mutants.

### Microscopic morphology

Hyphae are septate and branched, but no conidiophores are formed. One or two-celled arthroconidia (3–7 × 3–14 µm) are produced from hyphae. There are no empty cells between arthroconidia (Fig. 9.8). A pycnidial form very occasionally develops in old cultures. The pycnidia are large (100–300 µm in diameter). Pycnidial conidia are hyaline when young and with age develop 1–5 septa and a dark brown central area.

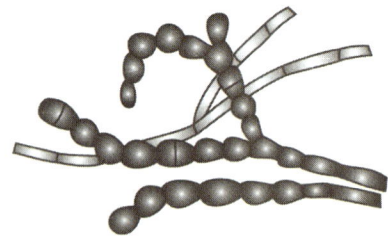

**Fig. 9.8.** *Neoscytalidium dimidiatum.*

## Alternaria spp.

*Alternaria* is a large genus composed mostly of

saprobic or plant pathogen species. More than 80 species of *Alternaria* have been identified. Human or animal infections are mostly caused by *A. alternata*, *A. chlamydospora*, *A. dianthicola*, *A. infectoria*, and *A. tenuissima*. They may occasionally cause phaeohyphomycosis most commonly in subcutaneous tissue, mycotic keratitis, paranasal sinusitis and dialysis-associated peritonitis.

### Colony morphology

Growth of *Alternaria* is rapid, with olivaceous to gray to black colonies. Growth matures within 5 days.

### Microscopic morphology

Hyphae are septate and dark. Conidiophores are erect, septate, of variable length, and sometimes have a zigzag appearance. Conidia are large (8–16 × 23–50 µm), brown in colour and have both transverse and longitudinal septations. They are borne singly or in chains. They are usually rather round at the end nearest the conidiophore while narrowing at the apex (Fig. 9.9).

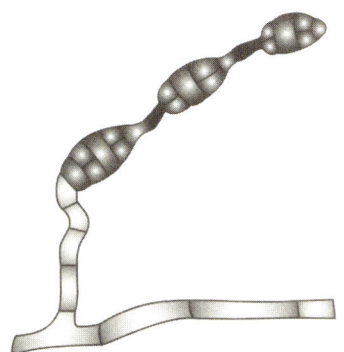

**Fig. 9.9.** *Alternaria* spp.

### Exserohilum spp.

This genus includes three human pathogens *E. rostratum*, *E. longirostratum*, and *E. mcginnisii*.

### Colony morphology

Growth is rapid and colonies are woolly and gray to black in colour. Reverse is black.

### Microscopic morphology

Hyphae are septate and dematiaceous. The conidiophores are dark and bent at the point where each conidium is formed. This produces a knobby, zigzag appearance. The conidia are brown, long, measure 14 × 80 µm or more, fusiform, appear thick-walled, and usually have 7–11 septa (Fig. 9.10).

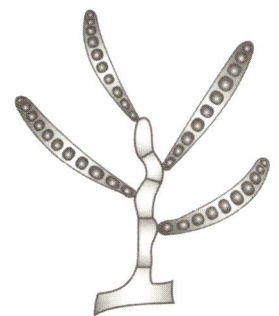

**Fig. 9.10** *Exserohilum rostratum*.

*E. rostratum* is the etiologic agent of keratitis, sinusitis, cutaneous and subcutaneous phaeohyphomycosis.

### Treatment

The usual treatment is excision. However, in disseminated phaeohyphomycosis it is impractical. The advent of azole and echinocandin classes of drugs has added to the available antifungal armamentarium. Older azole drugs, such as itraconazole, are very effective against dematiaceous fungi *in vitro*. In addition, many of the new azoles show good promise both *in vitro* and *in vivo*.

## Important Questions

1. Discuss pathogenesis and laboratory diagnosis of phaeohyphomycosis.
2. Write short notes on:
   (a) Cutaneous phaeohyphomycosis
   (b) Subcutaneous phaeohyphomycosis
   (c) Fungal sinusitis
   (d) Systemic phaeohyphomycosis
   (e) Cerebral phaeohyphomycosis.

## Multiple Choice Questions

1. Darkly pigmented septate hyphae in the tissue are seen in
   (a) aspergillosis.
   (b) penicilliosis.

(c) phaeohyphomycosis.
(d) hyalohyphomycosis.

2. Which of the following fungi is **not** a causative agent of phaeohyphomycosis?
   (a) *Cladophialophora bantiana*.
   (b) *Aspergillus fumigatus*.
   (c) *Ochroconis gallopava*.
   (d) *Wangiella dermatitidis*.

3. A biological safety cabinet must be used when handling
   (a) *Cladophialophora bantiana*.
   (b) *Ochroconis gallopava*.
   (c) *Wangiella dermatitidis*.
   (d) *Aspergillus fumigatus*.

4. Infection caused by phaeoid fungi, where the tissue morphology is mycelial, is known as:
   (a) chromoblastomycosis.
   (b) phaeohyphomycosis.
   (c) hyalohyphomycosis.
   (d) eumycetoma.

5. Which of the following forms of diseases is/are included in phaeohyphomycosis?
   (a) Cerebral abscess.
   (b) Fungal rhinosinusitis.
   (c) Subcutaneous cyst.
   (d) All of the above.

6. Which of the following is a neurotropic fungus?
   (a) *Trichophyton rubrum*.
   (b) *Cladophialophora bantiana*.
   (c) *Exophiala jeanselmei*.
   (d) *Scedosporium prolificans*.

7. Phaeohyphomycosis is caused by melanized mold which:
   (a) grows as hyphae in tissue.
   (b) grows as moniliform hyphae in tissue.
   (c) may produce yeast forms in tissue.
   (d) All of the above.

## ANSWERS TO MCQs

1. (c), 2. (b), 3. (a), 4. (b), 5. (d), 6. (b), 7. (d).

## Further Reading

1. Boggild AK, Poutanen SM, et al. Disseminated phaeohyphomycosis due to *Ochroconis gallopavum* in the setting of advanced HIV infection. *Med Mycol* 2006; 44: 777–82.
2. Borkar SA, Sharma MS, et al. Brain abscess caused by *Cladophialophora bantiana* in an immunocompetent host: need for a novel cost-effective antifungal agent. *Indian J Med Microbiol* 2008; 26: 271–4.
3. Brasch J, Busch JO, de Hoog GS. Cutaneous phaeohyphomycosis caused by *Alternaria infectoria*. *Acta Derm Venereol* 2008; 88: 160–1.
4. Cardoso SV, Campolina SS, et al. Oral phaeohyphomycosis. *J Clin Pathol* 2007; 60: 204–5.
5. Carter E, Boudreaux C. Fatal cerebral phaeohyphomycosis due to *Curvularia lunata* in an immunocompetent patient. *J Clin Microbiol* 2004; 42: 5419–23.
6. Revankar SG, Patterson JE, et al. Disseminated phaeohyphomycosis: review of an emerging mycosis. *Clin Infect Dis* 2002; 34: 467–76.
7. Revankar SG, Sutton DA, Rinaldi MG. Primary central nervous system phaeohyphomycosis: a review of 101 cases. *Clin Infect Dis* 2004; 38: 206–16.
8. Shivaswamy KN, Pradhan P, et al. Disseminated phaeohyphomycosis. *Int J Dermatol* 2007; 46: 278–81.

# CHAPTER 10

# Lobomycosis

Lobomycosis also known as Lobo's disease or Lacaziosis is a chronic localized mycosis of the skin and subcutaneous tissue, characterized by keloidal and sometimes verrucoid and ulcerated lesions. The disease was first recognized in 1931 by Jorge Lobo in a Brazilian human patient with cutaneous parakeloid lesions. It is caused by *Lacazia loboi* (formerly *Loboa loboi*), **an uncultivated fungal pathogen of humans and dolphins**.

*L. loboi* is currently classified as an **ascomycete fungus** in the order Onygenales and the family Ajellomycetaceae. This pathogen is restricted to Mexico, Central America, and South America. Sporadic and isolated cases have been described in Europe and North America. Cases in dolphins in the coast of France and USA with transmission to aquarium personnel have also been documented.

*L. loboi* has been known by various names such as: *Glenosporopsis amazonica*, *Glenosporella loboi*, *Paracoccidioides loboi*, *Blastomyces loboi*, *Loboa loboi* and *Lobomyces loboi*.

## Pathogenesis

*L. loboi* appears to be an aquatic saprophyte. It explains disease in aquatic mammals such as dolphin.

The disease mainly affects male patients from rural areas living or working in close contact with vegetation and aquatic environments. Most patients report having developed lesions after accidental trauma with plant thorns or insect bites, yet others do not recall trauma before the disease. Person-to-person spread, even with intimate contact, has not been reported. **It has not yet been successfully cultured *in vitro*.**

Lobomycosis is characterized by variably sized dermal nodules, either lenticular or plaques, which can attain the size of a small keloid-like cauliflower. They may be hyper- or hypopigmented and occasionally achromic. Any area of the body is potentially susceptible as infection commonly follow trauma. However, the most commonly affected areas include feet, legs, buttocks, face and the upper extremities and the disease is usually unilateral.

They spread slowly by peripheral extension with an active raised border, or by satellite lesions which may arise by autoinoculation. There is no marked lymphangitis and no visceral dissemination. Young lesions are sharply defined, with a smooth surface and elastic consistency. They are freely movable with the skin and are painless. Older lesions become verrucoid and may ulcerate. Clinically, the disease most closely resembles chromoblastomycosis. Microscopic examination of biopsy material will establish the diagnosis. The infection is not life-threatening and usually evolves very slowly sometimes over 20 or more years.

## Laboratory diagnosis

### 1. Wet mount

It is quick and easy. Scrape the lesion with a scalpel blade in order to obtain dermal tissue. Prepare wet mount preparation in 10% KOH and examine under microscope. It shows yeast-like unicellular, rounded, thick-walled cells which range from 6–12 μm in diameter and occur in chains of 2–10 cells connected by narrow, tube-like bridges (Fig. 10.1). Five to eight protoplasmic granules can also be observed within some of the yeast-like cells.

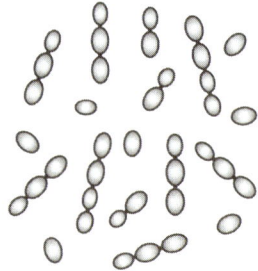

**Fig. 10.1.** *Lacazia loboi.*

Some cells with multiple budding closely resemble those of *Paracoccidioides brasiliensis*; however, the mother cells and the multiple daughter cells have the same diameter, a characteristic that helps to distinguish *L. loboi* from *P. brasiliensis*. Electron microscopic analysis of *L. loboi* shows thick chitinous yeast-like cell walls and an amorphous cytoplasmic content.

### 2. Histopathology

Histopathological examination of haematoxylin and eosin stained sections shows a granulomatous infiltrate constituted by histiocytes and numerous giant cells which are often clustered in small groups separated by interstitial tissue. The histiocytes and more often the multinucleated giant cells can be seen to have numerous phagocytosed thick-walled yeast-like cells clearly distinguishable by periodic acid-Schiff or Gomori methenamine silver (GMS) stains. Budding can be observed but hyphae are always absent. With GMS stain, *L. loboi* yeast-like cells are dark or have the appearance of empty cells.

### 3. Culture

There have been many attempts to culture *L. loboi*, but all have been unsuccessful.

## Treatment

There is no effective medical therapy for lobomycosis and where possible lesions may be excised.

 **Important Questions**

Discuss pathogenesis and laboratory diagnosis of lobomycosis.

### Multiple Choice Questions

1. Which of the following fungi causes keloidal and sometimes verrucoid and ulcerated lesions?
   (a) *Lacazia loboi.*
   (b) *Cladophialophora bantiana.*
   (c) *Ochroconis gallopava.*
   (d) *Wangiella dermatitidis.*

2. Which of the following fungi has **not** been successfully cultured *in vitro*?
   (a) *Lacazia loboi.*
   (b) *Cladophialophora bantiana.*
   (c) *Ochroconis gallopava.*
   (d) *Wangiella dermatitidis.*

3. Biopsied lesion tissue from a patient with lobomycosis, if minced and planted on medium, will:
   (a) grow as a yeast form at 37°C, only if 5% defibrinated sheep blood is added to brain-heart-infusion medium.
   (b) grow as the mold form on Sabouraud dextrose agar with cycloheximide at 25°C.
   (c) grow in biphasic blood culture bottle.
   (d) not yield growth because *Lacazia* cannot be cultivated.

### ANSWERS TO MCQs

1. (a), 2. (a), 3. (d).

**Further Reading**

1. Al-Daraji WI, Husain E, Robson A. Lobomycosis in African patients. *Br J Dermatol* 2008; 159: 234–6.
2. Camargo ZP, Baruzzi RG, et al. Antigenic relationship between *Loboa loboi* and *Paracoccidioides brasiliensis* as shown by serological methods. *Med Mycol* 1998; 36: 413–7.
3. Fonseca JJ, Lobomycosis. *Int J Surg Pathol* 2007; 15: 62–3.
4. Norton SA. Dolphin-to-human transmission of lobomycosis. *J Am Acad Dermatol* 2006; 55: 723–4.
5. Paniz-Mondolfi AE, Reyes Jaimes O, Davila Jones L. Lobomycosis in Venezuela. *Int J Dermatol* 2007; 46: 180–5.
6. Talhari C, Oliveira CB, et al. Disseminated lobomycosis. *Int J Dermatol* 2008; 47: 582–3.

# SECTION 4

# SYSTEMIC MYCOSES

**Chapter 11** Histoplasmosis
**Chapter 12** Blastomycosis
**Chapter 13** Coccidioidomycosis
**Chapter 14** Paracoccidioidomycosis

# CHAPTER 11

# Histoplasmosis

Histoplasmosis is an intracellular mycosis of reticulo-endothelial system involving lymphatic tissues, lungs, spleen, liver, adrenals, kidneys, skin, central nervous system and other organs of the body. It is caused by a dimorphic fungus, *Histoplasma capsulatum*. Taxonomically, *H. capsulatum* has been divided into three varieties – *H. capsulatum* var. *capsulatum*, *H. capsulatum* var. *duboisii*, and *H. capsulatum* var. *farciminosum*. Histoplasmosis caused by these fungi is known as histoplasmosis capsulati, histoplasmosis duboisii, and histoplasmosis farciminosi, respectively. Varieties *capsulatum* and *duboisii* differ in that in yeast phase they have different sizes, the *capsulatum* variety producing cells from 2–5 µm in diameter, and *duboisii* from 12–15 µm.

Classic histoplasmosis is the infection caused by *Histoplasma capsulatum* var. *capsulatum*. It is widely distributed throughout the world, occurring in some 60 temperate and tropical countries in the Americas, Africa and Australia. Infections with *duboisii* variety, known as African histoplasmosis or large-form histoplasmosis, have been reported only from Africa. The *farciminosum* variety is endemic in Africa, eastern Europe, the Middle East, Asia and the Far East. All the three varieties occur as saprophytes in the soil.

In India, histoplasmosis capsulati seems to be prevalent in the Gangetic delta. Panja and Sen reported the first case of disseminated histoplasmosis from Calcutta (now Kolkata) in 1954 and since then individual cases have been reported from various states. Histoplasmosis has been found to be endemic in West Bengal, and *H. capsulatum* has been isolated from the soil in Gangetic plain.

The genus *Histoplasma* was established in 1906 when Darling reported 3 fatal cases of a disseminated histoplasmosis in Panama which he had studied while looking for visceral leishmaniasis in that area. He erroneously considered it to be a protozoan closely related to the species of *Leishmania* but no kinetoplast was visible. In tissue sections, a clear space (halo) was seen between the protoplasmic mass and the cell wall. It led to the impression that it was capsulated organism. However, *Histoplasma* is neither a protozoan nor an encapsulated organism. In 1934, de Monbreum discovered dimorphism of *Histoplasma*. Emmons isolated *H. capsulatum* from soil in 1948.

*H. capsulatum* var. *capsulatum* grows in soil with high nitrogen content. The growth of the fungus appears to be most frequently associated with soil enriched by excreta of bats, chickens and other birds. This provides high nitrogen content. The organism has been isolated from bat caves, bird roosts, chicken houses and similar environments. Bat and bird excreta provides an excellent medium for enrichment of *H. capsulatum* var. *capsulatum*. Disturbances of such sites create aerosols laden with infectious propagules of *H. capsulatum* var. *capsulatum*. When inhaled, these aerosols result in infections varying in degree of severity depending on the size of the inoculum and the immunological status of the individuals involved.

Chickens are not susceptible to disseminated, progressive histoplasmosis under natural conditions. The apparent immunity of birds to systemic histoplasmosis may be dependent directly upon their body temperature (42–43°C) which is higher than the temperature at which the fungus can grow. Examination of autopsy and culture of many bats have demonstrated that histoplasmosis occurs in bats and the fungus is excreted in bat droppings from intestinal lesions.

In addition to humans, many animals (both wild and domestic) are susceptible to histoplasmosis. Some animals, including bats, may act as vectors to disseminate the organism in nature. From the soil, the conidia of *H. capsulatum* are airborne and these are inhaled leading to infection. Among humans, isolated cases and outbreaks of histoplasmosis capsulati almost invariably can be traced to sites associated with accumulation of bird and bat guanos in many parts of the world. No direct spread from man-to-man or animal-to-man has been reported.

For long time *H. capsulatum* was considered to be an asexual mold classified in the Fungi Imperfecti or Deuteromycetes. However, in 1972, Kwon-Chung discovered that *H. capsulatum* var. *capsulatum* was heterothallic and described its perfect state. It is an **Ascomycete** and was named *Emmonsiella capsulata*.

## Pathogenesis

Human infection with *H. capsulatum* var. *capsulatum* is usually acquired by inhalation of conidia and mycelial fragments of the fungus into the lungs. They lodge within the terminal bronchioles and alveoli. The organism changes from mycelial to yeast form cells, the form in which the *capsulatum* variety of *H. capsulatum* exists as a facultative intracellular parasite in the susceptible host. Alveolar macrophages phagocytose the organisms. They display less efficient antifungal activity and yeast forms multiply within them followed by lysis and the infection of new cells.

Following pulmonary infection, organisms spread through lymphatics to the regional lymph nodes and haematogenously to other organs. After low-inoculum exposure, the infection is asymptomatic in at least 90% of cases. Symptomatic patients develop fever, cough, and chest pain. X-ray chest shows mediastinal lymphadenopathy with adjacent infiltrate. Most patients recover in a few weeks, but some experience prolonged fatigue.

In heavy exposure, the lungs may be consolidated and the mycosis advances to an early fatal termination. The pulmonary manifestations may be less prominent, and hepatosplenomegaly, fever, anaemia, leucopenia, weight loss, and generalized lymphadenopathy (Fig. 11.1A, B & C) characterize the illness. Patient may also develop endocarditis, meningitis, adrenal insufficiency, hepatic insufficiency, solitary or multiple ulcerations of the mouth, pharynx, larynx, stomach, and small or large bowel, and papulonodular skin lesions (Fig. 11.1D).

Chronic, cavitary, pulmonary histoplasmosis capsulati occurs predominantly in adults. The pathologic findings typically resemble tuberculosis, with granulomas occasionally evolving to caseous necrosis. Disseminated infection is more common among individuals with underlying cell-mediated immunological defects, including those with HIV infection, and transplant recipients. Immuno-compromised persons with histoplasmosis have a higher mortality rate than those who are not immuno-suppressed.

Bone and joint infection by *H. capsulatum* is rare. Bone marrow involvement commonly occurs in cases of severe disseminated disease, but evidence of osteomyelitis is absent. *H. capsulatum* var. *capsulatum* may cause tenosynovitis and carpal tunnel syndrome. Approximately 10–20% of patients with progressive disseminated histoplasmosis have clinically apparent central nervous system involvement. Parenchymal mass lesions of the brain and spinal cord may account for 24–39% of cases of CNS disease. They may be single or multiple. Patients typically present with headache, and focal neurologic deficits. Diffuse encephalitis and meningitis may be seen in 16% and 40% patients respectively.

# Histoplasmosis

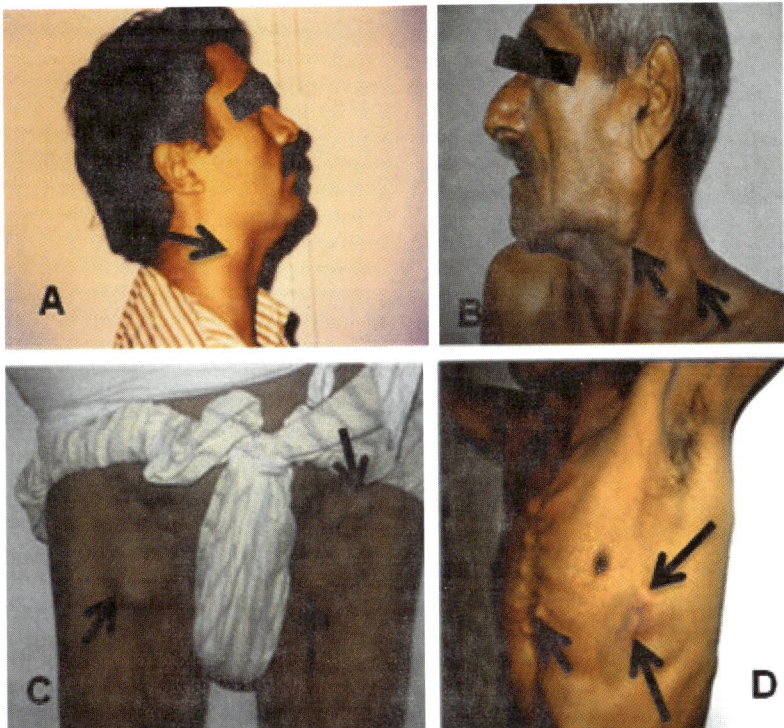

**Fig. 11.1.** Cervical (A and B), inguinal (C) lymphadenitis, and papulonodular skin nodules (D) caused by *H. capsulatum* var. *capsulatum*.

## Oral manifestations

The oral lesions appear as nodular, ulcerative or vegetative lesions on the buccal mucosa, gingiva, tongue, palate or lips. The ulcerated areas are usually covered by a nonspecific grey membrane and are indurated.

## Laboratory diagnosis

### Specimens

Sputum or bronchoalveolar lavage fluid, blood, urine, CSF, lymph node, and bone marrow samples.

### Direct examination

The diagnosis of histoplasmosis capsulati can be rapidly established by observation of the yeast phase by direct microscopic examination of specimens with special stains.

### Histopathology

*Histoplasma* is predominantly an intracellular parasite, growing within the cells of the reticuloendothelial system as an oval yeast 2–5 μm in diameter with budding on a narrow base. All phagocytic cells of the reticuloendothelial system are involved including those in the liver, spleen, lymph nodes and bone marrow, so that the cytoplasm is filled with masses of fungal cells. There is at first little tissue reaction, later necrosis takes place to be followed by granulomatous changes and fibrosis.

Less commonly, organisms may be observed by fungal staining of sputum, sterile body fluids, or peripheral blood smears. In disseminated histoplasmosis capsulati, the highest yield is from bone marrow (> 50%). With Giemsa or Wright stain, the cell wall and the cell protoplasm stain light blue and dark blue, respectively.

With haematoxylin and eosin (H&E) staining, only a central protoplasmic mass surrounded by a halo is seen (Fig. 11.2). **The so-called 'capsule' (halo) of *H. capsulatum* var. *capsulatum* is**

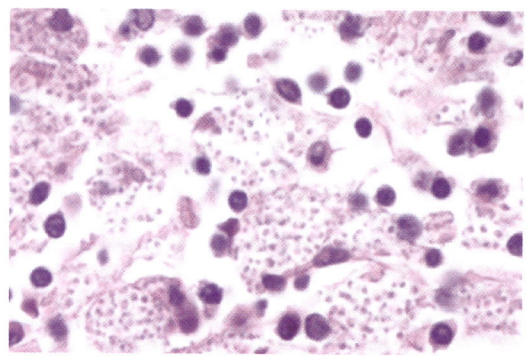

**Fig. 11.2.** Section of skin stained with haematoxylin and eosin (×400) showing *Histoplasma capsulatum* surrounded by clear halo filling the cytoplasm of phagocytes.

considered to be an artifact resulting from the shrinkage of the protoplasm within the cell wall. Only a dark staining can outline the cell wall. In the PAS stain, the wall is stained pink to purplish red with pallor coloured protoplasm filling the cell. In Gomori methenamine silver (GMS) stain, the cell wall stains intense black (Fig. 11.3). The yeast phase of *H. capsulatum* var. *capsulatum* should be carefully differentiated from other small yeasts and a few parasites:

- Yeast-like cells of *Penicillium marneffei* do not bud. They have a prominent transverse septum and reproduce by fission.
- Yeast cells of *Candida glabrata* are more variable in size, stain better with H&E and do not have a halo or pseudocapsule.

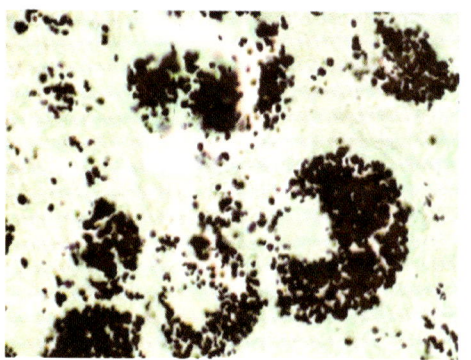

**Fig. 11.3.** Section similar to that demonstrated in Fig. 11.2 but stained with Gomori methenamine silver stain (×400). It shows black budding yeast cells.

- Mucicarmine staining for capsular material may be used to distinguish *Cryptococcus neoformans*, but capsule-deficient strains may be misidentified by this technique.
- *Sporothrix schenckii* causes a mixed suppurative and granulomatous reaction rather than the purely granulomatous reaction seen in histoplasmosis. In addition, in sporotrichosis, the yeast cells are often fewer.
- Endoconidia of *Coccidioides immitis* are rounder and do not bud and are accompanied by spherules.
- Intracellular parasites such as *Leishmania* spp. and *Trypanosoma cruzi* can be differentiated from *Histoplasma* in that they stain entirely with H&E, do not form a halo or pseudocapsule, do not reliably stain with special histologic fungal stains, and do not bud. In addition, amastigotes of *Leishmania* spp. and *Trypanosoma cruzi* possess kinetoplast which is absent in *Histoplasma*.
- Cells of *Toxoplasma gondii* packed within the histiocytes resemble the yeast cells of *H. capsulatum* var. *capsulatum* on H&E staining. *T. gondii* cells, however, are smaller than *H. capsulatum* var. *capsulatum* and also fail to stain with special fungus stains.
- The cyst forms of *Pneumocystis jirovecii* stained with GMS stain may superficially resemble *H. capsulatum* var. *capsulatum*. The cysts, however, do not bud, and they are almost always extracellular.

### Culture

Definitive diagnosis of histoplasmosis requires growth of the fungus from samples of body fluids or tissues. Cultures are most useful in patients with disseminated or chronic pulmonary histoplasmosis capsulati, being positive in 50–85% of cases. More than 75% of patients with disseminated disease have positive blood, bone marrow or urine cultures. However, in patients with other forms of histoplasmosis capsulati, culture is positive in only 10–15% of cases.

The clinical material is inoculated on Sabouraud dextrose agar and incubated at 25–30°C. Growth is slow. Mycelial forms usually mature within 15–20 days but may take up to 8 weeks. Colony is white to brown, or pinkish, with a fine, dense cottony texture.

The reverse is white, sometimes yellow or orange-tan. An enriched agar is the best growth medium.

In young cultures, septate hyphae are seen. They bear round to pear-shaped smooth or occasionally spiny microconidia (2–5 µm in diameter). They are sessile or stalked. After several weeks, large, thick-walled, round macroconidia (7–15 µm in diameter) form. They are tuberculate, knobby, or have short cylindrical projections. Occasionally, they may be smooth (Fig. 11.4A). The macroconidia of *H. capsulatum* var. *capsulatum* resemble those of *Sepedonium* species. However, latter does not produce microconidia and grows poorly or not at all at 37°C.

At 35–37°C on brain-heart-infusion agar, moist, white, yeast-like colonies may eventually form. These may require many generations. The yeast phase is inhibited by cycloheximide. Microscopically small, round or oval budding cells (2–3 × 3–5 µm) (Fig. 11.4B) and occasional abortive hyphae may be seen.

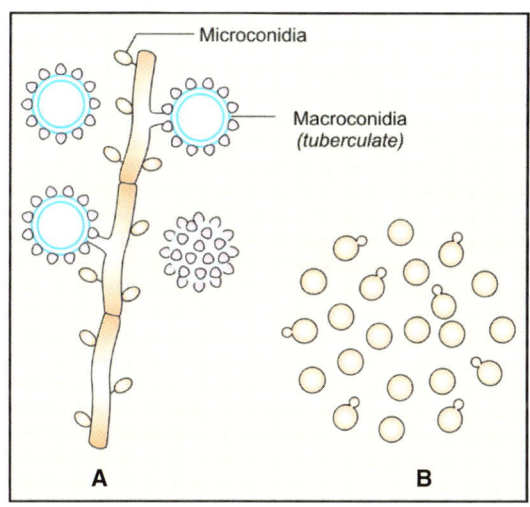

**Fig. 11.4.** *Histoplasma capsulatum*: mycelial phase (A); and yeast phase (B).

*Histoplasma* meningitis is difficult to diagnose, with CSF cultures being positive in no more than two-thirds of cases. The best results are obtained when large volumes of CSF (10–20 ml) are cultured on multiple occasions.

### Serological tests

Histoplasmosis capsulati may be diagnosed by immunodiffusion and complement fixation tests for detection of antibodies, and a radioimmunoassay and an enzyme immunoassay for demonstration of histoplasma polysaccharide antigen in serum and urine. The complement fixation test is performed with both histoplasmin and whole yeast cell antigens. Complement fixation titres of 1 : 8 or higher are found in most patients with active histoplasmosis capsulati, whereas titres of 1 : 32 or higher are more suggestive of active infection. Immunoglobulin M antibodies may be detected by latex agglutination test using histoplasmin as antigen. This semiquantitative test is used primarily for the presumptive diagnosis of acute histoplasmosis. It is less helpful for the detection of chronic infection.

*Histoplasma* polysaccharide antigen is found in blood, urine, and bronchoalveolar lavage fluid of more than 90% of individuals with disseminated histoplasmosis capsulati, in the urine of 75% of those with extensive pneumonitis, and in the cerebrospinal fluid of 25–50% of patients with meningitis caused by *H. capsulatum* var. *capsulatum*.

### Skin tests

Skin tests for histoplasmosis are not useful to establish a diagnosis because most patients in endemic zones have skin test reactivity to histoplasmin that is retained for years after infection, and patients with other fungal diseases give false positive results.

### Molecular methods

Molecular methods have been developed for diagnosis of histoplasmosis capsulati. DNA probes are commercially available and widely used reducing the time for definitive identification of positive cultures. *H. capsulatum* DNA may be detected in fixed paraffin-embedded tissue samples, blood, bronchial lavage fluids, bone marrow, and ophthalmic samples by polymerase chain reaction.

## HISTOPLASMA CAPSULATUM VAR. DUBOISII

*H. capsulatum* var. *duboisii* causes histoplasmosis duboisii or African histoplasmosis. The term African histoplasmosis correctly indicates that all cases have originated in the African continent but incorrectly suggests that the only histoplasmosis to occur in Africa is caused by *H. capsulatum* var. *duboisii*. Histoplasmosis caused by *H. capsulatum* var. *capsulatum* also occurs in Africa. It was first described in 1952 by Vanbreuseghem, named in 1960 by Ciferri and the disease caused by this fungus was fully described in 1964 by Cockshott and Lucas.

In 1994, Gugnani et al. isolated this fungus from soil collected from eastern Nigerian bat cave in the State of Anambara. Exposure to bat or bird droppings appears to be a risk factor for the acquisition of histoplasmosis duboisii. Infection is acquired by inhalation. The most common clinical manifestations in histoplasmosis duboisii involve skin, bone and subcutaneous tissues. However, pulmonary and disseminated infections may occur. Skin lesions may be papular, nodular, ulcerative or eczematoid. With the enlargement of nodular or papular lesions, the centre ulcerates.

Osteolytic lesions are commonly found in ribs, vertebrae, femur, tibia, humerus, skull and wrist. The granulation tissue from a vertebral lesion may cause compression of the spinal cord, resulting in paraplegia. Formation of subcutaneous abscesses from underlying bone lesions are common in histoplasmosis duboisii.

In patients with the disseminated form of histoplasmosis duboisii, multiple lesions are usually present in liver, spleen, lymph nodes, bone marrow and other visceral organs. Patient develops fever, anaemia, and loss of weight, and if untreated the disease may prove fatal. Several cases have been reported in patients with AIDS.

*H. capsulatum* var. *duboisii* is indistinguishable in its hyphal form in cultures incubated at temperature below 25°C from *capsulatum* variety. In parasitized tissues and in cultures on brain-heart-infusion agar incubated at 35–37°C it forms thick-walled (up to 1.5 µm) yeasts measuring 8–15 µm in diameter that are distinct from those of *H. capsulatum* var. *capsulatum* (2–5 µm in diameter). The yeast cells of *H. capsulatum* var. *duboisii* superficially resemble those of *Blastomyces dermatitidis* in size, but each cell is uninucleate, unlike the multinucleate cells of *B. dermatitidis*. In addition *H. capsulatum* var. *duboisii* buds by narrow base, while *B. dermatitidis* buds by broad base. *H. capsulatum* var. *duboisii* generally elicits a granulomatous inflammatory response, commonly associated with numerous giant cells that may contain abundant phagocytosed yeasts.

## HISTOPLASMA CAPSULATUM VAR. FARCIMINOSUM

*H. capsulatum* var. *farciminosum* causes epizootic lymphangitis, known as histoplasmosis farciminosi, in horses and mules. It is more common in tropical and subtropical regions than in temperate zones. It is endemic in some countries in the Mediterranean region, and in parts of Africa and Asia including India, Pakistan and Japan. Sporadic cases have been reported from other parts of the world.

The fungus causes subcutaneous and ulcerated lesions of the skin, particularly of the front legs and neck, and at the site of injury. The mycosis involves the lymphatics and may be disseminated to many organs. Noncutaneous lesions may occur in the mucous membranes and proliferate along the nasal septum to the pharynx, larynx, and trachea. Ocular involvement may also occur, especially in mules.

Diagnosis can be made by detection of the tissue-form cells of the dimorphic *H. capsulatum* var. *farciminosum*. The fungus in tissue is similar to *H. capsulatum* var. *capsulatum*. They measure 2.5–3.5 × 2.0–3.0 µm. These are found intracellular within phagocytes. Tissue sections can be stained with H&E, periodic acid-Schiff (PAS) or GMS staining.

*H. capsulatum* var. *farciminosum* can be cultured on a variety of fungal media including enriched SDA with 2.5% glycerol, and brain-heart-infusion agar with or without 5% sheep blood. This organism grows as a mycelium at cooler temperatures. The colonies grow slowly and develop in 2–8 weeks at 25°C. They are dry, granular, wrinkled and grayish-white, becoming brown as they age.

On microscopic examination, the hyphae are hyaline, septate, branched and pleomorphic. A variety of conidia including arthroconidia, blastoconidia and chlamydoconidia may be found, but *H. capsulatum* var. *farciminosum* does not produce the large, round, thick-walled macroconidia often seen in *H. capsulatum* var. *capsulatum* cultures.

# Histoplasmosis

Mycelial phase can be converted to yeast phase by growing the isolates at 37°C on brain-heart-infusion agar with or without 5% sheep blood. The yeast phase forms colonies that are flat, raised, wrinkled, white to grayish brown and pasty. Complete conversion occurs only after repeated serial transfers to fresh media.

## Treatment

For disseminated or localized forms of histoplasmosis capsulati oral itraconazole is highly effective including the treatment of the disease in AIDS patients, where long-term suppressive therapy is usually needed. Ketoconazole and fluconazole are alternatives. Amphotericin B is useful in patients with widespread and severe infections. In African histoplasmosis, itraconazole and ketoconazole are effective. In severe cases amphotericin B is an alternative. Solitary skin lesions may simply respond to excision without chemotherapy

### Important Questions

1. Discuss morphology, cultural characteristics, pathogenesis and laboratory diagnosis of *Histoplasma capsulatum* var. *capsulatum*.
2. Write short notes on:
   (a) Histoplasmosis duboisii
   (b) Histoplasmosis farciminosi
   (c) Differential diagnosis of histoplasmosis capsulati.

### Multiple Choice Questions

1. *Emmonsiella* is the generic name of perfect state of:
   (a) *Histoplasma capsulatum* var. *capsulatum*.
   (b) *Blastomyces dermatitidis*.
   (c) *Coccidioides immitis*.
   (d) *Sporothrix schenckii*.
2. Which of the following is intracellular mycosis of reticuloendothelial system?
   (a) Blastomycosis.
   (b) Histoplasmosis.
   (c) Coccidioidomycosis.
   (d) Mucormycosis.
3. Macroconidia of *Histoplasma capsulatum* var. *capsulatum* resemble those of:
   (a) *Trichophyton*.
   (b) *Microsporum*.
   (c) *Epidermophyton*.
   (d) *Sepedonium*.
4. Cycloheximide inhibits:
   (a) *Trichophyton rubrum*.
   (b) *Microsporum gypseum*.
   (c) *Epidermophyton floccosum*.
   (d) Yeast phase of *Histoplasma capsulatum*.
5. *Histoplasma* polysaccharide antigen may be detected in:
   (a) blood.
   (b) urine.
   (c) bronchoalveolar lavage fluid.
   (d) All of the above.
6. Which of the following fungi causes African histoplasmosis?
   (a) *Histoplasma capsulatum* var. *capsulatum*.
   (b) *Histoplasma capsulatum* var. *duboisii*.
   (c) *Histoplasma capsulatum* var. *farciminosum*.
   (d) None of the above.
7. Which of the following fungi **does not** produce large, round, thick-walled macroconidia?
   (a) *Histoplasma capsulatum* var. *capsulatum*.
   (b) *Histoplasma capsulatum* var. *duboisii*.
   (c) *Histoplasma capsulatum* var. *farciminosum*.
   (d) None of the above.
8. Mycelial phase of *Histoplasma capsulatum* var. *capsulatum* can be converted to yeast phase by growing the isolate at 37°C on:
   (a) brain-heart-infusion agar.
   (b) niger seed agar.
   (c) Sabouraud dextrose agar.
   (d) Cornmeal agar.
9. What do you find in the tease mount of *Histoplasma capsulatum* var. *capsulatum* cultured on Sabouraud dextrose agar at 30°C?
   (a) Arthroconidia.
   (b) Chlamydoconidia.
   (c) Budding yeast cells.
   (d) Tuberculate macroconidia.
10. A solitary pulmonary nodule may result from:
    (a) bronchogenic carcinoma.
    (b) tuberculosis.

(c) histoplasmosis.
(d) All of the above.
11. The perfect state of *Histoplasma capsulatum* is:
    (a) Basidiomycete.
    (b) Ascomycete.
    (c) Mucormycete.
    (d) None of the above.
12. Which of the following fungi produces macroconidia that may be mistaken for those of *Histoplasma capsulatum* var. *capsulatum*?
    (a) Sepedonium.
    (b) Trichophyton.
    (c) Epidermophyton.
    (d) Microsporum.
13. *Histoplasma capsulatum* var. *capsulatum* and *Blastomyces dermatitidis* can be differentiated because the latter fungus:
    (a) is difficult to convert to the yeast form.
    (b) has a larger yeast form with a broad-based bud.
    (c) produces tuberculate macroconidia.
    (d) All of the above are true.
14. *Histoplasma capsulatum* is:
    (a) a protozoan.
    (b) an encapsulated organism.
    (c) Both of the above.
    (d) Neither of the above.

## ANSWERS TO MCQs

1. (a), 2. (b), 3. (d), 4. (d), 5. (d), 6. (b), 7. (c), 8. (a), 9. (d), 10. (d), 11. (b), 12. (a), 13. (b), 14. (d).

**Further Reading**

1. Adderson E. Histoplasmosis. *Pediatr Infect Dis J* 2006; 25: 73–4.
2. Al-Agha OM, Mooty M, Salarieh A. Disseminated histoplasmosis. *Arch Pathol Lab Med* 2006; 130: 120–3.
3. Anand A. Diagnosis of systemic histoplasmosis in AIDS patients. *South Med J* 1993; 86: 844–5.
4. Arora B, Maheshwari M, Arora DR. Disseminated histoplasmosis presenting as skin nodule. *Brit J Med Res* 2016; 11: 1–5.
5. Assi M, McKinsey DS, et al. Gastrointestinal histoplasmosis in the acquired immunodeficiency syndrome: report of 18 cases and literature review. *Diagn Microbiol Infect Dis* 2006; 55: 195–201.
6. Guimaraes AT, Pizzini CV, et al. ELISA for early diagnosis of histoplasmosis. *J Med Microbiol* 2004; 53: 509–14.
7. Hindupur S, Despotovic V. Gastric histoplasmosis. *Lancet Infect Dis* 2006; 6: 60.
8. Kauffman CA. Diagnosis of histoplasmosis in immunosuppressed patients. *Curr Opin Infect Dis* 2008; 21: 421–5.
9. Kauffman CA. Histoplasmosis: a clinical and laboratory update. *Clin Microbiol Rev* 2007; 20: 115–32.
10. Manbon D, Simon S, Aznar C. Histoplasmosis diagnosis using a polymerase chain reaction method – application on human samples in French Guiana, South America. *Diagn Microbiol Infect Dis* 2007; 58: 441–4.
11. Naniwadekar A, Malhotra A. Gastrointestinal histoplasmosis. *J Gastroenterol Hepatol* 2008; 23: 668.
12. Wheat LJ, Kauffman CA. Histoplasmosis. *Infect Dis Clin N Am* 2003; 17: 1–19.
13. Wheat LJ. Current diagnosis of histoplasmosis. *Trends Microbiol* 2003; 11: 488–94.

# CHAPTER 12

# Blastomycosis

Blastomycosis, formerly known as **North American blastomycosis**, is a chronic infection of the lungs which may spread to the other tissues, particularly skin, bone and genitourinary tract. Chest radiograph may resemble that of tuberculosis or carcinoma. **Disseminated blastomycosis may develop in immunosuppressed patients including those with AIDS.** It is caused by *Blastomyces dermatitidis*, a dimorphic fungus. It is the imperfect stage (asexual form) of *Ajellomyces dermatitidis* (**an ascomycete**).

It was originally thought to be restricted to the North American continent where it extends from Canada, particularly Quebec, through the USA with occasional cases in Mexico and Central America. The largest number of cases is seen in the Mississippi valley. Central Kentucky is an endemic area. Blastomycosis is now known to be widely distributed in Africa, with the largest number of cases coming from Zimbabwe, and cases have been reported from the Middle East, India and Poland. Khan et al. (1982), from Delhi, isolated *B. dermatitidis* from the lungs of a bat. Subsequently, Randhawa et al. (1983) isolated the fungus from the bronchial aspirates of a patient in India. Jambhekar et al. (1988) reported a case of disseminated blastomycosis from Madhya Pradesh.

Gilchrist (1894) from Johns Hopkins Hospital in Baltimore first reported this disease in a patient with localized skin lesions, clinically diagnosed as scrofuloderma (cutaneous tuberculosis). He examined the tissue histologically but was unable to find tubercle bacilli. He saw 'numerous curious bodies' in tissue, which he thought were protozoa. Histopathological description was thorough and complete. Gilchrist called this disease process a protozoan dermatitis but expressed the opinion that the organisms were more probably of plant origin. In 1896, he was convinced that the causative agent was a 'blastomycete', a general term used at that time to refer to yeasts. The clinical entity was subsequently designated, to honour its discoverer, as **Gilchrist disease**.

Gilchrist and Stokes (1896) had the opportunity to see second patient and named the fungus *Blastomyces dermatitidis*. Tissue specimens were subjected to histopathology as well as culture. The culture from the diseased tissue grew in both their yeast and mycelial forms. They also observed that the mycelial form was not seen in tissues. The thermal basis for dimorphism was first described by Hamburger in 1907 by maintaining incubator at different temperatures. The gross colonial morphology and the microscopic characteristics of both forms were described. He converted the mycelial form of *B. dermatitidis* to the yeast form and vice versa simply by changing the temperature of incubation. The infection caused by *B. dermatitidis* showed substantial number of clinical manifestations in skin and hence the name of the species was described as *dermatitidis*. Subsequently, involvement of deeper structures and more disseminated nature of infection were recognized.

## Pathogenesis

The natural habitat of *B. dermatitidis* is the soil. It appears to survive best in moist acidic soils that contain a high nitrogen and organic content. Higher soil temperature and recent rainfall facilitate growth of the fungus. Occupational or recreational soil contact has been associated with outbreaks of infection. The incubation period has been estimated to be 4–6 weeks. Infection occurs in patients of all ages and both sexes, but cases usually occur in young to middle-aged adults and are more commonly reported in men than in women. African-American race and diabetes are risk factors for symptomatic disease. Next to humans, dogs are the most frequent animals infected with *B. dermatitidis*.

**The infectious particles of *B. dermatitidis* are its mycelial fragments and conidia.** The respiratory tract is the portal of entry for all forms of blastomycosis except direct transcutaneous inoculation. In the alveoli, the organism transforms into the yeast and induces an acute inflammatory response that includes neutrophils and macrophages, resulting in granuloma formation. It is relatively resistant to phagocytosis and killing. **Cell-mediated immunity is the principal host defence against the organism and is critical in preventing dissemination.** *B. dermatitidis* may also be transmitted by bites from an infected dog. Accidental inoculation through dog bites during examination or treatment is an occupational hazard of veterinarians. Human-to-human transmission does not normally take place.

## Clinical types

There are three clinical types of blastomycosis – pulmonary blastomycosis, disseminated extrapulmonary blastomycosis, and cutaneous blastomycosis.

### Pulmonary blastomycosis

The presentation of pulmonary blastomycosis may be asymptomatic or patient may develop a brief non-specific flu-like illness. The presentation may resemble bacterial pneumonia, tuberculosis, a fulminant adult respiratory distress-like syndrome and cancer.

### Disseminated extrapulmonary blastomycosis

Extrapulmonary sites of involvement include skin and soft tissues, bones, joints, genitourinary tract, central nervous system, liver, spleen, gastrointestinal tract, thyroid, pericardium and adrenal glands. Osseous sites, along with the skin, are among the most common loci of extrapulmonary blastomycosis, with the former being involved in 7–48% of cases of disseminated infection. Although any bone can be involved, the most common sites of osseous involvement include the lumbar and thoracic vertebrae; long bones (particularly the tibia); ribs; small bones of the hands, wrists, feet, and ankles; pelvis; facial bones, and skull. Joint infection is less frequent manifestation of extrapulmonary blastomycosis, occurring in 2.5–8% of patients with systemic disease.

Central nervous system involvement occurs in approximately 5% of patients with systemic blastomycosis. Disease manifestations may include chronic meningoencephalitis in one-third of patients, intracranial abscess (blastomycoma) in another one-third and spinal epidural or vertebral abscess in approximately 20%. In immunocompromised patients with blastomycosis the central nervous system is more likely to be affected. Central nervous system involvement may occur in up to 40% of patients with acquired immunodeficiency syndrome who acquire blastomycosis.

### Cutaneous blastomycosis

Cutaneous blastomycosis may be a primary transcutaneous disease or secondary to systemic infection. **Primary transcutaneous blastomycosis** is the result of the direct inoculations of *B. dermatitidis* into the skin. It may occur after accidental inoculation in the laboratory and after dog bites. Therefore, it is commonly seen as a solitary lesion. Cutaneous blastomycosis may originate as a subcutaneous nodule or be observed first as a papule or as a pustule which ulcerates. Generally, there is a sharp edge at the periphery of the lesion where invasive activity is occurring. It heals with scarring.

**Secondary cutaneous blastomycosis** occurs as a result of the haematogenous spread of infection from another focus, usually the lungs; therefore, the lesions are frequently multiple. Although cutaneous lesions result from disseminated blastomycosis, the initial pulmonary disease may not be obvious and cutaneous lesions may be the only presenting symptoms.

*B. dermatitidis* is uncommon as an opportunistic pathogen, but it causes more aggressive disease in persons with underlying cell-mediated immunological defects, such as those with HIV infection and transplant recipients. Immunocompromised persons with blastomycosis have a higher mortality rate than those who are not immunosuppressed.

## Oral manifestations

Oral lesions may resemble those of actinomycosis, although abscess formation is not usually as prominent. Tiny ulcers may be the chief feature. The oral lesion may be the primary lesion or secondary to lesions elsewhere in the body.

## Laboratory diagnosis

The diagnosis of blastomycosis can be made by demonstration of the fungus in the clinical specimens and confirmation by culture. The most common specimens from patients with suspected blastomycosis are sputum, bronchoalveolar lavage fluid, cerebrospinal fluid, urine, and lung biopsies. For suppurative cutaneous or visceral lesions, sample should be collected by aspiration.

### Direct examination

The fungus can be observed in direct calcofluor white, potassium hydroxide mounts or Gram stain of sputum, tissue, pus or scrapings as thick-walled, rounded, refractile, spherical yeasts with broad-based buds.

### Histopathology

Tissue and cytologic specimens can be examined with haematoxylin and eosin (H&E), Gomori methenamine silver (GMS), periodic acid-Schiff (PAS), Papanicolaou, and Giemsa stains.

The characteristic tissue response to *B. dermatitidis* is a combination of suppuration and epithelioid cell granulomatous reaction with giant cells. *B. dermatitidis* appears as yeast-like cells (3–30 µm in diameter; most commonly 8–15 µm). They are round to oval, with sharply defined refractile cell walls that are commonly referred to as "double contoured". The cytoplasm is often retracted from the rigid cell wall as a result of shrinkage during the fixation process, thus creating clear spaces, or "halos" in the fungal cells. Each yeast cell produces only one bud which is attached to the parent cell on broad base (average 4–5 µm). The bud characteristically grows to the same size as the parent cell before detaching. Budding *in vivo* may be relatively infrequent.

The broad bud base, which is sometimes as wide as the diameter of the cell, and the persistent attachment of the bud to the parent cell till it grows to the same size as the parent cell before detaching are two characteristics that distinguish *B. dermatitidis* from *Cryptococcus neoformans*, *Histoplasma capsulatum* var. *capsulatum*, *H. capsulatum* var. *duboisii* and *H. capsulatum* var. *farciminosum*. Mayer's mucicarmine stain aids in distinguishing small *Blastomyces* cells from *Cryptococcus*. In the latter the capsule stains bright carmine red, often with a spiny or scalloped appearance. Nuclear stains can be used to demonstrate the multinucleate status of *B. dermatitidis*, in contrast to *C. neoformans* and *H. capsulatum* which are uninucleate. *B. dermatitidis* can be further identified by direct fluorescent antibody (DFA) test.

### Culture

The specimen (pus, sputum, minced biopsy material or rarely blood) is inoculated on Sabouraud dextrose agar slants with antibacterial antibiotics. It is then incubated at 25–30°C for 3–4 weeks. When culture of yeast form is desired, the culture specimen is inoculated on brain heart infusion (BHI) agar or blood glucose cysteine agar and incubated at 37°C. Yeast form of *B. dermatitidis* is sensitive to cycloheximide; therefore, the media should not contain this antibiotic when the specimen is cultured at 37°C.

**Colony morphology:** On SDA at 25°C, growth matures within 14 days. Some strains are slower, therefore, cultures should be held for 8 weeks. Colonies at first are yeast-like, then prickly, and finally cottony with a white aerial mycelium. Old culture turns tan or brown. Reverse is tan. The conidia of the hyphal form, as for *H. capsulatum*, *Coccidioides immitis* and *Paracoccidioides brasiliensis*, are highly infectious when aerosolized. **Thus, the plating of specimens and culture should be performed within a biosafety cabinet.**

At 37°C on BHI agar and blood agar, colonies are cream to tan in colour, heaped or wrinkled, waxy in appearance.

**Microscopic morphology:** At 25–30°C on SDA, it shows delicate (1–2 μm in diameter), hyaline and septate hyphae with short or long conidiophores. Round or pear-shaped conidia (2–10 μm in diameter) develop at the apex of the conidiophore or directly on the hyphae (Fig. 12.1A). Older cultures have thick-walled chlamydoconidia.

On BHI agar and blood agar at 37°C, it forms yeast-like cells (8–15 μm in diameter) that bud on a broad base (4–5 μm wide) and appear to be thick-walled and double contoured. The bud often remains attached until it becomes the same size as the parent cell (figure of 8 morphology) (Fig. 12.1B).

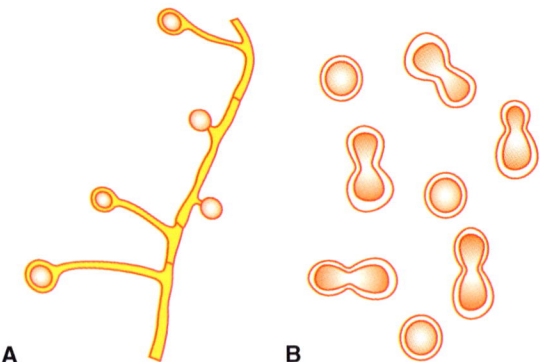

**Fig. 12.1.** *Blastomyces dermatitidis*: mycelial phase (A); yeast phase (B).

### Direct fluorescent antibody test

For rapid identification of yeast forms of the fungus direct fluorescent antibody test can be done. This technique may be applied to tissue sections or to a yeast form culture.

### Nucleic acid probes

A simplified test using nucleic acid probes has recently been developed for the identification of mycelial or yeast forms of *B. dermatitidis*. A single-stranded DNA probe is combined with a chemiluminescence label for detection. If the unknown organism is *B. dermatitidis*, the DNA probe will hybridize with the RNA of the target organism. The labelled DNA/RNA hybrid is then detected for identification of the fungus.

### Polymerase chain reaction (PCR)

A nested-PCR assay targeting the *WI-1* gene has been described for the detection of *B. dermatitidis* DNA in paraffin-embedded tissue.

### Serodiagnosis

- **Antibody detection:** *B. dermatitidis* antibodies can be detected by complement fixation test (CFT), immunodiffusion (ID) precipitin test and enzyme immunoassay (EIA). CFT becomes positive 2–3 months after the onset of symptoms. Both sensitivity and specificity of the CFT are poor. ID test may be positive in up to 80% of the patients with blastomycosis 2–3 weeks after the onset of symptoms. The sensitivity of this test is close to 100%. A positive test indicates recent or active disease. EIA test has a sensitivity of 100% and a specificity of 85.6%.
- **Antigen detection:** *B. dermatitidis* antigen can be detected by enzyme immunoassay (EIA). The *Blastomyces* antigen test is a microtitre plate-based double-antibody sandwich EIA to detect antigenuria and antigenemia in disseminated blastomycosis.

### Intradermal test

Delayed skin hypersensitivity to blastomycin (cell free culture-filtrate of mycelial phase) is unreliable as a diagnostic technique for blastomycosis.

### Treatment

Amphotericin B is still widely used for the treatment of widespread disseminated forms of blastomycosis.

# Blastomycosis

However, in most cases, itraconazole appears to be effective. It has the advantage that it can be given orally. Ketoconazole is an alternative therapy.

## Important Questions

Discuss pathogenesis and laboratory diagnosis of blastomycosis.

## Multiple Choice Questions

1. *Ajellomyces* is the generic name of perfect state of:
   (a) *Histoplasma capsulatum* var. *capsulatum*.
   (b) *Blastomyces dermatitidis*.
   (c) *Coccidioides immitis*.
   (d) *Sporothrix schenckii*.

2. Which of the following fungi is **not** thermally dimorphic?
   (a) *Cryptococcus neoformans*.
   (b) *Histoplasma capsulatum*.
   (c) *Coccidioides immitis*.
   (d) *Sporothrix schenckii*.

3. Which of the following fungi causes Gilchrist disease?
   (a) *Histoplasma capsulatum*.
   (b) *Coccidioides immitis*.
   (c) *Blastomyces dermatitidis*.
   (d) *Sporothrix schenckii*.

4. *Blastomyces dermatitidis* causes:
   (a) pulmonary blastomycosis.
   (b) disseminated extrapulmonary blastomycosis.
   (c) cutaneous blastomycosis.
   (d) All of the above.

5. In the yeast phase of which of the following fungi each yeast cell produces only one bud which is attached to the parent cell on broad base?
   (a) *Blastomyces dermatitidis*.
   (b) *Paracoccidioides brasiliensis*.
   (c) *Histoplasma capsulatum*.
   (d) *Sporothrix schenckii*.

6. Conidia and hyphal fragments of which of the following fungi are highly infectious when aerosolized?
   (a) *Histoplasma capsulatum*.
   (b) *Coccidioides immitis*.
   (c) *Paracoccidioides brasiliensis*.
   (d) All of the above.

7. Which of the following scientists demonstrated the dimorphic growth patterns of *Blastomyces dermatitidis*?
   (a) Emmons.
   (b) Sabouraud.
   (c) Conant.
   (d) Hamburger.

8. The characteristic/s of yeast form of *Blastomyces dermatitidis* in tissue is/are:
   (a) multiple budding.
   (b) broad-based bud.
   (c) polysaccharide capsule.
   (d) All are correct.

9. The disease of humans and dogs is caused by a dimorphic primary systemic fungal pathogen. The disease has a predilection to disseminate from lungs to the skin. KOH preparation from skin exudates or other infected sites shows a large yeast form with a broad-based bud. The etiologic agent is:
   (a) *Blastomyces dermatitidis*.
   (b) *Coccidioides immitis*.
   (c) *Histoplasma capsulatum*.
   (d) *Paracoccidioides brasiliensis*.

### ANSWERS TO MCQs

1. (b), 2. (a), 3. (c), 4. (d), 5. (a), 6. (d), 7. (d), 8. (b), 9. (a).

## Further Reading

1. Adams JS, Godin MS, Tsogas N. Disseminated blastomycosis. *Arch Otolaryngol Head Neck Surg* 2002; 128: 853–4.
2. Assalay RA, Hammersley JR, et al. Disseminated blastomycosis. *J Am Acad Dermatol* 2003; 48: 123–7.
3. Bedimo R, Weinstein J. Disseminated blastomycosis. *Clin Infect Dis* 2001; 33: 1706, 1770–1.
4. Bradsher RW Jr. Pulmonary blastomycosis. *Semin Respir Crit Care Med* 2008; 29: 174–81.
5. Bradsher RW, Chapman SW, Pappas PG. Blastomycosis. *Infect Dis Clin N Am* 2003; 17: 21–40.

6. Chakrabarti A, Slavin MA. Endemic fungal infections in the Asia-Pacific region. *Med Mycol* 2011; 49: 337–44.
7. Khan ZU, Randhawa HS, Lulia M. Isolation of *Blastomyces dermatitidis* from the lung of a bat, *Rhinopoma hardwickei hardwickei* Gray, in Delhi. *Sabouraudia* 1982; 20: 137–44.
8. Kauffman CA. Blastomycosis. *Curr Treat Option Infect Dis* 2000; 2: 481–5.
9. Oppenheimer M, Embil JM, et al. Blastomycosis of bones and joints. *South Med J* 2007; 100: 570–8.
10. Pappas PG. Blastomycosis. *Semin Respir Crit Care Med* 2004; 25: 113–21.
11. Randhawa HS, Khan ZU, Gaur SN. *Blastomyces dermatitidis* in India: first report of its isolation from clinical material. *Sabouraudia* 1983; 21: 215–21.
12. Randhawa HS, Chaturvedi VP, et al. *Blastomyces dermatitidis* in bats: first report of its isolation from the liver of *Rhinopoma hardwickei hardwickei* Gray. *Sabouraudia* 1985; 23: 69–76.
13. Walsh CM, Morris SK, et al. Disseminated blastomycosis in an infant. *Pediatr Infect Dis J* 2006; 25: 656–8.

# CHAPTER 13

# Coccidioidomycosis

Coccidioidomycosis, caused by **ascomycetous, soil dwelling molds**, *Coccidioides immitis* and *C. posadasii*, is a highly infectious disease. The two causative agents are phenotypically identical or very similar and the spectrum of disease they cause appears to be the same. It may be acute or benign, self-limiting respiratory disease or a chronic malignant, sometimes fatal infection involving the skin, bone, joints, lymph nodes, adrenals and central nervous system. The first recorded case of coccidioidomycosis was studied and reported by Posadas and by Wernicke in a series of papers published between 1892 and 1898. They described the disease in a considerable detail and they characterized the microorganism they found in the lesions as a protozoan.

As a result of its resemblance to the protozoan coccidia and severity of disease caused by it, the organism was named *Coccidioides immitis* (*Coccidia*, like; *im*, not; *mitis*, mild). The organism is endemic in the southwestern United States, northern Mexico, and scattered areas of Central and South America. *C. posadasii* is endemic in east and south of the Sierra Nevada range. With no clear clinical differences, both *C. immitis* and *C. posadasii* will be herein referred to as *C. immitis*. Skin tests have shown that the incidence of coccidioidomycosis in endemic areas may be as high as 95%. ***C. immitis* is probably the most virulent of all human mycotic pathogens.** It has been included as a **'select agent' of bioterrorism**.

## Pathogenesis

*C. immitis* exists as a saprophyte in the soil. The arthroconidia of the saprophytic phase are carried by wind and are inhaled by man and animals. A few arthroconidia may be sufficient to produce a naturally acquired respiratory infection. Pulmonary macrophages and neutrophils provide the initial host defence. Arthroconidia germinate to produce spherules filled with endoconidia (endospores), which is the characteristic tissue phase of the organism. At maturity, the spherules rupture and their endoconidia are released which develop to form new spherules in adjacent tissue or, following dissemination, in other organs of the body. The spherules become surrounded by neutrophils and macrophages, which lead to granuloma formation. Arthroconidia, endoconidia and spherules are resistant to killing by these cells. Rarely, traumatic introduction of the organism into the skin leads to infection and disease. Hyphal forms may be found in tissue section, particularly, if the affected site has been exposed to air. Human-to-human transmission of *C. immitis* ordinarily does not occur, but has followed transplantation of organs from individuals with coccidioidomycosis who served as donors.

### Primary pulmonary coccidioidomycosis

About 60% of the individuals infected by respiratory route are asymptomatic. Those who have had asymptomatic coccidioidomycosis are identifiable only by the acquisition of hypersensitivity to coccidioidin. These persons may have hilar or parenchymal healed and calcified lesions in addition to acquired hypersensitivity.

Forty per cent of the patients who develop symptoms develop acute febrile illness 7–28 days after exposure to the organism. Fever often exhibits diurnal variation and is associated with night sweats. Chest pain, often pleuritic and sometimes severe, occurs in 75% of cases. Patient may also develop cough, malaise, rash, sore throat, anorexia, weight loss, headache, arthralgia and/or myalgia.

Primary infection may be accompanied by a variety of **immune complex-mediated complications**, including an erythematous macular rash, erythema multiforme, and erythema nodosum. Acute infection usually resolves without therapy, although symptoms may persist for weeks. These patients are immune to exogenous reinfection as are those individuals who have incurred asymptomatic infections. About 10% of these patients will, however, be left with a pulmonary residual nodule or cavity.

### Disseminated coccidioidomycosis

Dissemination of coccidioidomycosis may occur by haematogenous spread of endoconidia from lungs to other organs. Dissemination can affect virtually any tissue and organ, although the gastrointestinal mucosal surface and endocardium have rarely been affected. Disseminated lesions may occur in skin, subcutaneous tissue, bones, joints and central nervous system. Progression may be slow or rapid or the patient may recover, except in cases of acute miliary dissemination and meningitis.

**Bone involvement** occurs almost exclusively as a result haematogenous dissemination. Two-fifths of cases are polyostotic. Any bone may be infected but the most common sites of involvement include the lumbar and thoracic vertebrae, followed by the tibia, skull, metacarpals, metatarsals, femur, and ribs. Joint space infection occurs in up to 25–30% of individuals with disseminated coccidioidomycosis.

**Central nervous system involvement** by *C. immitis*, which is most common, can take following forms:

- Subacute or chronic meningitis.
- Encephalitis.
- Parenchymal microscopic granulomas.
- Abscesses.
- Vascular occlusion with infarcts.

Subacute or chronic meningitis is the most common manifestation of CNS disease due to *C. immitis*. It occurs early in the disease process and is quite unusual after 2 years. Patient develops fever, weight loss, throbbing headache, nausea, vomiting, papilledema, disorientation, lethargy, confusion or loss of memory. Encephalitis is almost as common as meningitis.

Cell-mediated defences with T lymphocytes are central to the immune response. Disseminated infection occurs in immunocompromised patients with deficient cell-mediated immunity. **Coccidioidomycosis is one of the most frequent opportunistic infections among HIV-infected patients in southwestern USA.**

### Oral manifestations

The lesions of the oral mucosa and skin are proliferative granulomatous and ulcerated that are nonspecific in their clinical appearance. The lesions tend to heal by hyalinization and scar formation. Marked chronicity is often a feature of these lesions. Lytic lesions of the jaws may also occur.

### Laboratory diagnosis

#### Direct examination

Place bronchial washings, exudates, sputum, cerebrospinal fluid, pleural fluid, pericardial fluid or peritoneal fluid in a drop of 10–20% potassium hydroxide and examine with reduced illumination under a low power of the microscope. Demonstration of *C. immitis* particularly endosporulating spherules provides the most direct and secure method of diagnosis. Round spherules may be as small as 5 μm in diameter when immature (non-endosporulating) and grow to 30–100 μm or more in diameter upon maturity (endosporulating).

## Histopathology

Histopathological examination reveals granulomatous reaction in the presence of spherules (Fig. 13.1), and a predominantly suppurative reaction occurs in response to released endoconidia. Immature spherules stain well with periodic acid-Schiff (PAS) and Gomori methenamine silver (GMS) stains, but mature spherules are GMS variable and PAS negative due to the high phospholipid content of the mature cell wall. Endoconidia are round (2–5 μm in diameter) and uninucleate. They possess cell walls and cytoplasmic inclusions that are GMS and PAS positive. The spherules and endoconidia stain with haematoxylin and eosin (H&E) and are readily visible. Fragmented or empty ruptured spherules are common. When only endoconidia are seen, they may initially be confused with yeasts, but endoconidia do not bud.

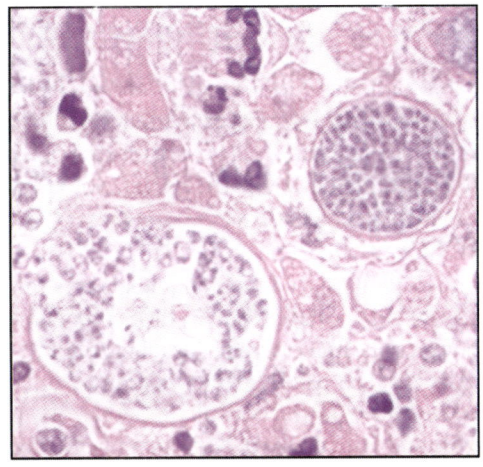

**Fig. 13.1.** Spherules of *Coccidioides immitis* containing endoconidia (H&E stain, ×400).

*Coccidioides* in the skin evokes a proliferative (pseudoepitheliomatous) response in the epidermis. The synovial membrane produces a villous response in coccidioidal arthritis. Bones have lytic lesions (occasionally proliferative). In old pulmonary lesions immature non-endosporulating spherules are often embedded in fibrocaseous material.

The differential microscopic diagnosis of endoconidia and small spherules includes atypical forms of *Blastomyces dermatitidis* and non-budding *Histoplasma capsulatum*, *Paracoccidioides brasiliensis*, *Candida glabrata*, and *Cryptococcus neoformans*. *Rhinosporidium seeberi* may be confused with larger spherules of *C. immitis*.

## Culture

Spread the pathologic material on Sabouraud dextrose agar (SDA) and blood agar slants and incubate these at 25°C and 37°C, respectively. *C. immitis* differs from other dimorphic fungi because under standard laboratory conditions it grows as a mold at 25°C as well as 37°C. Only when grown on special Converse medium with increased $CO_2$ at 37–40°C is the spherule or tissue phase formed *in vitro* (Fig. 13.2A). On SDA at 25°C or 37°C the growth of *C. immitis* appears in 3–5 days; and sporulation is seen 5–10 days after incubation. The colony often is at first moist, grayish, and membranous and soon develops a white, cottony aerial mycelium, which becomes gray or tan to brown with age. It may also be pinkish or yellow. Reverse is white to gray, sometimes yellow or brownish.

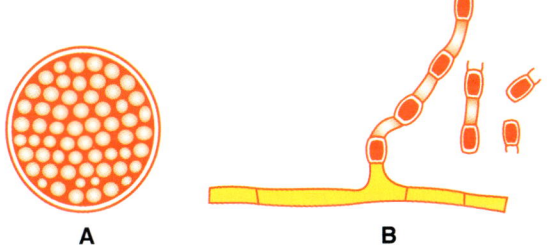

**Fig. 13.2.** *Coccidioides immitis*: (A) tissue phase; and (B) mycelial phase.

Because the arthroconidia are highly infectious and are readily airborne, therefore, **the cultures must be handled with great care and grown in tubes only, not in petri dishes**. Tubed growth should be wet down with sterile water before being handled. *C. immitis* **is probably the most virulent of all human mycotic agents. The inhalation of a few**

**arthroconidia produces primary coccidioidomycosis.** Handling and processing clinical specimens, and processing animal tissues are to be conducted using biosafety level 2 (BSL 2) practices. BSL 3 practices are to be used when propagating and manipulating sporulating cultures identified as *Coccidioides* species and for processing soil or other environmental materials known to contain infectious arthroconidia.

Microscopic examination shows septate, branched hyphae that produce thick-walled, barrel-shaped arthroconidia (3–4 × 3–6 μm). They characteristically alternate with smaller intervening empty cells (Fig. 13.2B). The walls of empty cells break easily and are characteristically present on either end of the freed conidia. Racquet hyphae are formed in young colonies. Arthroconidia are infectious particles. Careful microscopic examination should prevent confusion of arthroconidia of *C. immitis* with those of *Geotrichum candidum*. The latter do not possess alternating empty cells. **It is not necessary or advisable to prepare slide cultures of *C. immitis* and that method should be avoided.**

### DNA hybrid protection assay

Ribosomal RNA (rRNA) is extracted from the suspect organism and allowed to react with specific DNA from *C. immitis* to which is attached a potentially luminescent acridinium ester. If the rRNA is of coccidioidal origin, it will react with its complementary DNA, and this protects the ester linkage against hydrolysis, thus yielding luminescence.

### Serological tests

IgM antibodies may be present soon after infection or relapse but then wane. These can be detected by a complement fixation test, and tube precipitin (TP) test, in which serum is combined with a soluble antigen to form a precipitate. If the test is performed as a diffusion assay using agar, it is termed immunodiffusion tube precipitin (IDTP) test.

The anticoccidioidal IgG antibody appears later and remain positive for months. IgG antibodies are able to fix complement when combined with coccidioidal antigen, and can be detected by immunodiffusion complement fixation (IDCF) techniques. Rising titres of IgG are associated with progressive disease, while declining titres are associated with resolution. Patients with IDCF titres of ≥ 1 : 16 are more likely to have disseminated disease.

For the diagnosis of coccidioidomycosis, enzyme immunoassay has also been developed. A quantitative latex agglutination test using heat-treated coccidioidin as antigen is available. This test is simple and rapid to perform. It detects IgM antibodies and is more sensitive than the IDTP test in detecting early infection. However, it has a false positive rate of 5–10%, and the result should be confirmed using the IDTP and/or complement fixation test.

Cross reactions between antigens of *C. immitis* and those of other fungi are common, particularly with *Histoplasma capsulatum* and *Blastomyces dermatitidis*. Low titre complement-fixing antibody against *C. immitis* may be present in normal serum. It may represent remote, undiagnosed illness due to coccidioidomycosis or perhaps exposure to other fungi.

### Animal pathogenicity

Laboratory animals including mice, rats, rabbits, guinea pigs, and monkeys are very susceptible to experimental infection. Intraperitoneal injection of 10 viable particles (arthroconidia and hyphal fragments) from virulent strains can produce fatal disease within 20 days in mice, whereas with strains having low virulence, even 100 particles will not kill mice.

### Treatment

In primary pulmonary infection, no specific therapy apart from rest is necessary. In diffuse pneumonia, amphotericin B, itraconazole, posaconazole and voriconazole may be used. Severe meningeal infection can be treated with fluconazole, itraconazole, posaconazole and voriconazole. Non-meningeal infection can be treated with itraconazole, fluconazole, posaconazole and voriconazole.

 **Important Questions**

Discuss pathogenesis and laboratory diagnosis of coccidioidomycosis.

## Multiple Choice Questions

1. Which of the following fungi is a 'select agent' of bioterrorism?
   (a) *Histoplasma capsulatum*.
   (b) *Coccidioides immitis*.
   (c) *Paracoccidioides brasiliensis*.
   (d) *Blastomyces dermatitidis*.

2. Which of the following fungi is the most virulent of all human mycotic agents?
   (a) *Histoplasma capsulatum*.
   (b) *Coccidioides immitis*.
   (c) *Paracoccidioides brasiliensis*.
   (d) *Blastomyces dermatitidis*.

3. Which of the following fungi form spherules and endoconidia *in vivo*?
   (a) *Histoplasma capsulatum*.
   (b) *Coccidioides immitis*.
   (c) *Paracoccidioides brasiliensis*.
   (d) *Blastomyces dermatitidis*.

4. Which form/s of *Coccidioides immitis* is/are resistant to killing by pulmonary macrophages and neutrophils?
   (a) Arthroconidia.
   (b) Endoconidia.
   (c) Spherules.
   (d) All of the above.

5. Which of the following fungi shows septate, branched hyphae that produce thick-walled, barrel-shaped arthroconidia which alternate with smaller intervening empty cells?
   (a) *Geotrichum candidum*.
   (b) *Histoplasma capsulatum*.
   (c) *Blastomyces dermatitidis*.
   (d) *Coccidioides immitis*.

6. Which of the following organisms cause/s granulomatous meningitis?
   (a) *Cryptococcus neoformans*.
   (b) *Coccidioides immitis*.
   (c) *Mycobacterium tuberculosis*.
   (d) All of the above.

7. Which of the following statements is **true** about *Coccidioides* spherule?
   (a) It is the sexual stage of the species.
   (b) It is the infectious form of the species.
   (c) It is both the sexual stage and infectious form of the species.
   (d) It is neither the sexual stage nor the infectious form of the species.

8. What precautions should you take in processing a mold culture to protect yourself and other laboratory personnel against possible exposure to *Coccidioides* species?
   (a) Do not prepare slide culture.
   (b) Avoid the use of petri plates for culture.
   (c) Work in a certified BSL 3 cabinet.
   (d) All of the above.

## ANSWERS TO MCQs

1. (b), 2. (b), 3. (b), 4. (d), 5. (d), 6. (d), 7. (d), 8. (d).

## Further Reading

1. Ampel NM. Coccidioidomycosis in persons infected with HIV-1. *Ann NY Acad Sci* 2007; 1111: 336–42.
2. Anstead GM, Grabill JR. Coccidioidomycosis. *Infect Dis Clin N Am* 2006: 621–43.
3. Binnicker MJ, Buckwater SP, et al. Detection of *Coccidioides* species in clinical specimens by real-time PCR. *J Clin Microbiol* 2007; 45: 173–8.
4. Carmichael JK. Coccidioidomycosis in HIV-infected persons. *Clin Infect Dis* 2006; 42: 1059–60.
5. Catanzaro A. Coccidioidomycosis. *Semin Respir Crit Care Med* 2004; 25: 123–8.
6. Chang A, Tung RC, et al. Primary cutaneous coccidioidomycosis. *J Am Acad Dermatol* 2003; 49: 944–9.
7. Chiller TM, Galgiani JN, Stevens DA. Coccidioidomycosis. *Infect Dis Clin N Am* 2003; 17: 41–57.
8. de Aguiar Cordeiro R, Nogueira Brilhante RS, et al. Rapid diagnosis of coccidioidomycosis by nested PCR assay of sputum. *Clin Microbiol Infect* 2007; 13: 449–51.
9. Saubolle MA. Laboratory aspects in the diagnosis of coccidioidomycosis. *Ann NY Acad Sci* 1111: 301–14.
10. Wang CY, Jerng JS, et al. Disseminated coccidioidomycosis. *Emerg Infect Dis* 2005; 11: 177–9.
11. Warnock DW. *Coccidioides* species as potential agents of bioterrorism. *Future Microbiol* 2007; 2: 277–83.

# CHAPTER 14

# Paracoccidioidomycosis

Paracoccidioidomycosis, formerly known as **South American blastomycosis**, is a chronic progressive granulomatous infection caused by *Paracoccidioides brasiliensis*, a dimorphic fungus only known in its asexual state. In 1908, Lutz described a mycosis in a Brazilian patient with severe oral lesions. Lutz was able to isolate the causative agent in cultures in various media. He noted its dimorphic nature. As Lutz did not see endogenous sporulation, he considered the fungus to be different from *Coccidioides immitis*. Between 1909 and 1912, Alfonso Splendore, an Italian bacteriologist, observed new cases of the disease, and gave a more complete description of its causative agent and of the clinicohistopathological features of the disease.

Paracoccidioidomycosis has been reported from most Latin American countries, but the infection is most commonly found in Brazil, particularly in the state of Sao Paulo, Colombia and Argentina. The infection is not known in other countries.

The ecology of the endemic areas includes high humidity, rich vegetation, moderate temperatures, and acid soil. These conditions are found along rivers from the Amazon jungle to small indigenous forests in Uruguay. *P. brasiliensis* has been recovered from soil in these areas; however, its ecologic niche is not well established.

## Pathogenesis

The disease is thought to be acquired by inhalation of propagules from the filamentous phase of the infecting agent present in the nature. They reach the terminal bronchi and alveoli, convert into the yeast form in the lung parenchyma, which can subsequently disseminate to extrapulmonary sites. Cases are sporadic, neither epidemic outbreaks nor inter-human transmission have been reported.

Paracoccidioidomycosis is rare in children and young adults but is regularly diagnosed in men older than 30 years. Although, the rate of infection is equal in men and women, as shown by skin test with paracoccidioidin, progression towards symptomatic disease is more common in men. There has been an increase in the number of reports involving immunocompromised patients, including those with AIDS.

## Clinical features

Most primary infections are self-limited, diagnosed only by a reactive skin test. The organism has the ability to remain dormant for long periods of time and cause clinical disease at a later time when the host resistance is lowered. Patient complains of a persistent cough with purulent sputum, chest pain, weight loss, weakness, malaise, dyspnea and fever. Pulmonary lesions are nodular, infiltrative, fibrotic or cavitary. A paracoccidioidoma, a large cavitary mass, may also be seen. In approximately 25% of the patients, the lungs are the only organs affected.

If not diagnosed and treated, infection can disseminate to extrapulmonary locations including the skin and mucosa, lymph nodes (especially cervical), adrenals, liver, spleen, central nervous system, and bones. The cutaneous lesions, usually verrucous, ulcerative or granulomatous, occur around the mouth and nose and may affect lower limbs. These lesions may begin at the cutaneous-mucosal border by extension of the mucosal lesions and produce a deeply infiltrated lesion of the lip. Skin lesions may also begin from subcutaneous sites where the fungus is carried by circulating blood or lymph drainage. Occasionally, a solitary pustular lesion may be seen. It is assumed that the skin lesion may be primary and follow subcutaneous implantation of the fungus.

The conspicuous lesions of paracoccidioidomycosis are in the nasal or oral mucosa, the gingivae, sometimes in the conjunctivae or the anorectal mucosa. Patient develops ulcerated, painful mucosal lesions. The ulcers which spread slowly, have a granulomatous, sometimes mulberry-like base.

The lymphatics which drain the oronasal lesions, and eventually the entire lymphatic system, are invariably involved. Because the oronasal lesions appear early, the cervical lymph nodes are involved early in the course of the disease. They are enlarged, painful and may suppurate and drain through sinus tracts. Pus which is discharged contains many fungi.

The frequency of central nervous system involvement varies from 10–25% and manifests as seizures, hemiparesis, cerebellar signs, headache, hydrocephalus, paraesthesia or confusion.

The differential diagnosis of paracoccidioidomycosis includes tuberculosis, histoplasmosis, neoplastic disorders including lymphoma, leishmaniasis, Hansen's disease, and syphilis. Chest X-ray findings that favour tuberculosis and histoplasmosis include extensive calcification, pleural effusion, and apical localization.

## Laboratory diagnosis

### Specimens

Sputum, bronchoalveolar lavage fluid, crusts and granulomatous bases of ulcers, and pus especially from suppurating and draining lymph nodes, cerebrospinal fluid and tissue biopsy.

### KOH preparation

Place the specimen on a slide, mix it with a drop of 10% potassium hydroxide and examine under low power and high power of the microscope. Fungus cells are easily observed. They vary in size from recently separated buds 2–10 μm in diameter to mature cells 30–60 μm in diameter. The outstanding characteristic is the presence of multiple buds that are attached to the parent cell by narrow necks (Fig. 14.1A). Staining of wet preparations with lactophenol cotton blue, methylene blue, calcofluor white, or Gram stain can be helpful.

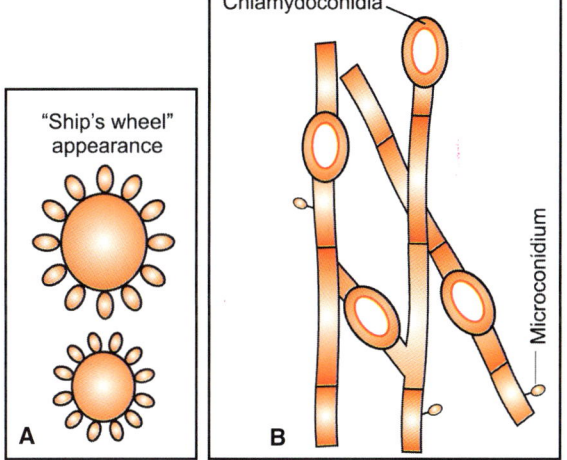

Fig. 14.1. *Paracoccidioides brasiliensis*: yeast phase (A); and mycelial phase (B).

The buds may be small and all approximately of the same size or fairly large and of unequal sizes and shapes. A large parent cell surrounded by small buds creates the **classic "ship's wheel" appearance**. Parent cells with fewer, but larger, buds are common, and single budding may also be seen. The presence of multiple budding distinguishes it from *Cryptococcus neoformans* and *Blastomyces dermatitidis*.

## SECTION 4 : Systemic Mycoses

### Histopathology

The histopathological features of paracoccidioidomycosis are similar to those of other systemic mycoses. It is characterized by a granulomatous reaction combined with pyogenic inflammation. Giant cells of the Langhans' and foreign body type are usually conspicuous. These cells very frequently contain the fungus. To establish the specific diagnosis of paracoccidioidomycosis on histopathologic material only, fungus cells showing typical peripheral budding must be identified. If the fungus is abundant, it may be identified by haematoxylin and eosin stain, but the special stains (such as Gomori methenamine silver, periodic acid-Schiff and Papanicolaou) demonstrate the cells much more effectively. When the disease is chronic, most of the fungal cells are found inside the giant cells, but free yeast cells predominate in disseminated cases.

### Culture

*P. brasiliensis* is thermally dimorphic fungus. To isolate and maintain the fungus in the parasitic or tissue form inoculate pathologic material on brain-heart-infusion (BHI) agar with antibacterial antibiotics, and incubate at 35–37°C. Cycloheximide should not be added into BHI agar for culturing the tissue form since the yeast cells are susceptible to the drug. To isolate the mycelial form, inoculate pathologic material on Sabouraud dextrose agar (SDA) with antibacterial antibiotics and cycloheximide, and incubate at 25–30°C. Fungus grows slowly and should be observed for 4 weeks.

At 35–37°C on BHI agar colony is heaped, cream to tan, moist, and soft, becoming waxy and yeast-like. Microscopically, it shows large, round, fairly thick-walled cells (5–50 μm in diameter) with single and multiple buddings (2–10 μm in diameter). The buds are attached to the mother cell by narrow necks and may almost completely surround the cell, giving the classic "ship's wheel" appearance (Fig. 14.1A).

At 25–30°C on SDA, the colony is white, heaped, compact, usually folded and almost glabrous or with short white aerial mycelium that often turns brown with age. Reverse is light or brownish. Microscopically, it shows septate, branched hyphae bearing intercalary and terminal chlamydoconidia. A few microconidia are sometimes observed along the hyphae (Fig. 14.1B). As the mycelial form is not characteristic, therefore, conversion of the mycelial form to the yeast phase is essential for identification. **Suspected cultures should be handled in a biologic safety cabinet.**

### Serology

Patients with paracoccidioidomycosis produce high amounts of anti-*P. brasiliensis* antibodies. These are long-lasting and generally correlate with the severity of the disease. With treatment serological titres tend to fall. They are useful for the diagnosis and treatment follow-up of patients. Antibodies may be detected by immunodiffusion, counterimmunoelectrophoresis, complement fixation test, indirect immunofluorescence, indirect haemagglutination test, enzyme-linked immunosorbent assay, dot blot and Western blotting.

### Treatment

The treatment of choice in most cases is itraconazole. Ketoconazole is an alternative. Patients with rapidly progressive and extensive infections may require amphotericin B.

### Important Questions

Discuss pathogenesis and laboratory diagnosis of paracoccidioidomycosis.

### Multiple Choice Questions

1. Which of the following dimorphic fungi shows multiple budding yeast cells?
   (a) *Paracoccidioides brasiliensis*.
   (b) *Coccidioides immitis*.
   (c) *Histoplasma capsulatum*.
   (d) *Sporothrix schenckii*.

2. Which of the following fungi is known only in its asexual state?
   (a) *Trichophyton rubrum*.
   (b) *Microsporum gyseum*.
   (c) *Histoplasma capsulatum*.
   (d) *Paracoccidioides brasiliensis*.

### ANSWERS TO MCQs

1. (a), 2. (d).

### Further Reading

1. Albuquerque CF, da Silva SH, Camargo ZP. Improvement of specificity of an enzyme-linked immunosorbent assay for diagnosis of paracoccidioidomycosis. *J Clin Microbiol* 2005; 43: 1944–6.
2. Benard G. An overview of the immunopathology of human paracoccidioidomycosis. *Mycopathologia* 2008; 165: 209–21.
3. Bethlem EP, Capone D, et al. Paracoccidioidomycosis. *Curr Opin Pulm Med* 1999; 5: 319–25.
4. Castro G, Martinez R. Disseminated paracoccidioidomycosis and coinfection with HIV. *N Engl J Med* 2006; 355: 2677.
5. de Almeida SM. Central nervous system paracoccidioidomycosis: an overview. *Braz J Infect Dis* 2005; 9: 126–33.
6. Deps PD, Neves MB, Pinto Neto LF. Paracoccidioidomycosis: an unusual presentation with a rapid progression. *Rev Soc Bras Med Trop* 2004; 37: 425–6.
7. Elias J Jr, dos Santos AC, et al. Central nervous system paracoccidioidomycosis: diagnosis and treatment. *Surg Neurol* 63 (Suppl. 1): S13–21.
8. Marques da Silva SH, Colombo AL, et al. Diagnosis of paracoccidioidomycosis by detection of antigen and antibody in bronchoalveolar lavage fluids. *Clin Vaccine Immunol* 2006; 13: 1363–6.
9. Restrepo A, Benard G, et al. Pulmonary paracoccidioidomycosis. *Seminar Respir Crit Care Med* 2008; 29: 182–97.

# SECTION 5

# OPPORTUNISTIC MYCOSES

**Chapter 15** Candidiasis
**Chapter 16** Cryptococcosis
**Chapter 17** Pneumocystosis
**Chapter 18** Penicilliosis marneffei
**Chapter 19** Aspergillosis
**Chapter 20** Mucormycosis
**Chapter 21** Hyalohyphomycosis

# CHAPTER 15

# Candidiasis

The genus *Candida* comprises about 200 species, of which about 20 have been associated with pathology in humans and animals. The major pathogenic species include *C. albicans*, *C. dubliniensis*, *C. glabrata*, *C. guilliermondii*, *C. kefyr*, *C. krusei*, *C. lusitaniae*, *C. parapsilosis* and *C. tropicalis*. *C. albicans* is round to oval yeast 3–6 μm in diameter. It produces budding cells, pseudohyphae, and true hyphae. This ability to simultaneously display several morphological forms is known as **polymorphism**. Although hyphae are likely to be produced during the process of tissue invasion, yeasts without hyphae may also occur in invasive disease, particularly in infections caused by non-*albicans Candida* species.

The history of candidiasis dates back to the fourth century B.C. when Hippocrates, in his book **Epidemics**, described oral aphtha (thrush) in two patients with other underlying disease. The first descriptions of thrush in modern medicine were made by Rosen von Rosenstein in 1771 and by Underwood in 1784, who identified the infection as a paediatric problem. Bennett isolated the fungus from sputum of a patient suffering from tuberculosis. Later on, it was isolated by other workers from vaginal infection, brain infection and systemic infection.

Medically important yeasts of the genus *Candida* are classified in the family Saccharomycetaceae, order Saccharomycetales, class Saccharomycetes, subphylum Saccharomycotina in the phylum Ascomycota.

## Pathogenesis

*Candida* is a human commensal, so that the source of infection is mostly endogenous. *Candida* spp. reside primarily in the gastrointestinal tract, but they are also commensals in the vagina, urethra, on the skin and under fingernails. *Candida* can be introduced from exogenous sources as well. These include introduction through various catheters and lines, or other indwelling prosthetic medical devices. This route leads to the development of deep-seated and systemic candidiasis as most of these therapeutic modalities are used primarily in compromised hosts whose defence systems are unable to combat the introduced pathogen.

- *C. albicans*, the species most often associated with human disease, is also recovered from fresh water, sea water and soil. Oral carriage rate may be higher in certain settings such as in HIV-infected patients with low CD4 counts, denture users with denture stomatitis, patients suffering from diabetes, patients receiving anticancer chemotherapy, and children.

**Predisposing factors** for candidiasis are AIDS, diabetes, iatrogenic immunosuppression, intravenous catheters, prolonged administration of antimicrobial agents, neutropenia, haematologic malignant diseases and burns. After *Candida* enters the blood stream, whether from exogenous or endogenous source, it adheres to the endothelial surface of the blood vessels, before dissemination into tissues.

Person-to-person transmission is not a predominant mechanism of pathogenesis in candidiasis. It occurs primarily in oral thrush of newborns acquired during birth from their mothers affected by vaginal infections, and rarely in sexual transmission from vaginitis patients to their male partners.

- *C. dubliniensis* is primarily associated with recurrent erythematous oral candidiasis in HIV-infected patients. It is also known, to a far lesser extent, to cause oral disease in non-HIV-infected individuals.
- *C. glabrata* causes infections usually occurring in the blood stream or urogenital tract and occasionally in the lungs and other sites.
- *C. parapsilosis* is a relatively frequent cause of endocarditis second only to *C. albicans* as a cause of *Candida* endocarditis.
- *C. lusitaniae* is an opportunistic pathogen in immunocompromised patients.
- *C. tropicalis*, *C. kefyr*, *C. guilliermondii*, and *C. krusei* are opportunistic pathogens, causing disease in patients:
  – with a breakdown in the body's immune system;
  – on prolonged treatment with antibiotics, corticosteroids, or cytotoxic drugs;
  – with intravenous catheters;
  – with diabetes mellitus; or
  – who are intravenous drug users.

## Virulence factors

Numerous virulence factors exist and may play different roles with differing sites and stages of a given infection. These include adhesin, enzymes, fungal surface hydrophobicity and phenotype switching.

### Adhesin

For colonization and tissue invasion adherence of *Candida* spp. to a wide range of tissue types and inanimate surfaces is essential. This is achieved by a combination of specific (ligand-receptor interaction) and non-specific (electrostatic charge) mechanisms. Mutants with reduced adherence exhibit decreased pathogenicity *in vivo*. Following attachment, *Candida* spp., particularly *C. albicans* grow in colonial communities and produce **'biofilms'**. The biofilms contain extracellular materials composed of proteins, carbohydrates, and other substances. Biofilms lead to poorer response of the pathogen in the biofilm to antimicrobials and the difficulties of the hosts' defence system to cope with the microbe, resulting in difficulties of eradication of infection.

### Enzymes

*Candida* spp. produce extracellular proteinases, phospholipases, lipases and hydrolytic enzymes. These are important virulence factors.

### Fungal surface hydrophobicity

Hydrophobicity of the cell surface of *C. albicans* plays an important role in the adhesion of the organism to eukaryotic cells and inert surfaces. **Blastoconidia of *C. albicans* are hydrophilic, but the germ tube formation is associated with a significant rise in the cell surface hydrophobicity.**

### Phenotype switching

Phenotype switching is the ability of organisms of a single strain to switch to different colony phenotype. Due to this ability, *C. albicans* can grow in variety of morphological forms, ranging **from budding yeast to filamentous pseudohyphae and true hyphae**. Such switching enables adaptation to different or changing conditions in the host facilitating its ability to survive, invade tissues and escape host defences.

Transformation into the hyphal form is observed during an active infection. It is believed that phospholipase concentrated at the hyphal tip may be related to the greater invasiveness of this form as compared to the yeast. In addition, the hyphae, being larger than the yeast form, are more resistant to phagocytosis. Thus morphological change contributes to the increased pathogenic potential of the fungus.

## Clinical features

*Candida* species can cause a range of clinical forms, from superficial manifestations involving skin, nails, and mucosal surfaces to deep-seated infections involving various internal organs and to disseminated disease (Table 15.1).

**Table 15.1.** Clinical forms of candidiasis

1. **SUPERFICIAL INFECTIONS**
   I. **Cutaneous infections**
      - Candidal intertrigo
      - Interdigital candidiasis
      - Perianal (diaper) rash
      - Candids
      - Chronic mucocutaneous candidiasis
   II. **Nail infections**
      - Paronychia
      - Onychomycosis
   III. **Mucosal infections**
      - Oral candidiasis
        – Acute pseudomembranous and acute atrophic candidiasis (oral thrush)
        – Chronic atrophic and hyperplastic candidiasis (denture stomatitis)
        – Angular cheilitis
      - Vaginal candidiasis
2. **DEEP INFECTIONS**
   - Candidiasis of gastrointestinal tract
     – Esophagitis
     – Gastrointestinal candidiasis
   - Candidiasis of liver, spleen and other organs
   - Candidiasis of respiratory system
   - Candidiasis of cardiovascular system
   - Renal and urinary tract candidiasis
     – Lower urinary tract infection
     – Renal infection
   - Central nervous system candidiasis
   - Ocular *Candida* infection
   - Bone and joint *Candida* infection
3. **DISSEMINATED CANDIDIASIS AND CANDIDEMIA**

## SUPERFICIAL INFECTIONS

Superficial infections result from invasion of the superficial layers of skin and/or mucosae by the microorganism. These infections are characterized by the formation of a grayish plaque, surrounded by edema, which on histopathological examination consists of the infecting microorganisms, neutrophils, and cell debris.

### Cutaneous infections

The major symptoms discussed under this head are:
- Candidal intertrigo
- Interdigital candidiasis
- Perianal (diaper) rash
- Candids
- Chronic mucocutaneous candidiasis.

### Candidal intertrigo

It is the most common clinical form of the cutaneous infection, as *Candida* spp. readily colonize skin folds, particularly in moist and macerated sites. These may include groin, perineum, gluteal folds, umbilicus, axillae, inframammary folds or interdigital spaces. Lesions may be erythematous, with vesicles and pustules, in combination with pruritis. Obesity, diabetes mellitus, various endocrine disturbances, HIV infection and steroid therapy are predisposing factors.

### Interdigital candidiasis

In this form the skin folds between the fingers of the hand are macerated and itching. This condition is associated with excessive exposure to moisture, and thus seen particularly among dishwashers.

### Perianal (diaper) rash

This occurs in infants wearing diapers. It causes rash in the perianal area and on the buttocks.

### Candids

Sterile, grouped, vesicular lesions resembling dermatophytids may be found beyond the limits of infected lesions. They probably represent allergic responses to circulating fungal antigens.

### Chronic mucocutaneous candidiasis (CMC)

It is a rare condition in which susceptible individuals develop superficial *Candida* infections as a result of variable defects in T lymphocyte responsiveness to the fungus. It is characterized by the presence of persistent lesions, with high rate of recurrence, starting in early childhood and possibly persisting throughout the individual's lifetime. Lesions can be seen on various skin sites. CMC may appear in a generalized form or may be localized and assume a form of hyperkeratotic lesions – *Candida* granuloma.

### Nail infections

The syndromes discussed under this head are:

- Paronychia
- Onychomycosis

### Paronychia

It is chronic swelling and inflammation of the nail fold usually affecting the nails of the hands and less frequently those of the feet.

### Onychomycosis

It is an invasive infection of the fingernails. As in paronychia, it is more often seen in nails of the hands. Infected nails may become discoloured, eroded, brittle, detached from the nail bed, and painful.

### Mucosal infections

Involvement of mucosal surfaces by *Candida* is the most frequent clinical manifestation of candidiasis. The syndromes discussed under this head are:

- Oral candidiasis
- Vaginal candidiasis

### Oral candidiasis

Candidiasis of oral mucosa is a disease recognized since antiquity. Very old, very young and very ill persons are more susceptible to oral candidiasis. In the mouth, carbohydrate levels are important; food debris, likely to be present in the mouth of severely ill patients with inadequate oral hygiene may be as significant as diabetic saliva. It has gained renewed significance more recently as an infection frequently seen in AIDS patients and in other conditions. *C. albicans* is the most frequently isolated etiological agent of oral candidiasis. Additional *Candida* spp., such as *C. glabrata*, *C. tropicalis*, *C. parapsilosis* and *C. guilliermondii* are also implicated in oral candidiasis. Oral candidiasis can be clinically classified into:

- acute pseudomembranous and acute atrophic candidiasis (oral thrush)
- chronic atrophic and hyperplastic candidiasis (denture stomatitis)
- angular cheilitis.

### Acute pseudomembranous and acute atrophic candidiasis

**Acute pseudomembranous candidiasis** is also known as **oral thrush**. It occurs predominantly in patients with systemic or local immunosuppression. Immunosuppressed individuals at risk include newborns with birth asphyxia, malnourished or diabetic patients, patients with HIV infections, and those receiving corticosteroid or cytotoxic chemotherapy.

The tongue, soft palate, buccal mucosa and other oral surfaces are characteristically covered with discrete or confluent patches of a cream-white to gray pseudomembrane (Fig. 15.1) composed of hyphae and yeasts of *C. albicans*. The lesions, particularly when covering larger areas, may be painful. They may spread to the mucosa of esophagus (Fig. 15.2), as seen in significant number of AIDS patients, and cause dysphagia.

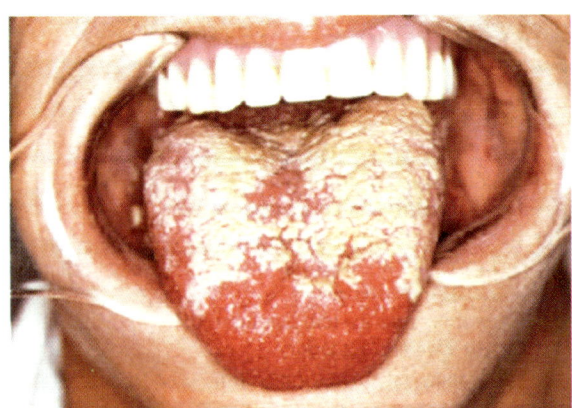

**Fig. 15.1.** Oral candidiasis (oral thrush).

# Candidiasis

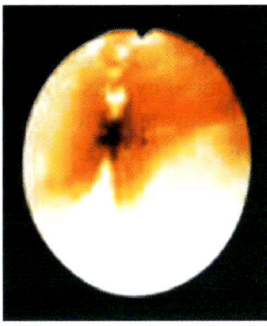

**Fig. 15.2.** Esophageal candidiasis.

**Oropharyngeal and esophageal candidiasis is the commonest opportunistic fungal disease in HIV-infected patients worldwide.** The occurrence of oropharyngeal or esophageal candidiasis is recognized as an indicator of immune suppression and is most often observed in patients with CD4+ cell counts < 200/μl. Antiretroviral treatment has led to a dramatic decline in the prevalence of mucosal candidiasis.

**Acute atrophic candidiasis** is characterized by painful erythematous mucosa, particularly on the tongue, which can be associated with loss of the tongue papillae, affecting food intake. It may follow the acute pseudomembranous form with the disappearance of the pseudomembranous lesions.

## Chronic atrophic and hyperplastic candidiasis or denture stomatitis

Denture stomatitis has been well recognised as a complication of wearing dentures. It is a chronic inflammatory condition caused by the trauma of ill-fitting dentures or possibly by an allergic response to denture material with a superimposed *Candida* infection.

## Angular cheilitis

*Candida* may cause red fissured lesions that crack and crust at the folds of the corners of the mouth. It may accompany other clinical forms of oral candidiasis, such as denture stomatitis or oral thrush.

## Vaginal candidiasis

Candidal vulvovaginitis is a common genital complaint in women. This affects primarily young and middle-aged females, particularly during their active reproductive life. Around 75% experience at least one episode of this condition during their lifetime. Severe forms of vaginal candidiasis may be associated with use of oral contraceptives, corticosteroids or antibiotics, diabetes and pregnancy. Besides *C. albicans*, *C. glabrata* and *C. tropicalis* are the most frequently isolated *Candida* spp. both from vulvovaginitis patients and from healthy carriers.

Patient complains of vulvovaginal pruritus, discharge which can be thick and curd-like or thin, and dyspareunia. The lesions on the mucosal surface are basically adherent plaques. Sexual transmission to a male partner is known. In the male, infection presents as a balanitis with erythema on the penis.

## DEEP INFECTIONS

*Candida* spp. may cause deep infections of several parenchymatous organs. These infections are characterized by microabscesses. Microscopically, these reveal blastoconidia, pseudohyphae, true hyphae (in case of *C. albicans*), neutrophils and mononuclear cells, and a necrotic centre. In chronic infections granulomata with giant cells and lymphocytes may be formed.

### Candidiasis of gastrointestinal tract

The syndromes discussed under this head are:

- esophagitis
- gastrointestinal candidiasis

### Esophagitis

Patient complains of painful dysphagia with nausea and/or vomiting. Endoscopy of esophageal mucosa shows white patches which resemble those of oral candidiasis (Fig. 15.2). Esophagitis may be associated with presence of oral candidiasis. However, it may also present as a separate clinical entity without oral involvement. **Esophageal candidiasis remains one of the most common AIDS-defining illnesses.**

### Gastrointestinal candidiasis

Candidiasis can involve any site of gut. These lesions may progress to haematogenous infection, obstruction or even perforation. The pathology of candidal infection of the lower gut ranges from mucosal ulceration with or without pseudomembrane to exophytic lesions. Pseudomembranes are composed of a mixture of yeasts and pseudohyphae embedded in necrotic debris and fibrin. Pseudohyphae may extend beyond the muscular layer and reach the serosa.

### Candidiasis of the liver, spleen and other organs

*C. albicans* and other species may cause candidiasis of liver, spleen, gall bladder, pancreas and peritoneum. Hepatosplenic candidiasis is seen primarily in leukemics. Fungal elements can be seen in the biopsied tissues from liver and spleen.

### Candidiasis of respiratory system

*C. albicans* may cause pneumonia. It is commonly seen in patients with haematogenous candidiasis. *Candida* empyema occurs among patients with severe underlying diseases, particularly cancer. Diagnosis requires the isolation of *Candida* spp. from an exudative pleural effusion. *C. albicans* may also cause laryngitis, epiglottitis and mediastinitis.

### Candidiasis of cardiovascular system

*Candida* spp. can cause clinical manifestations in pericardium, myocardium or endocardium with endocarditis being the best known clinical entity. It can be caused by *C. albicans* and other species, such as *C. parapsilosis* and *C. tropicalis*. *Candida* endocarditis resembles bacterial endocarditis. It may, however, have a more prolonged onset; e.g., in post-surgery patients it may become apparent months later. Patient presents with fever, heart murmur, splenomegaly, congestive heart failure and anaemia. *Candida* endocarditis is characterized by large vegetations from which emboli may be released.

### Renal and urinary tract candidiasis

This syndrome is discussed under following heads:
- lower urinary tract infection
- renal infection

### Lower urinary tract infection

Candidal infection of lower urinary tract (cystitis) is frequently seen in association with indwelling catheters. They may originate from gastrointestinal tract or genital flora. It occurs more often in females and diabetics. Symptoms are similar to those observed with bacterial cystitis. Cystoscopy reveals soft, pearly white, elevated patches with hyperemic and friable mucosa underneath.

### Renal infection

Renal candidiasis is secondary to haematogenous candidiasis. It is characterized by microabscess formation, mostly evident in the cortex of the kidneys.

### Central nervous system candidiasis

Central nervous system infections by *Candida* spp. are rare, and present as meningitis or abscesses. Most susceptible individuals are AIDS patients and premature infants. *Candida* meningitis may present acutely but more typically has a subacute course with evolution over 2–4 weeks. Patients have fever, headache, diminished consciousness, lethargy and confusion. Meningeal signs may be present. Invasion of arteries at the base of the brain can occur and result in vasculitis with thrombosis. Microabscesses present like cerebral mass lesions with seizures and neurological focal signs including hemiparesis, aphasia, and visual field defects. They occur most commonly at the parieto-occipital level. Patients develop a progressive increase in intracranial pressure.

### Ocular Candida infection

*Candida* spp. can affect both the outer and inner eye. Infection may originate from haematogenous dissemination or from direct fungal introduction, the former, generally results in inner eye infection, and the latter in clinical manifestations of the outer parts of the eye. Both categories of eye involvement are caused by *C. albicans* and some other *Candida* spp., such as *C. parapsilosis*, *C. krusei* and *C. glabrata*. Outer eye infections include conjunctivitis, keratitis, blepharitis and lacrimal canaliculitis. Such infections follow some ocular trauma, surgery or even the use of contact lenses.

### Bone and joint Candida infection

*Candida* osteomyelitis is rare and usually occurs via haematogenous seeding, but it may also result from inoculation during surgery or trauma or from contiguous infected ulcers in diabetic patients. Candidal osteomyelitis is most commonly due to *C. albicans* but it may also be caused by *C. parapsilosis*, *C. tropicalis* and *C. glabrata*. A wide variety of candidal species have been reported to cause joint infection, including *C. albicans*, *C. glabrata*, *C. guilliermondii*, *C. krusei*, *C. parapsilosis* and *C. tropicalis*.

## DISSEMINATED CANDIDIASIS AND CANDIDEMIA

Disseminated candidiasis may be defined as multi-organ infection with possible candidemia. *Candida* infection may involve central nervous system, liver, spleen, kidneys, heart, eyes or other organs and systems. It occurs mainly in cancer patients, particularly those with acute leukemia, in patients post-surgery, particularly gastrointestinal and cardiac surgery, transplant patients, particularly bone marrow transplants and burn patients.

### Laboratory diagnosis

*Specimens*

Scrapings from mucosal, dermal or nail lesions, sputum, bronchial aspirate, pus, swabs, etc.

*Direct examination*

Place the specimen in a drop of 10% KOH, warm gently over a small flame and examine under microscope. All species of *Candida* form round to oval budding yeast cells, 3–6 μm in diameter.

They occur singly, in chains, or in small loose clusters. Most species, when invading tissue, form both pseudohyphae and true hyphae. Pseudohyphae are actually chains of blastoconidia that have elongated and have not separated from one another. They can be recognized by distinct constrictions at the septa; also, pseudohyphal branching will only occur at the site of a septation. True hyphae have no, or only slight constrictions at the septa, and there is often no septation at the initiation of a branch. Blastoconidia develop along the sides of both types of hyphae (Figs. 15.3 and 15.4). *C. glabrata* is unique in that it is slightly smaller (2–5 μm in diameter) than the other species of *Candida*, and it does not

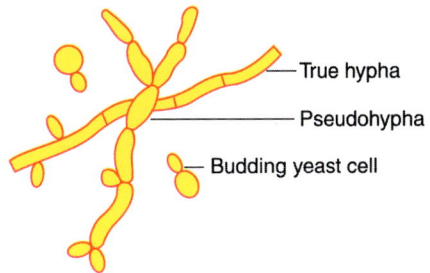

**Fig. 15.3.** Budding yeast cells, pseudohyphae and true hyphae of *Candida albicans*.

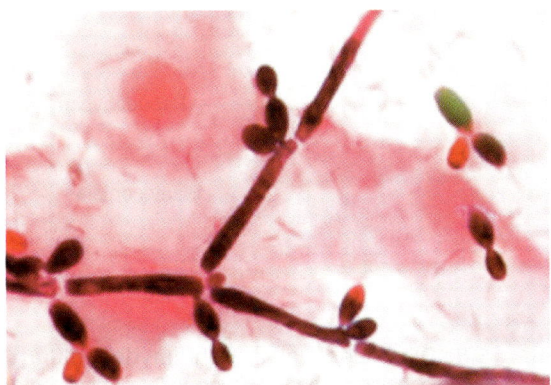

**Fig. 15.4.** Vaginal smear showing budding yeast cells, true hyphae and epithelial cells (PAS stain, ×400).

produce hyphal forms. For species identification culture is required.

*Histopathology*

In systemic infections, *Candida* spp. most commonly elicit an acute suppurative inflammation composed of polymorphonuclear as well as mononuclear cells. Granulomas only rarely occur. *Candida* spp. are also known to invade blood vessels and produce infarcts.

*Culture*

**Candida albicans:** For isolation in culture spread pathological material on slants of SDA with chloramphenicol and incubate at 30°C. It grows rapidly. Growth matures in 3 days. Colonies are cream-coloured, pasty and smooth. On enriched media (e.g., blood agar or chocolate agar), extensions commonly called "feet" develop at the border of the colony. Lactophenol cotton blue preparation and Gram-stained smears show round to oval budding yeast cells (3.5–7 × 4–8 µm) and pseudohyphae. Rarely true hyphae may also be seen. On cornmeal-Tween 80 agar at 25°C for 72 hours, pseudohyphae (and some true hyphae) form with clusters of round blastoconidia at the septa. Large thick-walled, usually single terminal chlamydoconidia are characteristically formed (Fig. 15.5). Chlamydoconidia formation is inhibited at 30–37°C.

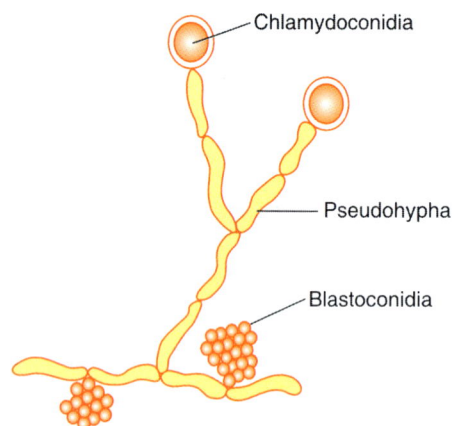

Fig. 15.5. Blastoconidia and chlamydoconidia of *Candida albicans* on cornmeal-Tween 80 agar incubated at 25°C for 72 hours.

After incubation in sheep, horse or normal human serum for about 90 minutes at 37°C yeast cells of *C. albicans* begin to form germ tubes (Fig. 15.6). Germ tube test is also positive in *C. dubliniensis*. All other species are negative for this test. **Germ tubes are the beginning of true hyphae and appear as filaments that are not constricted at their points of origin on the parent cell. If the filaments are constricted at their points of origin, they are pseudohyphae, not germ tubes** (Fig. 15.6).

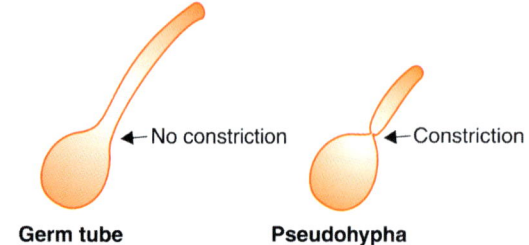

Fig. 15.6. Germ tube and pseudohypha of *Candida albicans*.

*Candida dubliniensis:* Cultural characteristics of *C. dubliniensis* are similar to those of *C. albicans*. However, in *C. dubliniensis* large, thick-walled terminal chlamydoconidia characteristically form in pairs or small clusters (as opposed to *C. albicans* which usually produces terminal chlamydoconidia singly).

Microscopic characteristics of *Candida* spp. other than *C. albicans* and *C. dubliniensis* on cornmeal-Tween 80 agar incubated at 25°C for 72 hours are given in Table 15.2.

Table 15.2. Microscopic characteristics of *Candida* spp. other than *C. albicans* and *C. dubliniensis* on cornmeal-Tween 80 agar incubated at 25°C for 72 hours

| Organism | Cultural characteristics on cornmeal-Tween 80 agar incubated at 25°C for 72 hours |
|---|---|
| *C. tropicalis* | Blastoconidia are borne singly or in very small groups along pseudohyphae. True hyphae may also be present. |
| *C. parapsilosis* | Blastoconidia singly or in small clusters, are seen along relatively short, curved pseudohyphae. Large hyphal elements, called giant cells, are occasionally seen. |
| *C. lusitaniae* | Microscopically, it resembles *C. parapsilosis* but it differs in its ability to ferment cellobiose and usually to assimilate rhamnose. |
| *C. guilliermondii* | Fairly short, fine pseudohyphae with clusters of blastoconidia at septa. True hyphae are not produced. |
| *C. glabrata* | Only small (2–3 × 3.5–4.5 µm) oval yeast cells with single terminal budding. No pseudohyphae are formed. |
| *C. krusei* | Pseudohyphae with elongated blastoconidia forming a cross-matchsticks or treelike blastoconidia. |

### Biochemical reactions

Species identification of *Candida* spp. can be carried out by fermentation and assimilation reactions (Table 15.3).

General characters of medically important yeasts and schematic outline of procedures for identification of yeast isolates are given in Table 15.4 and Flowchart 15.1.

## Table 15.3. Fermentation and assimilation reactions of *Candida* spp.

| | Fermentation of | | | | Assimilation of | | | | | | | | | | | | |
|---|---|---|---|---|---|---|---|---|---|---|---|---|---|---|---|---|---|
| | Glucose | Maltose | Sucrose | Lactose | Glucose | Maltose | Sucrose | Lactose | Galactose | Melibiose | Cellobiose | Inositol | Xylose | Raffinose | Trehalose | Dulcitol | KNO₃ |
| C. albicans / C. dubliniensis | + | + | – | – | + | + | v | – | + | – | – | – | + / – | – | + / – v | – | – |
| C. glabrata | + | – | – | – | + | – | – | – | – | – | – | – | – | – | + | – | – |
| C. guilliermondii | + | – | + w | – | + | + | + | – | + | + | + | – | + | – | + | + | – |
| C. kefyr | + | – | + | + | + | – | + | + | + | – | + | – | + v | + | – | – | – |
| C. lusitaniae | + | – | v | – | + | + | + | – | + | – | + | – | + | – | + | – | – |
| C. parapsilosis | + | – | – | – | + | + | + | – | + | – | – | – | + | – | + | – | – |
| C. tropicalis | + | + | + v | – | + | + | + v | – | + | – | + v | – | + | – | + | – | – |

+, positive; –, negative; v, species or strain variation; w, weak

## Table 15.4. General characters of medically important yeasts

| Genus | Blastoconidia or buds | Arthroconidia | Pseudohyphae | True hyphae | Chlamydoconidia | Germ tube |
|---|---|---|---|---|---|---|
| Cryptococcus | + | – | – | – | – | – |
| Torulopsis | + | – | – | – | – | – |
| Pityrosporum | + | – | – | – | – | – |
| Rhodotorula | + | – | – | – | – | – |
| Candida | + | – | + | + | + | + |
| Trichosporon | + | + | + | + | – | – |
| Geotrichum | – | + | – | + | – | – |

+, positive; –, negative

## Serological diagnosis

Serological diagnosis of candidiasis is based on detection of the humoral immune response as expressed in antibody production, and detection of fungal antigens. **Antibodies to *Candida*** detected by the agglutination technique, which generally represent antimannan antibodies can be found in healthy individuals or in those with superficial infections. Therefore, this test is not useful in the diagnosis of deep-seated candidiasis. On the other hand, tests determining the presence of antibodies against *Candida* internal antigens, which, it is assumed, are released into the patient's body fluids, primarily during invasive infection, could be more discriminatory and therefore more useful for diagnosis. *Candida* antibodies can be detected by immunodiffusion, counterimmunoelectrophoresis, latex agglutination and ELISA.

**Detection of *Candida* antigens** in body fluids is an important diagnostic tool, particularly in immunocompromised patients who have difficulties in mounting antibodies at a detectable level. Antigen is generally detected in serum and other body fluids such as urine by latex agglutination and ELISA.

**Flowchart 15.1.** Schematic outline of procedures used for identification of yeast isolates

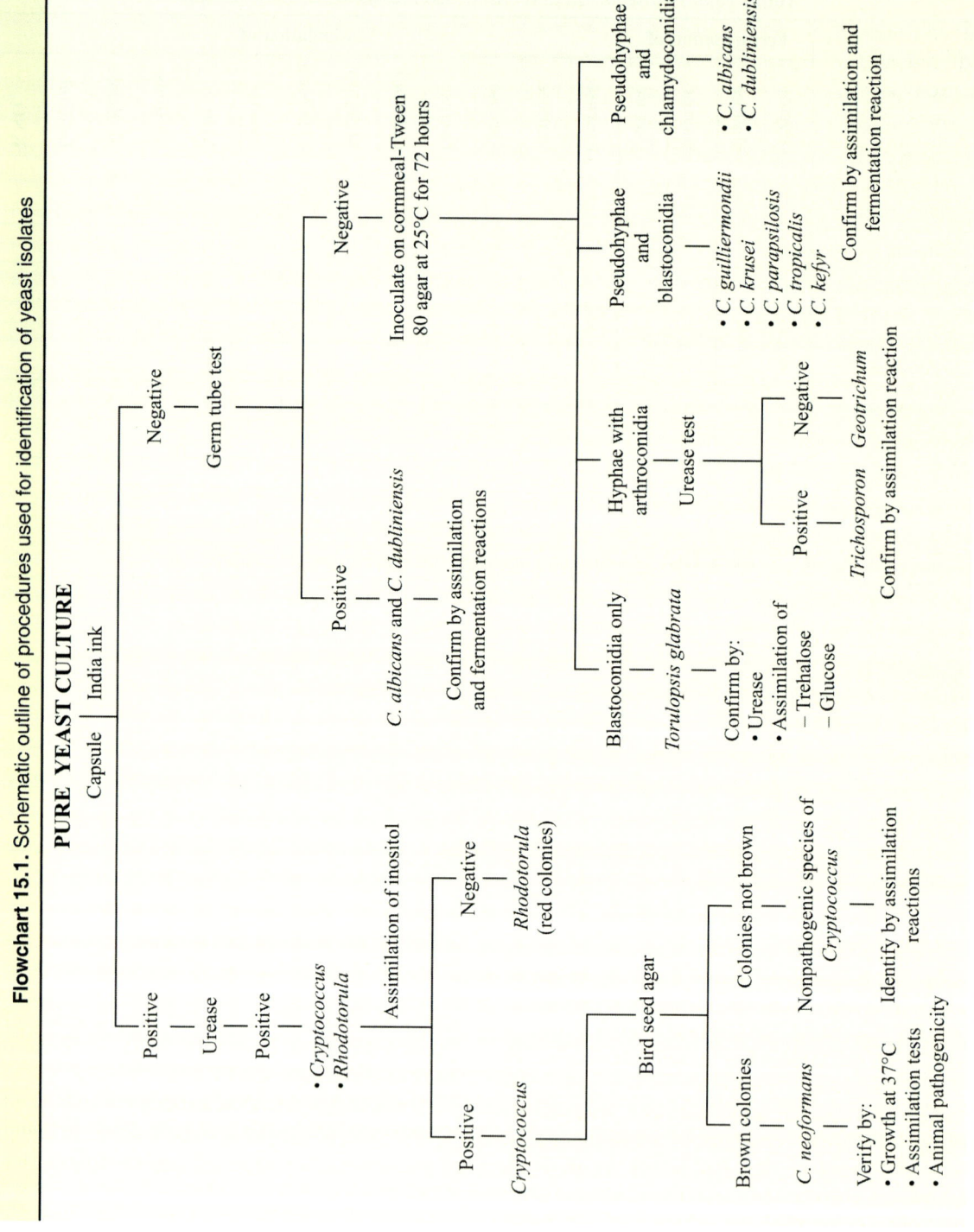

# Candidiasis

## Skin test

The skin test may be performed to evaluate **cell-mediated immunity** *in vivo* by a skin test to measure delayed type of hypersensitivity to candidal antigen. *In vitro* assays such as lymphocyte transformation may also be done to assess the immune competence of the patient.

## Detection of fungal metabolites

Candidal metabolite arabinitol is released into patient's body fluids by most of the pathogenic *Candida* spp. except *C. krusei* and *C. glabrata*. It can be detected by **gas-liquid chromatography**, and the more recent techniques involving enzymatic-fluorometric measurements.

## Treatment

The polyene antibiotics, amphotericin B, nystatin and natamycin are highly effective against *Candida* species and most other yeast pathogens. Of these drugs, only amphotericin B is used systemically, and this must be given by intravenous infusion. The other important group of agents effective against *Candida* are imidazoles. Clotrimazole, miconazole and econazole are the best known. The most useful treatments are with the two triazoles, fluconazole and itraconazole.

## Important Questions

1. Discuss pathogenesis and laboratory diagnosis of candidiasis.
2. Write short notes on:
   (a) Virulence factors of *Candida albicans*
   (b) Superficial infections caused by *Candida albicans*
   (c) Deep and disseminated infections caused by *Candida albicans*
   (d) Oral candidiasis
   (e) Fermentation and assimilation reactions of *Candida* spp.

## Multiple Choice Questions

1. In addition to *Candida albicans*, which of the following *Candida* species cause/s oral candidiasis?
   (a) *Candida glabrata*.
   (b) *Candida tropicalis*.
   (c) *Candida guilliermondii*.
   (d) All of the above.
2. Which of the following infections caused by *Candida albicans* is one of the most common AIDS-defining illness?
   (a) Esophagitis.
   (b) Vaginal candidiasis.
   (c) Angular cheilitis.
   (d) Onychomycosis.
3. Which of the following species of *Candida* **does not** produce hyphal forms?
   (a) *Candida glabrata*.
   (b) *Candida tropicalis*.
   (c) *Candida parapsilosis*.
   (d) *Candida guilliermondii*.
4. Which of the following *Candida* species **does not** form true hyphae?
   (a) *Candida albicans*.
   (b) *Candida dubliniensis*.
   (c) *Candida tropicalis*.
   (d) *Candida guilliermondii*.
5. Which of the following *Candida* species ferments lactose?
   (a) *Candida tropicalis*.
   (b) *Candida kefyr*.
   (c) *Candida glabrata*.
   (d) *Candida albicans*.
6. Which of the following *Candida* species assimilates raffinose?
   (a) *Candida tropicalis*.
   (b) *Candida kefyr*.
   (c) *Candida glabrata*.
   (d) *Candida albicans*.
7. Which of the following yeasts **does not** form blastoconidia?
   (a) *Geotrichum*.
   (b) *Rhodotorula*.
   (c) *Torulopsis*.
   (d) *Pityrosporum*.
8. Which of the following yeasts forms pseudohyphae?
   (a) *Geotrichum*.
   (b) *Trichosporon*.

(c) *Candida*.
(d) *Rhodotorula*.

9. Which of the following yeasts forms true hyphae?
   (a) *Torulopsis*.
   (b) *Pityrosporon*.
   (c) *Geotrichum*.
   (d) *Rhodotorula*.

10. Which of the following yeasts forms germ tubes?
    (a) *Cryptococcus*.
    (b) *Rhodotorula*.
    (c) *Geotrichum*.
    (d) *Candida*.

11. Which of the following yeasts forms chlamydoconidia?
    (a) *Cryptococcus*.
    (b) *Candida*.
    (c) *Geotrichum*.
    (d) *Trichosporon*.

12. Which of the following yeasts forms arthroconidia?
    (a) *Torulopsis*.
    (b) *Pityrosporon*.
    (c) *Rhodotorula*.
    (d) *Trichosporon*.

13. Which of the following yeasts is capsulated?
    (a) *Cryptococcus*.
    (b) *Candida*.
    (c) *Torulopsis*.
    (d) *Trichosporon*.

## ANSWERS TO MCQs

1. (d), 2. (a), 3. (a), 4. (d), 5. (b), 6. (b), 7. (a), 8. (c), 9. (c), 10. (d), 11. (b), 12. (d), 13. (a).

### Further Reading

1. Arora B, Kalra R, et al. Incidence of trichomoniasis, candidiasis and herpes simplex infection of female genital tract. *The Indian Practitioner* 1993; XLVI: 711–4.
2. Arora DR, Saini S, Aparna GN. Evaluation of germ tube test in various media. *Indian J Pathol Microbiol* 2003; 46: 124–6.
3. Benjamin DK Jr, Garges H, Steinbach WJ. *Candida* bloodstream infection in neonates. *Semin Perinatol* 2003; 27: 375–83.
4. Blot SI, Vandewonde KH, De Waele JJ. *Candida* peritonitis. *Curr Opin Crit Care* 2007; 13: 195–9.
5. Capoor MR, Nair D, et al. Emergence of non-*albicans Candida* species and antifungal resistance in a tertiary care hospital. *Jpn J Infect Dis* 2005; 58: 344–8.
6. Carvalho A, Costa-De-Oliveira S, et al. Multiplex PCR identification of eight clinically relevant *Candida* species. *Med Mycol* 2007; 45: 619–27.
7. Chakrabarti A, Das A. Emergence of non-*albicans Candida* species. *J Int Med Sci Acad* 2004; 17: 186–9.
8. Chakrabarti A, Rao P, et al. *Candida* in acute pancreatitis. *Surg Today* 2007; 37: 207–11.
9. Chapman RL, Faix RG. Invasive neonatal candidiasis: an overview. *Semin Perinatol* 2003; 27: 352–6.
10. Chi HW, Yang YS, et al. *Candida albicans* versus non-*albicans* bloodstream infections: the comparison of risk factors and outcome. *J Microbiol Immunol Infect* 2011; 44: 369–75.
11. Dimopoulos G, Karabinis A, et al. Candidemia in immunocompromised and immunocompetent critically ill patients: a prospective comparative study. *Eur J Clin Microbiol Infect Dis* 2007; 26: 377–84.
12. Ellepola AN, Morrison CJ. Laboratory diagnosis of invasive candidiasis. *J Microbiol* 2005; 43: 65–84.
13. Eschenbach DA. Chronic vulvovaginal candidiasis. *N Engl J Med* 2004; 351: 851–2.
14. Guo F, Yang YS, et al. Invasive candidiasis in intensive care units in China: a multicentre prospective observational study. *J Antimicrob Chemother* 2013; 68: 1660–8.
15. Henriques M, Azeredo J, Oliveira R. *Candida albicans* and *Candida dubliniensis*: comparison of biofilm formation in terms of biomass and activity. *Br J Biomed Sci* 2006; 63: 5–11.
16. Kauffman CA. Candidura. *Clin Infect Dis* 2005; 41 (Suppl. 6) S371–6.
17. Kojic EM, Darouiche RO. *Candida* infections of medical devices. *Clin Microbiol Rev* 2004; 17: 255–67.
18. Kuebrich CT. Chronic vulvovaginal candidiasis. *N Engl J Med* 2004; 351: 2554–6.

19. Pappas PG. Invasive candidiasis. *Infect Dis Clin N Am* 2006; 20: 485–506.
20. Rowen JL. Mucocutaneous candidiasis. *Semin Perinatol* 2003; 27: 406–13.
21. Sims CR, Ostrosky Zeichner L, Rex JH. Invasive candidiasis in immunocompromised hospitalized patients. *Arch Med Res* 2005; 36: 660–71.
22. Sobel JD. Pathogenesis of recurrent vulvovaginal candidiasis. *Curr Infect Dis Rep* 2002; 4: 514–9.
23. Sobel JD. The emergence of non-*albicans Candida* species as causes of invasive candidiasis and candidemia. *Curr Infect Dis Rep* 2006; 8: 427–33.
24. Spence D. Candidiasis (vulvovaginal). *Clin Evid* 2005; 14: 2200–15.
25. Steinbach WJ, Roilides E, et al. Results from a prospective international, epidemiologic study of invasive candidiasis in children and neonates. *Pediatr Infect Dis* 2012; 31: 1252–7.
26. Vazquez JA, Sobel JD. Mucosal candidiasis. *Infect Dis Clin N Am* 2002; 16: 793–820.
27. Wu JQ, Zhu LP, et al. Epidemiological risk factors for non-*Candida albicans* candidemia in non-neutropenic patients at a Chinese teaching hospital. *Med Mycol* 2011; 49: 552–5.

# CHAPTER 16

# Cryptococcosis

Cryptococcosis is an acute, subacute or chronic fungal infection caused by encapsulated **basidiomycetous yeast**, *Cryptococcus neoformans*. It is most frequently recognized as a disease of the central nervous system, although the primary site of infection is the lungs. The disease occurs sporadically throughout the world.

*C. neoformans* has become a major human pathogen and a common infection in immunocompromised hosts. It has emerged as an important cause of illness and death in human immunodeficiency virus-infected people.

Prior to acquired immunodeficiency syndrome (AIDS) era, cryptococcosis was a rare disease, but with the onset of AIDS pandemic, the incidence has increased considerably. Presently, with the availability of an effective highly active antiretroviral therapy (HAART), the incidence of this disease in the developed world has decreased considerably. However, due to non-availability or unaffordability of the HAART in developing countries (especially certain African and Asian countries), this disease still continues to be a major problem in HIV-infected population. Recent studies from Southeast Asia reported that *Cryptococcus* was 2nd or 3rd most common species isolated from blood of HIV-positive individuals.

The first case of cryptococcosis was reported in 1894 by Busse who named the fungus *Saccharomyces hominis*. In the same year, but separately, Sanfelice cultured the yeast from peach juice. He demonstrated its pathogenicity in experimental animals and named the fungus *Saccharomyces neoformans*. A few more reports of isolation of this fungus from humans and animals appeared, and then in 1901 Vuillemin renamed the yeast *Cryptococcus hominis* to distinguish it from *Saccharomyces* spp. because it did not form ascospores. *C. neoformans* is now considered the most valid name based on priority since Sanfelice first proposed the species name in 1894. In 1976, Kwon-Chung discovered and characterized the sexual stage of this basidiomycete and the teleomorph was named *Filobasidiella neoformans*.

## MYCOLOGY

At least 19 species of genus *Cryptococcus* have been described, but few are recognized as causing infection in humans. The predominant pathogen is *C. neoformans*, but two other species, *C. albidus* and *C. laurentii* have been reported to rarely cause disease in humans. *C. neoformans* is a round or oval encapsulated yeast, measuring 4–10 µm in diameter in clinical specimens, and having a capsule ranging in size from 1 to > 30 μm. In specimens isolated from nature, organisms tend to be smaller and poorly encapsulated.

On the basis of antigenic differences in the capsular polysaccharide, five serotypes (A, B, C, D and an hybrid AD) have been identified which have been grouped in three varieties – var. *neoformans* (serotypes D and AD), var. *grubii* (serotype A) and var. *gattii* (serotypes B and C). *C. neoformans* var. *neoformans* and var. *grubii* are responsible for the majority of clinical infections in immunocompromised hosts while var. *gattii* causes disease primarily in immunocompetent hosts. Since there are considerable genetic differences among the varieties, it has been suggested that they should be considered separate species.

*C. neoformans* is ubiquitous in the soil. Soil contaminated with pigeon, chicken, or turkey droppings, in which the pH is alkaline and the nitrogen concentration is increased, promotes organism replication and it apparently provides a reservoir of the organisms. *C. neoformans* does not appear to infect the birds, probably because of their high body temperature, but survives passage through their gut. In moist or desiccated pigeon excreta, they survive for more than two years. Their survival is enhanced by increased humidity.

## VIRULENCE FACTORS

*C. neoformans* has several means by which it escapes the host's defences, to survive and multiply inside the host. Factors that contribute to the virulence of the fungus are (i) its ability to grow at 37°C, (2) to produce a thick polysaccharide capsule and release soluble products into the blood stream, and (3) to synthesize melanin. Other virulence factors include urease, phospholipase, proteases and mannitol production.

### 1. Ability to grow at 37°C

For survival in the human host the ability to grow at 37°C is essential. Mutants of *C. neoformans* that cannot grow well at 37°C are avirulent even when they possess capsules. Except for *C. neoformans*, and occasionally *C. laurentii* and *C. albidus* isolates, other species cannot grow at 37°C and are considered to be nonpathogenic for humans. The varieties *gattii* and *neoformans* appear to be more sensitive to high temperatures than var. *grubii*, and at 40°C most strains of var. *gattii* and *neoformans* lose viability within 24 hours.

### 2. Capsule

The capsule is an important virulence determinant of *C. neoformans*. Infections caused by capsule-free or poorly encapsulated strains are associated with less severe disease. The capsule, as well as the soluble polysaccharide released from the yeast cells during infection, plays a significant role in pathogenicity as it protects the yeast cell from phagocytosis and from cytokines induced by the phagocytic process, and suppresses both cellular and humoral immunity. The capsular material can be released from the yeast and extrudes into various tissues such as blood and CSF. **It is this antigen that is detected by the cryptococcal antigen test which is so effective for diagnosis.**

### 3. Melanin production

*C. neoformans* possesses a unique enzyme, phenoloxidase, which has been identified as a lactase. This enzyme participates in the conversion of diphenolic compounds into melanin. The production of this pigment by a simple biochemical pathway is both a means for identifying *C. neoformans* in the laboratory and also a major virulence factor. This enzyme is bound to the cell membrane and catalyses the reaction in the presence of phenolic compounds, including catecholamines. This ability was first observed in agar containing a *Guizotia abyssinica* seed extract and subsequently in medium containing caffeic acid extracted from the seeds, and iron compounds.

**Melanin is deposited in cell walls**, conferring a brown colour to the yeast cells. It promotes cell integrity and increases its negative charge, protecting them from phagocytosis. Melanin prevents *in vitro* T cell response and cytokine secretion, and reduces antibody-mediated phagocytosis. Other functions include protection from oxidants and host oxidative killing, from temperature extremes, UV light, amphotericin B and microbicidal peptides. Melanin is essential for extrapulmonary dissemination as it allows survival of yeast inside the alveolar macrophages and their transport into the lymph nodes and subsequently into the bloodstream.

## PATHOGENESIS

Cryptococcosis is usually acquired by inhalation of aerosolized yeast cells. Animal-to-human and human-to-human transmission of the disease has not been reported. In nature, yeast cells are minimally encapsulated, small dry and easily aerosolized and reach the alveolar spaces. The size of the poorly encapsulated yeast cells in the environment is less than 3 μm in diameter. It is compatible with alveolar deposition. In the alveoli they gradually rehydrate and acquire their characteristic polysaccharide capsule. Development of disease largely depends on the competence of the host's cellular defences, and the number and virulence of the inhaled yeast cells.

Most patients with cryptococcosis have evidence of some underlying immunocompromising condition. The most common of these underlying conditions worldwide is AIDS, followed by prolonged treatment with corticosteroids, organ transplantation, malignancies and sarcoidosis. The commonest form of the cryptococcosis is a mild, self-limiting pulmonary infection. Dissemination of infection may lead to the involvement of CNS, skin, mucosa, bone and other organs.

## IMMUNE RESPONSE

Once the yeasts arrive in the alveoli, the earliest immune response elicited is composed of alveolar macrophages. Macrophages can ingest the yeast but have limited efficacy in eliminating the fungus. However, they are effective in producing proinflammatory monokines (interferon-α, interleukin-6) for the recruitment of neutrophils, monocytes, NK cells and T cells from the bloodstream into the lungs. The recruited cells are effective in killing the yeasts by intracellular and extracellular mechanisms. Intracellular killing occurs through lysosomal fusion, phagosomal acidification, sequestration of iron and enzymatic degradation of fungal proteins. Extracellular killing is mediated by antifungal peptides and nitric oxide.

## CLINICAL MANIFESTATIONS

### Pulmonary cryptococcosis

In the immunocompetent host, inhalation of the fungus leads to a variety of clinical features. Patient may develop asymptomatic or mildly symptomatic pulmonary disease. It may resolve spontaneously or result in an encapsulated lung nodule. Patients who develop progressive pulmonary cryptococcosis usually present with chronic cough, low grade fever, chest pain, scant mucoid or blood-tinged sputum, malaise, and weight loss.

Immunocompromised patients with cryptococcal pneumonia may have a more rapid symptomatic clinical course than that seen in immunocompetent hosts and dissemination frequently occurs.

### Central nervous system cryptococcosis

*Cryptococcus neoformans* varieties *neoformans* and *gattii* are strongly neurotropic and tend to disseminate from a primary pulmonary focus to the CNS, primarily invading the leptomeninges. The infection may also extend to the brain's parenchyma to form massive lesions or mucoid cysts. Cryptococcal meningoencephalitis is the most frequently encountered manifestation of cryptococcosis. The term 'meningoencephalitis' is more appropriate than meningitis since the underlying brain parenchyma is often involved. Signs and symptoms include headache, fever, meningismus, visual disturbances, abnormal mental status and seizures.

### Ocular cryptococcosis

In patients with disseminated cryptococcosis ocular involvement with *C. neoformans* is not a rare event. Patient develops keratitis, papilledema, scotoma, chorioretinitis and ocular palsy, which often lead to irreversible visual loss.

### Osseous cryptococcosis

Cryptococcosis of bone causes osteomyelitis. It is an uncommon but severe infection. The vertebrae and bony prominences are the most involved sites. The infection may be acquired by haematogenous spread from a self-limited pulmonary or lymph node localization, or may originate from contiguous skin lesion.

### Cutaneous cryptococcosis

Cutaneous cryptococcosis usually results from the haematogenous dissemination of the infection. However, primary cutaneous lesions following a direct inoculation of the fungus into the skin have been reported. The cutaneous lesions may be papules, acneform pustules or subcutaneous abscesses which ulcerate. The ulcers may be solitary or multiple and may resemble carcinoma, rodent ulcer or gumma.

### Oral cryptococcosis

Oral involvement has been reported as the presenting feature of the infection in a number of patients, especially associated with HIV infection. Lesions may be found on the tongue, gingiva, hard and soft palate, pharynx, buccal mucosa, and tonsils. They are typically seen as ulcers or nodules of granulation tissue. Lesions on the buccal mucosa may have a thrush-like appearance. Ulcerating lesions may be found on the lateral border of the tongue with rolled, elevated borders with minimal inflammation present and marked induration beyond the border of the ulcer.

### Other foci of infection

In disseminated cryptococcosis, any organ or tissue may have foci of infection. Infection of prostate gland does not cause symptoms of prostatitis, but these yeasts have been isolated from prostate tissue and blood after urological procedures. Seminal fluid and urine collected after prostatic massage have been found to contain cryptococci. *C. neoformans* may cause penile ulcer and a vulval lesion. Occasionally, lymph nodes may be the only apparent site of the infection. The cervical or supraclavicular lymph nodes are the most involved.

## LABORATORY DIAGNOSIS

***C. neoformans* is a true yeast. Both in tissues, and in culture at room temperature as well as at 37°C, only budding yeasts are seen.** Diagnosis is established by demonstration of budding yeast cells in CSF, sputum, pus, brain tissue, etc. by direct microscopy and culture, and by serological tests for capsular antigen.

### Direct microscopy

The clinical specimens are collected as per the site involved particularly CSF, sputum, pus, brain tissue, etc. Place **a drop of India ink** on a clean glass slide, add and mix with it a drop of CSF or other body fluid and, under reduced light, look for the spherical cells of *C. neoformans* and their enveloping capsule (Fig. 16.1).

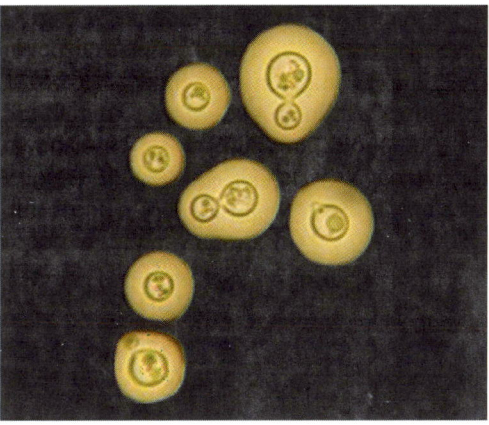

**Fig. 16.1.** An India ink wet mount (×400) of *Cryptococcus neoformans* showing encapsulated budding yeast cells.

The ink's carbon particles do not penetrate the capsule which appears as a clear halo surrounding the yeast cells. If fungus is not found upon immediate examination, centrifuge CSF at 3000 rpm for 10 minutes and carefully withdraw the sediment with a pipette for microscopic examination and culture. India ink examination of CSF is the most rapid test for diagnosing cryptococcal meningitis. Cryptococci may be distinguished from lymphocytes and artifacts by the presence of clear refractive cell walls and characteristic buds. In addition, the halo that may be present around the lymphocytes progressively reduces and disappears in 5–10 minutes. Sputum, pus and brain tissue should be examined after digestion in potassium hydroxide.

Sputum or pus should be mixed with **10% potassium hydroxide** before examination. In a properly prepared specimen, pus cells and partially digested cellular debris delineate the capsule which is resistant to potassium hydroxide.

*C. neoformans* may not be recognized in dried smear preparation of biologic samples because the fungal cells collapse, become crescent-shaped and stain irregularly. Gram staining is variable, varying from intensely purple to shades of pink.

### Histopathology

The histopathological examination of biopsy specimen can be done by **staining with Mayer's mucicarmine, periodic acid-Schiff, Gomori** methenamine silver and haematoxylin and eosin staining.

In immunocompetent patients, *C. neoformans* evokes a mixed suppurative and granulomatous reaction or purely a granulomatous reaction with various degrees of necrosis. Chronic pulmonary infection results in formation of residual granuloma (**cryptococcoma**). Healing is by fibrosis, generally without calcification. In immunocompromised patients, the reaction may be minimal or absent. In this case, the yeasts proliferate abundantly creating mucoid "cystic" lesions packed with round encapsulated cryptococci. These are seen most frequently in the brain.

The yeast cells are round or oval with thin walls, 4–10 μm in diameter, vary in size within the microscopic field, bud on a narrow base and characteristically produce thick capsules, but cells relatively deficient in capsular material sometimes occur. Capsules should be suspected when the yeast cells do not appear to touch one another because of the surrounding mucopolysaccharide capsular material. Tissue stained with Mayer's mucicarmine show the capsule as bright carmine red, often with a spiny or scalloped appearance (Fig. 16.2). Drying, fixing, and staining may cause the yeast cells to collapse or become crescent-shaped. The mucicarmine stain may also colour the cell walls of *Rhinosporidium seeberi*

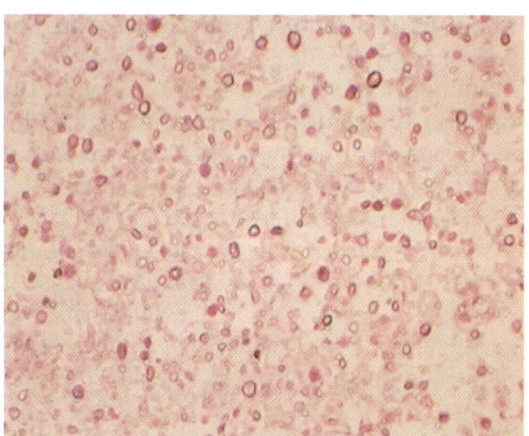

**Fig. 16.2.** Cryptococci stained with Mayer's mucicarmine stain (×400). The capsule is stained bright carmine red in colour.

and *Blastomyces dermatitidis*. With GMS stain the cryptococcal yeast cell but not the capsule is stained.

## Culture

Cryptococci can be cultured from biologic samples on Sabouraud dextrose agar. Chloramphenicol (0.05 mg/ml) can be incorporated in the medium to inhibit growth of bacterial contaminants, but do not use cycloheximide because this inhibits *C. neoformans*. As only a few yeast cells may be present at the site of infection, pellets from centrifuged CSF and other biologic fluids should be cultured.

Colonies are flat or slightly heaped, shiny, moist, and usually mucoid with smooth edges. Colour is cream at first later becoming tannish. *C. neoformans* grows equally well at 25°C and 37°C, and incubation at 37°C inhibits other species of the genus.

*C. neoformans* possesses the enzyme phenol oxidase, and testing for its presence is another means of accurate identification. This can be done by culturing the suspected yeasts on special agars such as niger seed agar, bird seed agar and caffeic acid agar and looking for the black colonies. *C. neoformans* breaks down caffeic acid to melanin. *Candida*, *Rhodotorula*, *Geotrichum*, and *Trichosporon* species do not break down caffeic acid to melanin

Bronchial secretions and urine, especially from AIDS patients, are often contaminated by *Candida* spp. which masks or inhibits the growth of cryptococcal cells. A selective medium, inositol agar with chloramphenicol, has been developed to inhibit *Candida* growth and enhance isolation of *Cryptococcus* spp. On this medium pallets from centrifuged bronchial secretions and urine can be inoculated. Inositol, as the unique carbon source, is assimilated by *Cryptococcus* spp. but not by *Candida* spp. that may be present in biologic fluids. After 3–5 days of incubation, *Cryptococcus* colonies can be recognized among the pinpoint *Candida* colonies.

*Cryptococcus* yeast cells usually grow on conventional isolation media with small or no capsule. They can be easily identified as *Cryptococcus* spp. as they do not produce hyphae or pseudohyphae, are not fermentative, assimilate inositol and hydrolyze urea. Schematic outline of procedures used for identification of yeast isolates is given in Flowchart 15.1.

## Biochemical reactions

*C. neoformans* can assimilate dextrose, maltose, sucrose, galactose, inositol, xylose, trehalose and dulcitol. It does not assimilate lactose, melibiose and $KNO_3$. Assimilation of cellobiose and raffinose is variable. All species of *Cryptococcus* lack fermentative ability.

## Serodiagnosis

Detection of polysaccharide antigen of *C. neoformans* in body fluids is highly effective for a rapid and accurate diagnosis. The titre is highest in serum, intermediate in CSF and lowest in urine. Bronchoalveolar lavage fluid may also be tested for cryptococcal antigen. The most frequently used test is the slide agglutination using latex particles coated with polyclonal or monoclonal antibodies. A positive serum antigen test at a dilution of 1 : 4 is strongly suggestive of cryptococcal infection. A titre of $\geq 1 : 8$ is indicative of active disease. Higher antigen titres indicate more severe infection and a falling titre is a good prognostic sign.

## Treatment

Amphotericin B with or without flucytosine for 7–14 days, followed by long-term oral maintenance with fluconazole 200–400 mg/day. Itraconazole is an alternative for long-term therapy.

### Important Questions

1. Discuss mycology, pathogenesis and laboratory diagnosis of cryptococcosis.
2. Write short notes on:
   (a) Virulence factors of *Cryptococcus neoformans*
   (b) Clinical manifestations of cryptococcosis.

### Multiple Choice Questions

1. *Cryptococcus neoformans* belongs to which of the following phyla?
   (a) Ascomycota.
   (b) Basidiomycota.
   (c) Glomeromycota.
   (d) None of the above.
2. *Filobasidiella* is the generic name of teleomorph of which of the following fungi?
   (a) *Cryptococcus neoformans.*
   (b) *Blastomyces dermatitidis.*
   (c) *Histoplasma capsulatum.*
   (d) *Trichophyton rubrum.*
3. Which of the following is **not** a virulence factor of *Cryptococcus neoformans*?
   (a) Ability to form pseudohyphae.
   (b) Ability to grow at 37°C.
   (c) Ability to form capsule.
   (d) Melanin production.
4. Which of the following fungi is strongly neutrotropic?
   (a) *Candida albicans.*
   (b) *Cryptococcus neoformans.*
   (c) *Histoplasma capsulatum.*
   (d) *Blastomyces dermatitidis.*
5. Which of the following fungi forms black colonies on niger seed agar?
   (a) *Geotrichum.*
   (b) *Trichosporon.*
   (c) *Candida albicans.*
   (d) *Cryptococcus neoformans.*
6. Which of the following fungi assimilates inositol?
   (a) *Cryptococcus neoformans.*
   (b) *Rhodotorula.*
   (c) *Candida albicans.*
   (d) *Candida guilliermondii.*
7. In which of the following fungal infections, detection of antigen in serum or cerebrospinal fluid is frequently used for the diagnosis of causative agent?
   (a) Cryptococcosis.
   (b) Candidiasis.
   (c) Coccidioidomycosis.
   (d) Blastomycosis.
8. Urease test is positive in:
   (a) *Trichophyton mentagrophytes.*
   (b) *Trichosporon* spp.
   (c) *Cryptococcus neoformans.*
   (d) All of the above.

9. Headache in an AIDS patient suggests the possibility of:
   (a) cryptococcosis.
   (b) toxoplasmosis.
   (c) intracranial lymphoma.
   (d) All of the above.
10. Which of the following fungi is found in pigeon droppings?
    (a) *Candida albicans*.
    (b) *Cryptococcus neoformans*.
    (c) *Coccidioides immitis*.
    (d) *Blastomyces dermatitidis*.
11. Which of the following tests would be relevant for mycological examination of CSF?
    (a) India ink preparation of centrifuged pallet.
    (b) *Cryptococcus* latex agglutination test for antigen on supernatant after centrifugation.
    (c) Culture of centrifuged pallet on Sabouraud dextrose agar.
    (d) All of the above.
12. A CSF specimen arrives in mycology laboratory. How would you proceed to detect, recover, and identify a fungus in the specimen?
    (a) Centrifuge and plant the specimen on Sabouraud dextrose agar.
    (b) Plant a drop of sediment on Bird seed agar.
    (c) Centrifuge and place a drop of sediment in an India ink preparation.
    (d) All of the above.

## ANSWERS TO MCQs

1. (b), 2. (a), 3. (a), 4. (b), 5. (d), 6. (a), 7. (a), 8. (d), 9. (d), 10. (b), 11. (d), 12. (d).

### Further Reading

1. Bicanic T, Harrison TS. Cryptococcal meningitis. *Br Med Bull* 2005; 72: 99–118.
2. Bisson GP, Molefi M, et al. Early versus delayed antiretroviral therapy and cerebrospinal fluid fungal clearance in adults with HIV and cryptococcal meningitis. *Clin Infect Dis* 2013; 56: 1165–73.
3. Chayakulkeeree M, Perfect JR. Cryptococcosis. *Infect Dis Clin N Am* 2006; 20: 507–44.
4. Chuang YM, Ho YC, et al. Disseminated cryptococcosis in HIV-uninfected patients. *Eur J Clin Microbiol Infect Dis* 2008; 27: 307–10.
5. Day JN, Chau TT, et al. Combination antifungal therapy for cryptococcal meningitis. *N Engl J Med* 2013; 368: 1291–302.
6. Dimino-Emme L, Gurevitch AW. Cutaneous manifestations of disseminated cryptococcosis. *J Am Acad Dermatol* 1995; 32: 844–50.
7. Enache-Angoulvant A, Chandenier J, et al. Molecular identification of *Cryptococcus neoformans* serotypes. *J Clin Microbiol* 2007; 45: 1261–5.
8. Feldman C. Cryptococcal pneumonia. *Clin Pulm Med* 2003; 10: 67–71.
9. Ito-Kuwa S, Nakamura K, et al. Serotype identification of *Cryptococcus neoformans* by multiplex PCR. *Mycoses* 2007; 50: 277–81.
10. Jarvis JN, Harrison TS. Pulmonary cryptococcosis. *Semin Respir Crit Care Med* 2008; 29: 141–50.
11. Leal AL, Faganello, et al. *Cryptococcus* species identification by multiplex PCR. *Med Mycol* 2008; 46: 377–83.
12. Lin X, Heitman J. The biology of the *Cryptococcus neoformans* species complex. *Annu Rev Microbiol* 2006; 60: 69–105.
13. Lortholary O, Nunez H, et al. Pulmonary cryptococcosis. *Semin Respir Crit Care Med* 2004; 25: 145–57.
14. Park BJ, Wannemuehler KA, et al. Estimation of the current global burden of cryptococcal meningitis among persons living with HIV/AIDS. *N Engl J Med* 2013; 368: 1291–302.
15. Perfect JR, Casadevall A. Cryptococcosis. *Infect Dis Clin N Am* 2002; 16: 837–74.

**CHAPTER 17**

# Pneumocystosis

*Pneumocystis* is an **ascomycetous fungus** that causes life-threatening pulmonary infection in debilitated and immunocompromised individuals. *Pneumocystis* pneumonia (PCP) is the most important opportunistic infection in HIV-infected patients. *Pneumocystis* is also a significant cause of morbidity and mortality in non-HIV associated immunosuppressed patients (transplantation, malignancy, connective tissue disease).

The organism was first described in Brazil by Carlos Chagas in 1909. It was originally thought to be a protozoan parasite and was given the name *P. carinii* in 1914.

Sequence analysis of the 16S-like ribosomal RNA gene as well as protein-encoding genes has revealed that the members of the *Pneumocystis* genus are fungi of the class Pneumocystidiomycetes rather than protozoons as was once thought. Like other fungi *Pneumocystis* has:

1. Cyst wall ultrastructure similar to that of fungal cell wall.
2. Lamellar cristae in the mitochondria (protozoans have tubular cristae).
3. Formation of intracystic bodies resembling the formation of ascospores by the ascomycetes.

The yeast-like fungi in the genus *Pneumocystis* are extracellular, host-obligate, host-specific, and typically restricted to the lung tissues of mammals, although extrapulmonary manifestations have been reported. Once known collectively by the single genus and species "*Pneumocystis carinii*" it is now clear that the organism first identified as "*Pneumocystis carinii*" is actually a collection of many species within the genus *Pneumocystis* that likely number in the hundreds to thousands. Almost every mammal examined to date appears to harbour at least one species of *Pneumocystis* that is not found in any other mammal. Five *Pneumocystis* species have been formally described according to the International Code of Botanical Nomenclature – *P. carinii* and *P. wakefieldiae* infect rats, *P. murina* infects mice, *P. oryctolagi* infects rabbits, and *P. jirovecii* infects human beings.

## MORPHOLOGY

The terminology used to describe the various life cycle stages of *Pneumocystis* bears remnants of its earlier classification as a protozoan parasite. Three developmental forms of *P. jirovecii* are generally recognized – trophozoite or trophic form, precyst or sporocyte and cyst or ascus.

### Trophozoite or trophic form

The trophozoite of *P. jirovecii* is the smallest of the life cycle stages of the organism. It ranges in size from 1–4 µm and is ellipsoidal in shape when unfixed preparations are viewed by light microscopy. After fixation it may appear amoeboid in shape. It is thought to reproduce by binary fission. Trophozoites are unicellular. They stain with Giemsa stain but not with stains designed to complex with the cell wall such as Gomori methenamine silver stain (GMS). Trophozoites are believed to be infectious propagules, spread by droplet aerosols.

### Precyst or sporocyte

The precyst is recognized as an intermediate stage of the sexual phase of reproduction leading to cyst development. It is presumed that a mating event first occurs to provide a zygote that initiates sporogenesis. Precyst is smaller than the mature cyst (5–8 µm in diameter) and is frequently oval in shape. In contrast to the trophozoites, the precyst forms contain a rigid cell wall and may be visualized with GMS and other fungal cell wall stains. The precyst stage contains nuclei that are at varying stages of nuclear division (2–8 nuclei), but have not yet been compartmentalized into individual conidium structures.

### Cyst or ascus

The cyst is the end product of sporogenesis. It has a rigid cell wall that excludes stains such as Giemsa and may be visualized with cell wall complexing stains such as GMS (Fig. 17.1). Under light microscopy, the cyst appears as a spherical, cup-shaped or crescent-shaped object 8 µm in diameter. Some cysts may appear empty or collapsed whereas others contain focal thickenings of the cyst wall. The mature cyst contains eight conidia. The conidia measure 1–2 µm in diameter. The cyst wall consists of three layers as visualized by electron microscopy, and is composed of β-1,3-glucan, chitin, melanin and other complex polymers.

*P. jirovecii* is an atypical fungus because:
- it is unable to be continuously cultivated *in vitro* unlike most pathogenic fungi;
- *Pneumocystis* spp. are host-specific and do not cross-infect other species;
- PCP is a communicable disease via the respiratory route; and
- it is not susceptible to amphotericin B or to azole antifungal drugs.

## LIFE CYCLE

The life cycle of *Pneumocystis* in lungs comprises of an asexual phase of cell division by the apparent haploid trophic form and sexual phase (sporogenesis) leading to the production of a thick-walled reproductive cyst (ascus) containing eight intracystic bodies (conidia). The asexual reproduction of the trophic forms appears to resemble binary fission, rather than budding, a process used by many but not all yeasts.

In sexual cycle opposite mating types fuse and undergo karyogamy, resulting in a diploid zygote. The zygote then undergoes meiosis resulting in four nuclei. Additional postmeiotic mitosis increases the number of nuclei to eight. The nuclei are compartmentalized by invagination of the inner plasma membrane, resulting in eight intracystic bodies (conidia). Each contains a single nucleus, a rounded mitochondrion, rough endoplasmic reticulum and numerous ribosomes. Conidia may be spherical, banana-shaped, or irregular. Once mature, conidia are extruded from the ascus (cyst) probably through a pore. Expulsion of conidia may be facilitated by residual fluid from the ascus, leaving behind a collapsed, empty ascus remnant. The conidia then differentiate into eight haploid trophic forms. They escape into the extracellular alveolar space and may resume vegetative growth and reproduce by fission as trophic forms.

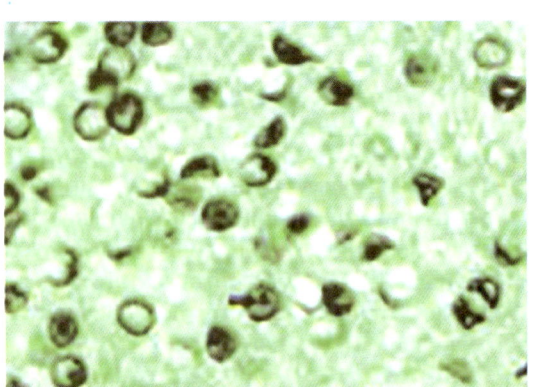

**Fig. 17.1.** Intra-alveolar clusters of non-budding cysts of *Pneumocystis jirovecii* stained by Gomori methenamine silver stain (×400) in an AIDS patient suffering from *Pneumocystis jirovecii* pneumonia.

Although organisms may be observed within macrophages as a result of the host response to the infection, there is no evidence for an intracellular phase in the life cycle of *Pneumocystis*.

## PATHOGENESIS

*Pneumocystis* is ubiquitous throughout nature, infecting a variety of warm-blooded animals. Most potential reservoirs of *P. jirovecii* are children and both symptomatic and asymptomatic immunocompromised individuals. *P. jirovecii* is carried in the respiratory tracts of asymptomatic individuals with mild immunosuppression induced by HIV or malignancy or connective tissue disorders, and in pregnant women. These groups of patients may be important in the human-to-human transmission of *P. jirovecii*.

Pneumocystosis is probably acquired through droplet infection. Trophic forms of *Pneumocystis* adhere tightly to type I alveolar cells and proliferate in lungs of immunocompromised host. The exuberant host inflammatory response causes injury to the alveolar epithelium with denudation of the basement membrane and subsequent hypertrophy of alveolar type II cells. An increase in alveolar capillary membrane permeability occurs. This leads to interstitial edema and the filling of the alveolar spaces with masses of organisms, alveolar macrophages, desquamated alveolar epithelial cells and polymorphonuclear leucocytes.

*P. jirovecii* causes pneumonia in immunocompromised patients; dissemination is rare. In the absence of immunosuppression, it does not cause disease. Until the AIDS epidemic, human disease was confined to interstitial plasma cell pneumonitis in malnourished infants and immunosuppressed patients. Prior to introduction of effective chemoprophylactic regimens, it was a major cause of death among AIDS patients. Chemoprophylaxis has resulted in a dramatic decrease in the incidence of pneumonia, but infections are increasing in other organs, primarily the spleen, lymph nodes and bone marrow.

*P. jirovecii* pneumonia generally occurs in HIV-infected patients with CD4+ lymphocyte count < 200/µl. Incidence of *P. jirovecii* pneumonia is 0.5% in patients with CD4+ lymphocyte counts of 200–350/µl. Patients with PCP frequently present with dyspnea, nonproductive cough, inability to breathe deeply, chest tightness, and night sweats. A low-grade fever (e.g., 38.5°C) and tachypnea are often present. Haemoptysis and sputum production is rare. The chest radiograph may show diffuse, symmetrical, interstitial infiltrates. Focal infiltrates, lobar consolidation, cavities, and nodules are less common. The incidence of *Pneumocystis* organisms in sites other than the lung has been reported in 1–3% of postmortem examinations of patients with pulmonary *P. jirovecii* infections.

## LABORATORY DIAGNOSIS

To establish the diagnosis of *P. jirovecii* pneumonia, specimens of bronchoalveolar lavage, lung biopsy or induced sputum (by administration of a saline mist to induce production of sputum) are stained by Gomori methenamine silver (GMS), Giemsa and calcofluor white and examined for the presence of cysts or trophozoites. The Papanicolaou stain, frequently used for staining cytopathological specimens, can demonstrate the foamy exudate surrounding the organisms, although the organisms stain poorly.

With Giemsa stain, all forms of the organism are stained, which permits rapid assessment of the total organism burden. The nuclei appear reddish-purple in contrast to the light blue cytoplasm. The cyst wall excludes the dye and appears as a circumscribed clear zone around the cyst contents. Organisms can also be demonstrated by immunofluorescent techniques, using fluorescein-tagged monoclonal antibodies against surface antigens of both cysts and trophic forms. ***P. jirovecii* cannot be cultured.**

### Polymerase chain reaction (PCR)

PCR-based detection of *P. jirovecii* DNA has been shown to have greater sensitivity and specificity for the diagnosis of PCP from respiratory specimens than conventional (Giemsa or GMS) microscopic methods.

### Serologic tests

A presumptive serodiagnosis can be made in suspected cases of *P. jirovecii* infections. Complement fixation titres of 1 : 4 or higher usually indicate active disease. Latex agglutination tests for *P. jirovecii* are positive in only about one-third of patients with known disease.

## TREATMENT AND PROPHYLAXIS

Acute cases of *P. jirovecii* pneumonia can be treated with trimethoprim-sulphamethoxazole or pentamidine isethionate. Trimethoprim-sulphamethoxazole is the drug of first choice for prophylaxis. It can be given either as a daily dose (one single or double-strength tablet) or one double-strength tablet three times weekly. Azole and polyene antifungal drug are not active against *P. jirovecii*.

 **Important Questions**

Discuss morphology, life cycle, pathogenesis and laboratory diagnosis of pneumocystosis.

### Multiple Choice Questions

1. *Pneumocystis jirovecii* belongs to which of the following phyla?
    (a) Basidiomycota.
    (b) Ascomycota.
    (c) Glomeromycota.
    (d) None of the above.
2. *Pneumocystis jirovecii* is a:
    (a) sporozoan.
    (b) flagellate.
    (c) ciliate.
    (d) fungus.
3. The asexual reproduction of the trophic forms of *Pneumocystis jirovecii* appears to resemble:
    (a) binary fission.
    (b) budding.
    (c) splitting.
    (d) pseudohyphae.
4. *Pneumocystis jirovecii* is carried in the respiratory tracts of asymptomatic individuals with:
    (a) mild immunosuppression induced by HIV.
    (b) malignancy.
    (c) connective tissue disorders.
    (d) All of the above.
5. *Pneumocystis jirovecii* can be cultured on:
    (a) Sabouraud dextrose agar.
    (b) brain heart infusion agar.
    (c) blood agar.
    (d) None of the above.
6. Which of the following is **not** a protozoan?
    (a) *Leishmania donovani*.
    (b) *Toxoplasma gondii*.
    (c) *Trypanosoma cruzi*.
    (d) *Pneumocystis jirovecii*.
7. Which of the following species of *Pneumocystis* causes infection in humans?
    (a) *carinii*.
    (b) *wakefieldiae*.
    (c) *murina*.
    (d) *jirovecii*.

### ANSWERS TO MCQs

1. (b), 2. (d), 3. (a), 4. (d), 5. (d), 6. (d), 7. (d).

 **Further Reading**

1. Agarwal R, Reddy C, et al. It's *Pneumocystis jirovecii* not *Pneumocystis carinii*. Chest 2006; 129: 498.
2. Bandt D, Monecke S. Development and evaluation of a real-time PCR assay for detection of *Pneumocystis jirovecii*. Transpl Infect Dis 2007; 9: 196–202.
3. Bellamy R. Pneumocystis pneumonia in people with HIV. Clin Evid 2006; 15: 982–95.
4. Castro JG, Manzi G, et al. Concurrent PCP and TB pneumonia in HIV infected patients. Scand J Infect Dis 2007; 39: 1054–8.
5. Crothers K, Beard CB, et al. Severity and outcome of HIV-associated *Pneumocystis* pneumonia containing *Pneumocystis jirovecii* genotype associated dihydropteroate synthase gene mutations. AIDS 2005; 19: 801–5.
6. Daly KR, Huang L, et al. Antibody response to *Pneumocystis jirovecii* major surface glycoprotein. Emerg Infect Dis 2006; 12: 1231–7.
7. Daly KR, Koch J, et al. Enzyme linked immunosorbent assay and serologic responses to *Pneumocystis jirovecii*. Emerg Infect Dis 2004; 10: 848–54.

8. Flori P, Bellete B, et al. Comparison between real-time PCR, conventional PCR and different staining techniques for diagnosing *Pneumocystis jirovecii* pneumonia from bronchoalveolar lavage specimens. *J Med Microbiol* 2004; 53: 603–7.
9. Luks AM, Neff MJ. *Pneumocystis jirovecii* pneumonia. *Respire Care* 2007; 52: 59–63.
10. Rabodonirina M, Vaillant L, et al. *Pneumocystis jirovecii* genotype associated with increased death rate of HIV-infected patients with pneumonia. *Emerg Infect Dis* 2013; 19: 21–8; quiz 186.
11. Shankar SM, Nania JJ. Management of *Pneumocystis jirovecii* pneumonia in children receiving chemotherapy. *Paediatr Drugs* 2007; 9: 301–9.
12. Sritangratanakul S, Nuchprayoon S, Nuchprayoon I. *Pneumocystis* pneumonia: an update. *J Med Assoc Thai* 2004; 87 (Suppl. 2): S309–17.
13. Stringer JR. Pneumocystis. *Int J Med Microbiol* 2002; 292: 391–404.
14. Thomas CF Jr, Limper AH. *Pneumocystis* pneumonia. *N Engl J Med* 2004; 350: 2487–98.
15. Wakefield AE. *Pneumocystis carinii. Br Med Bull* 2002; 61: 175–88.
16. Wazir JF, Ansari NA. *Pneumocystis carinii* infection: update and review. *Arch Pathol Lab Med* 2004; 128: 1023–7.

# CHAPTER 18

# Penicilliosis marneffei

There are more than 250 described species of the genus *Penicillium*. They occur as saprophytes in the soil and decomposing organic debris. **P. marneffei is the only species of genus *Penicillium* which is pathogenic dimorphic fungus.** It was first isolated in 1956 from bamboo rats in Vietnam. The first human case occurred in 1959. Segretain accidentally got inoculated his finger by a needle used to inoculate hamsters. Nine days later, a small nodule appeared at the site, followed by lymphangitis and axillary adenopathy. Subsequently, Segretain isolated the causative fungus from himself and gave its description. In 1960, he named the fungus *Penicillium marneffei* in honour of Hubert Marneffe, the then Director of the Pasteur Institute of Indochina.

The first spontaneous infection in a human case was reported in 1973 in an American Minister with Hodgkin's disease. He had travelled in Southeast Asia one year before. The second case of natural human infection was also reported from the USA in a 59-year-old man who had travelled extensively in the Far East. Disseminated *P. marneffei* infections began to be observed in 1988-89 in AIDS patients who had travelled to or were living in Southeast Asia. The disease caused by *P. marneffei* is known as **penicilliosis marneffei**.

## EPIDEMIOLOGY AND PATHOGENESIS

Penicilliosis marneffei is an infection endemic in Southeast Asia (Thailand, Vietnam, Myanmar, Hong Kong, Laos, Malaysia, Singapore, Taiwan, the Manipur State of India and the Guangxi province of China). Imported cases have been reported in Europe and the USA. The infection is more common in the immunosuppressed population mostly HIV-infected patients. **Penicilliosis marneffei is the third most common AIDS-defining illness (after tuberculosis and cryptococcosis) in Chiang Mai province of Thailand.**

The natural habitat of *P. marneffei* is probably soil. The route of acquisition of the fungus has not yet been definitely established. Like other dimorphic fungal pathogens that produce conidia in their saprophytic habitats in nature, the infection is thought to occur through inhalation of the conidia or through cutaneous inoculation. The organisms are engulfed by macrophages, in which they multiply intracellularly and transform into yeast. *Melanin is produced by both conidia and yeast. It may act as a virulence factor.*

The reticuloendothelial system is predominantly involved. It causes deep-seated infection that can be disseminated predominantly in immunocompromised (HIV-infected) patients. Most cases of penicilliosis marneffei are observed in patients who have CD4+ lymphocyte count < 100/μl. Disseminated disease is thought to be universally fatal, if untreated. In the immunocompetent host, the cell-mediated immune response is prominent with the formation of epithelioid granuloma.

## CLINICAL FINDINGS

Penicilliosis marneffei occurs mainly in adults. However, cases have also been reported in children with or without AIDS, living in endemic areas. Patient develops fever, anaemia, leucopenia, thrombocytopenia, weight loss, diarrhoea, hepatosplenomegaly, generalized lymphadenopathy, cough and pulmonary infiltrates. Skin lesions occur in over 50% of cases. They are small papules, ulcers or molluscum-like lesions. They are usually widely scattered on the face and trunk. Left untreated, this infection is fatal.

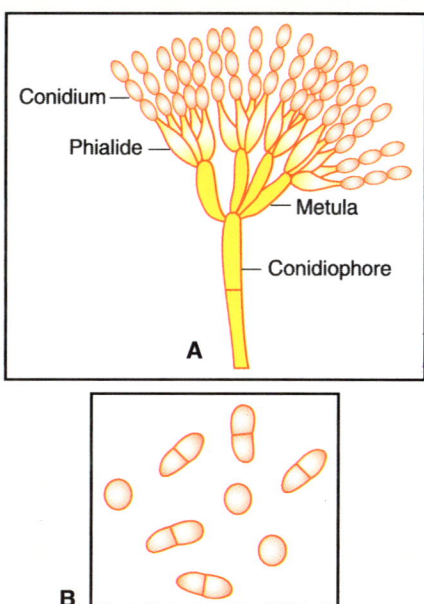

**Fig. 18.1.** *Penicillium marneffei:* mycelial phase (A) and yeast-like phase (B).

## MYCOLOGY

Sabouraud dextrose agar (SDA) supports the growth of *P. marneffei* and demonstrates thermal dimorphism. Cycloheximide inhibits growth. At 25–30°C on SDA growth matures within 3 days. It produces rapidly growing **greenish-yellow sporulating colonies, with a pink or red centre and dark green edges**. A characteristic brick-red pigment is released into the medium.

Microscopically, at 25–30°C, structures typical of the genus *Penicillium* develop, i.e., smooth conidiophores with 4–5 terminal metulae, each metula bearing 4–6 phialides. Conidia are ellipsoidal to globose (2–3 μm), smooth walled, often with prominent disjunctors, and arranged in short chains. The terminal conidia of the conidial chains are sometimes larger than the ones beneath them, which is a characteristic of *P. marneffei* (Fig. 18.1A).

At 35–37°C on SDA or brain heart infusion agar, colony is soft, white to tan, dry and yeast-like. Conversion from mold to yeast-like form may take up to 14 days. Hyphae first become shorter, develop more septa and branches, and cease to produce conidia. They eventually fragment at the septa, producing single-celled round to oval arthroconidia (2.5–5 μm in length). This form is referred to as yeast-like cells. Buds are not produced. The arthroconidia continue to reproduce by fission and in so doing may elongate to 8–9 μm (Fig. 18.1B).

## HISTOPATHOLOGY

The host response to *P. marneffei* invasion mainly involves the mononuclear phagocytic cells of the lung and the reticuloendothelial system. *P. marneffei* yeast-like cells are engulfed by histiocytes where they proliferate within the phagosomes. As the lesion progresses, central necrosis develops, with infiltration of neutrophils and formation of abscesses. Granulomas slowly evolve in the lung and may lead to fibrosis and cavitation. In contrast to histoplasmosis, calcification does not usually occur. In the severely immunocompromised patient, the inflammatory response may be minimal or absent. Special stains such as periodic acid-Schiff (PAS) or Gomori methenamine silver (GMS) are essential to distinguish penicilliosis marneffei from tuberculosis and other systemic mycoses as the fungi stain poorly with haematoxylin and eosin (H&E).

## LABORATORY DIAGNOSIS

### Microscopic examination

Clinical specimens include bone marrow aspirate, buffy coat of blood, lymph node aspirate or biopsy, liver biopsy, skin biopsy, skin scrapings, sputum, bronchoalveolar lavage pellets, pleural fluid, cerebrospinal fluid, pharyngeal ulcer scrapings, palatal papule scrapings, urine and stool. Impression smears and histopathological sections are stained with H&E, PAS and GMS.

Microscopic examination reveals oval yeast-like cells, 2.5–5 μm in length. They multiply within histiocytes in tissue or within monocytes in blood or bone marrow. Budding does not occur. A prominent central septum forms, and reproduction is by fission. Outside the histiocytes, yeast cells are up to 8 μm in length. These may have several septa, and are often curved to be sausage-shaped. They must be differentiated from *Leishmania donovani*, *Pneumocystis jirovecii* and *Histoplasma capsulatum* var. *capsulatum*.

*P. marneffei* gives a false impression of having a capsule when stained with H&E. Therefore, they can very closely mimic *H. capsulatum* var. *capsulatum*, especially when intracellular. However, the two organisms multiply differently. *P. marneffei* replicates by fission, instead of budding, and the considerable variation in size and shape of the extracellular yeasts makes *P. marneffei* easily distinguishable from the budding tissue-form cells of *H. capsulatum* var. *capsulatum*.

A specific indirect fluorescent antibody examination of histological sections has been described.

### Culture

*P. marneffei* can be isolated from various clinical specimens particularly bone marrow, skin biopsy and blood (for cultural characteristics see above). Handling and culture of specimens possibly containing *P. marneffei* should be performed with care, avoiding inhalation of conidia from sporulating mold culture or accidental injection into the skin. **Biosafety level 2 practices and facilities are recommended for propagating and manipulating cultures known to contain *P. marneffei*.**

### Serodiagnosis

Penicilliosis marneffei infection may be diagnosed by detection of IgG antibodies in the sera of patients by an **indirect fluorescent antibody test**, using conidia and yeast cells as antigens. **Latex agglutination, ELISA and immunodiffusion tests** can be used for detection of *P. marneffei* antigens in body fluids of the patients. Antigens may be detected in urine as well as serum.

### Treatment

In severe cases amphotericin B is necessary. However, there is usually a good response to itraconazole 200–400 mg/day, but this may have to be given for a long period to prevent relapse.

**Important Questions**

Discuss mycology, pathogenesis and laboratory diagnosis of *Penicillium marneffei*.

**Multiple Choice Questions**

1. Which of the following fungi is thermally dimorphic?
   (a) *Penicillium marneffei*.
   (b) *Penicillium commune*.
   (c) *Penicillium citrinum*.
   (d) *Penicillium griseofulvin*.

2. Yeast-like form of which of the following fungi divides by fission and not by budding?
   (a) *Sporothrix schenckii*.
   (b) *Penicillium marneffei*.
   (c) *Histoplasma capsulatum*.
   (d) *Blastomyces dermatitidis*.

3. Which of the following fungi give/gives a false impression of having a capsule?
   (a) *Histoplasma capsulatum*.
   (b) *Penicillium marneffei*.
   (c) Both of the above.
   (d) None of the above.

4. Which of the following is/are AIDS-defining illness/es?
   (a) Tuberculosis.
   (b) Cryptococcosis.
   (c) Pneumocystitis marneffei.
   (d) All of the above.

### ANSWERS TO MCQs

1. (a), 2. (b), 3. (c), 4. (d).

### Further Reading

1. Cristofaro P, Mileno MD. *Penicillium marneffei* infection in HIV-infected travellers. *AIDS Alerts* 2006; 21: 140–2.
2. Hortung TK, Chimbayo D, et al. Etiology of suspected pneumonia in adults admitted to a high-dependency unit in Blantyre, Malawi. *Am J Trop Med Hyg* 2011; 85: 105–12.
3. Jayanetra P, Nitiyanant P, et al. Penicilliosis marneffei in Thailand: report of five human cases. *Am J Trop Med Hyg* 1984; 33: 637–44.
4. Kullavanijaya P. Penicilliosis in AIDS. *J Dermatol* 2001; 28: 667–70.
5. Lim D, Lee YS, Chang AR. Rapid diagnosis of *Penicillium marneffei* infection by fine needle aspiration cytology. *Clin Pathol* 2006; 59: 443–4.
6. Lo Y, Tintelnot K, et al. Disseminated *Penicillium marneffei* infection in an African AIDS patient. *Trans Roy Soc Trop Med Hyg* 2000; 94: 187.
7. Lu PX, Zhu WK, et al. Acquired immunodeficiency syndrome associated disseminated *Penicillium marneffei* infection: report of 8 cases. *Chin Med J* 2005; 118: 1395–9.
8. Tsunemi Y, Takahashi T, Tamaki T. *Penicillium marneffei* infection diagnosed by polymerase chain reaction from the skin specimen. *J Am Acad Dermatol* 2003; 49: 344–6.
9. Ungpakorn R. Cutaneous manifestations of *Penicillium marneffei* infection. *Curr Opin Infect Dis* 2000; 13: 129–34.
10. Wortman PD. Infection with *Penicillium marneffei*. *Int J Dermatol* 1996; 35: 393–9.

# CHAPTER 19

# Aspergillosis

There are more than 200 species of *Aspergillus* to which humans are constantly exposed. However, approximately 19 species have been associated with human disease (aspergillosis), which is worldwide in occurrence. Of these, over 95% of all infections are caused by *A. fumigatus*, *A. flavus* and *A. niger*. Several additional species of clinical importance include *A. nidulans*, *A. terreus*, *A. oryzae*, *A. ustus* and *A. versicolor*. *A. fumigatus* causes most cases of both invasive and non-invasive aspergillosis. Allergic forms of the disease appear to be almost exclusively caused by *A. fumigatus*. *A. flavus*, *A. niger*, *A. terreus* and *A. nidulans* cause invasive aspergillosis, and *A. flavus* and *A. niger*, in addition, also cause aspergilloma. After *Candida* spp., *Aspergillus* spp. are the second most common genus recovered from positive fungal cultures in hospitalized patients, but positive cultures alone may not indicate a pathogenic process. Pathogenic species of *Aspergillus* share some properties not found in other species which confer on them an intrinsic pathogenic advantage. These are:

- Ability to grow efficiently at 37°C.
- Production of proteolytic enzyme.
- Ability to digest elastin.
- Antigens with protease activity.

Most species of *Aspergillus* reproduce asexually. However, some species, in addition to their asexual reproduction, have characteristic of reproducing sexually by formation of ascospores, which typifies **Ascomycetes**.

## PATHOGENESIS

*Aspergillus* spp. cause aspergillosis. It is caused by inhalation of conidia or mycelial fragments which are present on vegetation (especially nuts and grains), decaying matter, soil and air. Inhalation of the conidia of *Aspergillus* spp. can give rise to a number of different clinical forms of aspergillosis, depending upon the immunological status of the host. Atopic subjects may develop **asthma**. In non-atopic subjects, the presence of damaged lung tissue may result in the growth of a fungus ball (**aspergilloma**). Inhalation of massive doses of the conidia may lead to **alveolitis**.

### Disease spectrum

*Aspergillus* induces a wide range of clinical syndromes ranging from colonization to acute invasive disease:

*1. Allergic bronchopulmonary aspergillosis (ABPA)*

This is seen in atopic individuals with elevated IgE levels. Following inhalation of spores, the fungus grows within the lumen of the bronchioles. Some patients may expectorate mucus plugs containing *Aspergillus* hyphae which may be seen in smear or may be isolated from sputum. Patient develops bronchial allergic reactions to inhaled *Aspergillus* conidia. Repeated allergic reactions in bronchi cause bronchiectasis. Patient suffers from breathlessness, fever and malaise after a few hours of exposure. ABPA may also occur in patients with cystic fibrosis.

### 2. Intracavitary aspergilloma (fungus ball)

Aspergilloma represents a non-invasive (saprophytic) form of aspergillosis. This usually develops in pre-existing pulmonary cavities such as in tuberculosis or cystic disease. The inhaled conidia enter a cavity, germinate and produce abundant hyphae. Aspergilloma is defined as a fungal ball caused by an *Aspergillus* species; a mass of fungal hyphae embedded in a matrix of cell debris and fibrin, contained in a preexisting pulmonary cavity. The cavity wall may become thickened and gradually the fungus ball may lie freely in the cavity.

Fungus balls are usually located in the upper lobes. Less frequently, they occur in the apical segments of the lower lobes. Patients are often asymptomatic, but may present with chronic cough, malaise, and weight loss. Haemoptysis is the most common symptom, occurring in 50–80% of cases. It may occasionally be massive and life-threatening.

Fungus ball may also develop in maxillary sinus and occasionally in the ethmoid, sphenoid and frontal sinuses. It is only saprophytic colonization without invasion of the lung or sinus mucosa.

### 3. Acute invasive pulmonary aspergillosis

Acute invasive pulmonary aspergillosis is most commonly caused by *A. fumigatus* in human, but other species such as, *A. flavus, A. nodulans*, and *A. terreus*, have also been implicated. This occurs in severely immunocompromised individuals who are on immunosuppressive drugs, cytotoxic drugs, corticosteroids, broad-spectrum antibiotics and AIDS patients. There is a widespread growth of the fungus in lung tissue that disseminates to involve other organs particularly kidneys and brain. The disease has poor prognosis. Invasive aspergillosis is a common hospital-acquired fungal infection.

This type of infection may present in several forms. A bronchopneumonia with solitary or multiple infiltrates and fever is the common manifestation of acute invasive pulmonary aspergillosis. Lobar pneumonia resembling bacterial infection may also occur. Another manifestation is haemorrhagic pulmonary infarction caused by invasion and thrombosis of a large pulmonary artery. Patient develops sudden onset of fever, and a pleural friction rub. The *Aspergillus* infection may extend by invasive growth into neighbouring organs and structures, e.g., the mediastinum, ribs, vertebrae, oesophagus, and pericardium.

Conidia of *A. fumigatus* can, because of their small size (< 5 µm) and aerodynamic properties, bypass the upper respiratory tract defences and may reach distal regions of the lung. They adhere to pulmonary epithelial cells, and are readily endocytosed. Within the epithelial cells, the conidia germinate to form hyphae, which grow by apical extension and escape from the epithelial cells. The emergent hyphae penetrate the abluminal surface of endothelial cells and cause endothelial cell damage. Hyphal fragments disseminate haematogenously and adhere to the luminal endothelial cell surface before invading these cells. Luminal invasion results in endothelial cell damage and extravascular invasion of deep organs.

*Aspergillus* infection of the upper respiratory tract can involve the gingiva and hard palate. Primary oral aspergillosis typically involves the marginal gingiva or palate. The patient is usually granulocytopenic and complains of severe gingival pain with associated fever. The infection begins as violaceous lesion in the marginal gingiva in the absence of surrounding oedema. Within a few days, the lesion progresses to necrotic ulcers covered with pseudomembranes. The infection rapidly spreads to involve alveolar bone and facial muscles.

### 4. Paranasal Aspergillus granuloma

In this condition, there is colonization of paranasal sinuses by *A. flavus* and *A. fumigatus*. There is no evidence of invasion of the sinus, although pressure necrosis of the sinus may occur. Paranasal *Aspergillus* granuloma is a slowly progressive condition. It is most common in tropics, where *A. flavus* is the most common cause, although cases have been reported from temperate climates. Affected individuals usually complain of longstanding symptoms of nasal obstruction and headache. Generally, only one sinus is involved with *Aspergillus* spp., most commonly the maxillary sinus. The others, in decreasing order of frequency, are the ethmoid, sphenoid, and frontal sinuses.

Chronic granulomatous sinusitis (primary paranasal *Aspergillus* granuloma) is a slowly progressive invasive syndrome characterized by florid granulomatous inflammation. Invasion of the cavernous sinus, orbit and brain is frequently seen, and erosion of bone is common. The ethmoid sinuses are invariably involved and a pansinusitis, subsequently, develops in a majority of patients.

### 5. Endocarditis

*Aspergillus* may sometimes cause endocarditis in immunosuppressed patients and those who have undergone open-heart surgery. This condition also has a poor prognosis. It has also been described as a complication of parenteral nutrition and drug addiction. The aortic and mitral valves are most frequent sites of infection. Vegetations tend to be large and friable with a propensity for embolization.

Myocardial infection with abscess formation or mural vegetations may occur as a result of haematogenous dissemination.

### 6. Cerebral aspergillosis

Brain is the most important organ affected in disseminated aspergillosis apart from the lungs. It leads to focal neurological deficits including hemiparesis, focal seizures, and cranial nerve palsy.

### 7. Keratitis

*Aspergillus* spp. are an occasional etiologic agent of this locally invasive infection of the cornea following a penetrating injury or corneal surgery. *Aspergillus* keratitis is occupationally associated with agricultural workers. This infection is characterized by ocular pain and rapid vision loss. *Aspergillus* spp. are an infrequent cause of fungal keratitis in contact lens wearers who are not compliant with proper antiseptic cleaning procedure.

### 8. Otomycosis

Otomycosis refers to the growth of *Aspergillus* spp. (usually *A. niger* or *A. fumigatus*) within the external auditory canal. The fungus grows on cerumen, epithelial scales and detritus deep in the external canal. The resulting plug of mycelium and debris cause irritation, pruritus and impairment of hearing. *Aspergillus* spp. may invade the external auditory canal of immunocompromised patients, extending into contiguous bone or even brain. The lesion of aspergillosis is dry, and the occurrence of exudate and foul odour indicates bacterial etiology.

The dermatophytes may invade the ear canal, usually by extension of facial dermatophytosis. In addition to *Aspergillus* spp., *Penicillium* spp., *Scedosporium apiospermum*, *Candida albicans*, *C. tropicalis*, *C. krusei* and *Malassezia sympodialis* may also cause otomycosis.

### 9. Cutaneous aspergillosis

Cutaneous aspergillosis may be classified into primary and secondary infection. Primary cutaneous aspergillosis may arise at catheter insertion sites. It has been reported in neonates and in patients with HIV/AIDS and prolonged neutropenia. The lesion begin as erythematous to violaceous, oedematous, indurated plaques that evolve into necrotic ulcers covered with a black eschar. In about 5% of patients with aspergillosis, haematogenous spread of infection gives rise to cutaneous lesions. These may be single or multiple, well-circumscribed, maculopapular lesions which become pustular. They evolve into necrotic ulcers covered with a black eschar.

## LABORATORY DIAGNOSIS

Diagnosis may be made by microscopic examination and by culture.

### Direct examination

### KOH preparation

10% KOH preparation of sputum, bronchoalveolar lavage, fine needle aspirates, transbronchial biopsy and other biopsies reveal non-pigmented septate hyphae, 3–6 μm in diameter with characteristic dichotomous branching (i.e., each branch is approximately equal in width to the originating parent hypha) at 45° angles. The hyphae have a tendency to branch repeatedly. *A. terreus* is unique in having the ability to produce conidia along the hyphae *in vivo* during invasive infection. Addition of calcofluor white enhances visibility when viewed under a fluorescence microscope. In a majority of pulmonary and disseminated lesions, only hyphal forms are seen.

- In allergic aspergillosis there is usually abundant fungus in the sputum and mycelial plugs may also be present.
- In aspergilloma, fungus may be difficult to find in sputum smear.
- In invasive aspergillosis, sputum smear is often negative.

### Histopathology

The most reliable method for the diagnosis of acute invasive aspergillosis is the examination of stained tissue sections. Histological sections can be stained with haematoxylin and eosin (H&E), periodic acid-Schiff (PAS), and Gomori methenamine silver (GMS) and examined for characteristic hyphae (Figs. 19.1 and 19.2). In chronic lesions, short, distorted hyphae may be as wide as 12 µm. Conidial heads (vesicles, phialides, and conidia) may occasionally form in areas exposed to air, e.g., in pulmonary cavities, and ear or skin infections (Fig. 19.3).

Many other fungi appear similar to the aspergilli in tissue or other clinical specimens; however, there are subtle differences:

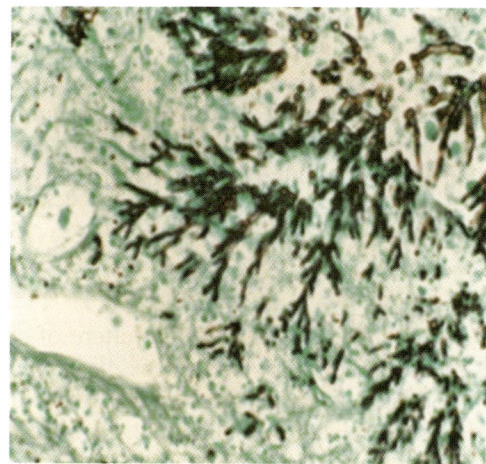

**Fig. 19.2.** Section stained by Gomori methenamine silver stain (×400). The hyphae of *Aspergillus* are stained black in colour.

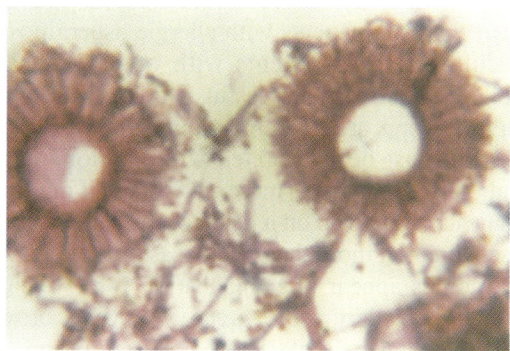

**Fig. 19.3.** Conidial heads (vesicles, phialides and conidia) of *Aspergillus* in a pulmonary cavity (H&E stain, ×400).

- **Mucorales** have hyphae that are nonseptate, are commonly broader (up to 25 µm in diameter), show random branching, often appear collapsed and twisted, are irregular and non-parallel, and usually stain lighter with GMS than do the aspergilli.
- **Candida spp.** show budding yeast cells, hyphae and pseudohyphae. These can be differentiated from *Aspergillus* spp. by the presence of budding yeast cells and distinct constrictions at the septa of pseudohyphae of *Candida* spp. However, when the hyphae of *Aspergillus* are cut on cross-section, they may be mistaken for non-budding yeast cells.

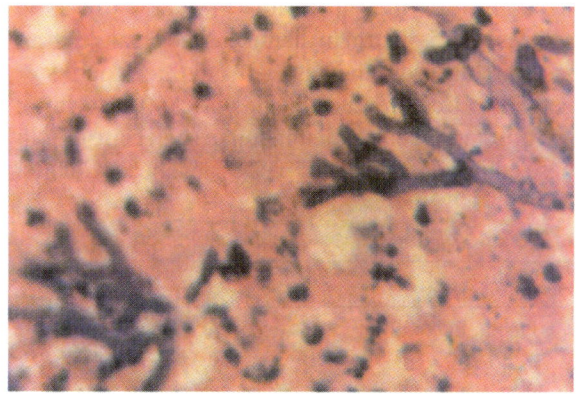

**Fig. 19.1.** Aspergillosis showing septate hyphae with characteristic dichotomous branching in haematoxylin and eosin staining (×400).

## SECTION 5 : Opportunistic Mycoses

Invasive aspergillosis is characterized by acute inflammation (neutrophils) and necrotic debris. In severely neutropenic patients, the acute inflammatory response is greatly reduced. Occasionally, a granulomatous response occurs. *Aspergillus* has a predilection for invading blood vessels causing blockage of blood vessels, tissue death and necrosis (infarction).

### Culture

*Aspergillus* can be recovered from culture of sinus tissue, other tissue biopsy specimens, heart valves, and appropriate ophthalmologic samples. The clinical material is inoculated on Sabouraud dextrose agar without cycloheximide. It can be incubated at any temperature from that of room to 45°C. Temperatures of 37°C and above are favourable for *A. fumigatus* and will inhibit growth of many fungal contaminants. The fungus may be recovered from sputum specimens from patients with allergic aspergillosis, but cultures from patients with other forms of aspergillosis are less successful. Moreover, because *Aspergillus* spp. are commonly found in the air, their isolation must be interpreted with caution. Their isolation from sputum is more convincing if multiple colonies are obtained on a plate, or the same fungus is recovered on more than one occasion.

Colonies appear after incubation for 1–2 days producing powdery white, green, yellowish, brown or black colonies (Table 19.1). *Aspergillus* spp. do not require specific biohazard precautions in the laboratory, although culture material should be handled in a biosafety cabinet to avoid dispersal of the dry spores throughout the environment and cross contamination of other cultures. The isolate is identified on the basis of growth characteristics and microscopic morphology. Lactophenol cotton blue mount shows branching and septate hyphae. From the latter arise conidiophores, the ends of which are expanded to form vesicles. The vesicle bears one or two layers of phialides which, in turn, bear conidia, **the inner layers of phialides are called metulae**. The length and width of the conidiophores, the size and contour of the vesicle, the arrangement of the phialides and the colour, size, and chain-length of the conidia are features used in making species identifications.

### Aspergillus fumigatus

*A. fumigatus* is thermotolerant and grows and sporulates up to 48°C and also below 20°C. The colonies of *A. fumigatus* are granular to cottony and usually have some shades of **green, green-grey or green-brown pigmentation**. Reverse is pale to light yellow. Microscopically, the conidiophores are smooth, relatively short (usually less than 300 µm long), the vesicles are 20–30 µm in diameter, club-shaped and covered on **upper two-thirds** with only **a single row of phialides** arising directly from the vesicle (**uniseriate**), giving rise to long chains of spherical to slightly ovoid conidia that tend to sweep towards the central axis (Fig. 19.4A). Conidia measure 2–3.5 µm in diameter.

### Aspergillus flavus

The colonies of *A. flavus* are granular to woolly and have some shade of **yellow or yellow-brown**. Reverse is usually yellowish to tan. Microscopically, the conidiophores are long (400–800 µm), the vesicles are 25–45 µm in diameter. The phialides may arise directly from the vesicle from three-fourths or the entire circumference of the vesicle (**uniseriate**), or from sterile cells called metulae (**biseriate**). Both these conditions may exist in the same head. Conidia

**Table 19.1.** Colony colour on Sabouraud dextrose agar in *Aspergillus* species of medical importance

| Species | Surface | Reverse |
| --- | --- | --- |
| A. fumigatus | Green, green-grey or green-brown | Pale to light yellow |
| A. flavus | Yellow or yellow-brown | Yellowish to tan |
| A. niger | Black with white border | White to cream |
| A. terreus | Cinnamon buff, brown or orange-brown | Yellow to tan |
| A. nidulans | Dark green to dark olive-buff | Buff, brownish orange or deep reddish purple |

# Aspergillosis

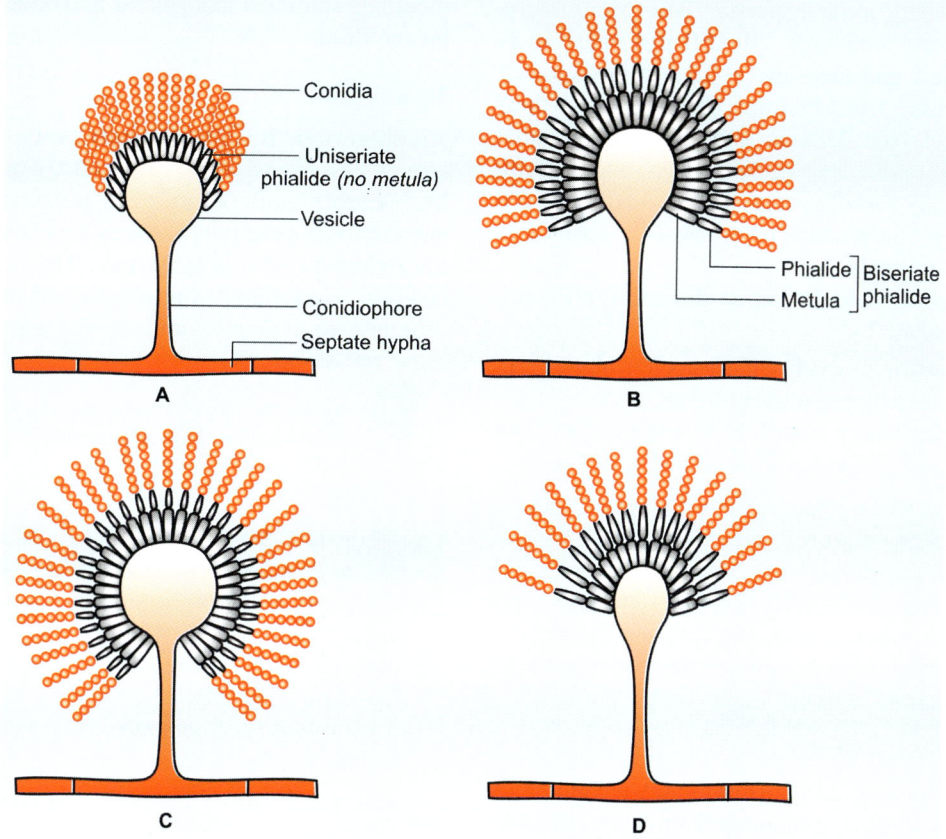

Fig. 19.4. *Aspergillus* spp. (A) *A. fumigatus*, (B) *A. flavus*, (C) *A. niger*, (D) *A. terreus*.

are spherical, 3–6 µm in diameter smooth, or slightly roughened with maturity and form long chains (Fig. 19.4B).

## Aspergillus niger

The surface of the colonies of *A. niger* is covered by a dense aggregate of **jet black conidia**. Thalus is composed of long, white to cream, erect hyphae. The reverse is white to cream. Microscopically, the vesicles are globose and measure 30–75 µm in diameter. Phialides arise from metulae (**biseriate**) around entire vesicle, with metulae twice as long as the phialides. Conidiation is extremely profuse, to the extent that the **vesicles are obscured by dense aggregates** of 4–5 µm diameter, spherical, black conidia that become roughened with maturity (Fig. 19.4C).

## Aspergillus terreus

The colonies of *A. terreus* are **cinnamon buff, brown or orange-brown**, texture velvety or powdery. Reverse is yellow to tan. Microscopically, the vesicles are relatively small (10–20 µm in diameter) flask-shaped or hemispherical. Phialides arise from metulae (**biseriate**) on the upper half only. The proximal, primary phialides (metulae) are shorter (5–8 µm) than the secondary phialides (8–12 µm). Conidia are smooth, elliptical, measure 2–2.5 µm in diameter (Fig. 19.4D).

## Aspergillus nidulans

*A. nidulans* may rarely be recovered from cases of human infections. The colonies are dark green to dark olive buff, cottony to granular in consistency, and may have radial folds. The reverse is buff, brownish orange or deep reddish purple. Microscopically, conidiophore measures 70–150 μm, vesicle is hemispherical and measures 8–12 μm in diameter. Phialides arise from metulae (**biseriate**) on their upper half surface. Metulae and phialides are equal in length. Conidia are globose, rough, and 3–4 μm in diameter. *A. nidulans* may form sexually derived **ascospores** contained within sac-like structures called **cleistothecia**.

It is imperative to determine clinical significance of fungal isolate by:
- demonstrating hyphae in fresh clinical material,
- demonstrating hyphae in tissue, and
- isolating heavy growth from a single specimen or the same species from multiple specimens.

Fungal culture of at least three serial sputum specimens is recommended whenever fungal infection is suspected. Most convincing evidence of aspergillosis is provided by recovery of organisms from normally sterile sites, such as lung tissue from biopsy, and by histopathologic demonstration of hyphal elements in tissue.

### Serological diagnosis

Immunodiffusion, counterimmunoelectrophoresis and enzyme-linked immunosorbent assay (ELISA) are widely used for detection of antibodies in the diagnosis of all forms of aspergillosis, particularly aspergilloma and allergic bronchopulmonary aspergillosis. In invasive aspergillosis antigen can be detected by ELISA and latex agglutination. This is helpful in establishing early diagnosis.

### Skin tests

Skin tests with *A. fumigatus* antigen are useful in the diagnosis of allergic aspergillosis. Those with allergic bronchopulmonary aspergillosis give an immediate type I reaction and may also give a delayed type IV reaction.

### Detection of Aspergillus DNA by polymerase chain reaction (PCR)

PCR is a useful tool to aid in the diagnosis of invasive aspergillosis. *Aspergillus* DNA has been detected in CSF samples by nested PCR assay. Various other clinical specimens have been analyzed by PCR, including sputum, whole blood, and bronchoalveolar lavage fluid.

### Treatment

Amphotericin B, until recently, was the drug of choice for invasive aspergillosis. The triazoles, itraconazole, voriconazole and posaconazole have anti-*Aspergillus* activity and they have revolutionized the treatment of this syndrome. The three echinocandins – caspofungin, micafungin and anidulafungin – demonstrate *in vitro* and *in vivo* activity against *Aspergillus* spp.

 **Important Questions**

Discuss pathogenesis and laboratory diagnosis of aspergillosis.

## Multiple Choice Questions

1. Most cases of both invasive and non-invasive aspergillosis are caused by:
   (a) *Aspergillus flavus*.
   (b) *Aspergillus niger*.
   (c) *Aspergillus fumigatus*.
   (d) *Aspergillus terreus*.

2. Allergic forms of disease is caused by:
   (a) *Aspergillus fumigatus*.
   (b) *Aspergillus flavus*.
   (c) *Aspergillus niger*.
   (d) All of the above.

3. Which of the following properties is/are found in pathogenic *Aspergillus* species?
   (a) Ability to grow efficiently at 37°C.
   (b) Production of proteolytic enzyme.
   (c) Ability to digest elastin.
   (d) All of the above.

4. Some species of *Aspergillus*, in addition to their asexual reproduction, have characteristic of reproducing sexually by formation of:
   (a) basidiospores.
   (b) ascospores.
   (c) zygospores.
   (d) blastoconidia.

5. Non-pigmented septate hyphae are seen in histological sections stained with haematoxylin and eosin in:

(a) mucormycosis.
(b) aspergillosis.
(c) phaeohyphomycosis.
(d) chromoblastomycosis.

6. A blue-green mold is isolated from a clinical specimen. Microscopically its asexual reproductive structure is a conidiophore, brush-like, simple or branched, with clusters of phialides producing chains of conidia. Vesicle is not formed. Which of the following is likely to be its identity?
   (a) *Aspergillus fumigatus*.
   (b) *Aspergillus flavus*.
   (c) *Aspergillus nodulans*.
   (d) *Penicillium* spp.

7. Which of the following is a preferred medium for isolation of *Aspergillus* spp. from a nonsterile site specimen?
   (a) Brain heart infusion agar.
   (b) Malt extract agar.
   (c) Sabouraud dextrose agar with chloramphenicol.
   (d) Bird seed agar.

## ANSWERS TO MCQs

1. (c), 2. (d), 3. (d), 4. (b), 5. (b), 6. (d), 7. (c).

### Further Reading

1. Almyroudis NG, Holland SM, Sehgal BH. Invasive aspergillosis in primary immunodeficiencies. *Med Mycol* 2005; 43 (Suppl. 1): S247–59.
2. Arora B, Arora DR, Bhatia JN, Jain K. *Aspergillus* granuloma of maxillary sinus – A case report. *Indian J Pathol Microbiol* 1979; 22: 217–19.
3. Buchheidt Hummel M. *Aspergillus* polymerase chain reaction (PCR) diagnosis. *Med Mycol* 2005; 43 (Suppl. 1): S139–45.
4. Chakrabarti A, Chatterjee SS, et al. Invasive aspergillosis in developing countries. *Med Mycol* 2011; 49 (Suppl 1): S35–S47.
5. de Aguirre L, Hurst SF, et al. Rapid differentiation of *Aspergillus* species from other medically important opportunistic molds and yeasts by PCR-enzyme immunoassay. *J Clin Microbiol* 2004; 42: 3495–504.
6. Denning DW, Pleury A, Cole DC. Global burden of chronic pulmonary aspergillosis as a sequel to pulmonary tuberculosis. *Bull World Health Organ* 2011; 89: 864–72.
7. Dimopoulos G, Piagnerelli M, et al. Disseminated aspergillosis in intensive care unit patients: an autopsy study. *J Chemother* 2003; 15: 71–5.
8. Dupont B, Richardson M, et al. Invasive aspergillosis. *Med Mycol* 2005; 38 (Suppl. 1): S215–24.
9. Gabal MA, el-Sherif AM, et al. A polymerase chain reaction 'PCR' for a quick diagnosis of aspergillosis. *Mycoses* 1999; 42: 515–20.
10. He H, Ding L, et al. Clinical features of invasive bronchopulmonary aspergillosis in critically ill patients with chronic obstructive respiratory diseases: a prospective study. *Crit Care* 2011; 15: R5.
11. Herbrecht R, Natrajan-Ame S, et al. Invasive pulmonary aspergillosis. *Semin Respir Crit Care Med* 2004; 25: 191–202.
12. Hinrikson HP, Hurst SF, et al. Molecular methods for the identification of *Aspergillus* species. *Med Mycol* 2005; 43 (Suppl. 1): S129–37.
13. Hizel K, Kokturk N, et al. Polymerase chain reaction in the diagnosis of invasive aspergillosis. *Mycoses* 2004; 47: 338–42.
14. Hope WW, Walsh TJ, Denning DW. Laboratory diagnosis of invasive aspergillosis. *Lancet Infect Dis* 2005; 5: 609–22.
15. Khan Zu, Kortom M, et al. Bilateral pulmonary aspergilloma caused by an atypical isolate of *Aspergillus terreus*. *J Clin Microbiol* 2000; 38: 2010–4.
16. Khatri ML, Stefanato CM, et al. Cutaneous and paranasal aspergillosis in an immunocompetent patient. *Int J Dermatol* 2000; 39: 853–6.
17. Khoo SH, Denning DW. Invasive aspergillosis in patients with AIDS. *Clin Infect Dis* 1994; 19 (Suppl. 1): S41–8.
18. Malnick SD, Shtalrid M, Landau Z. Early diagnosis of invasive aspergillosis. *Lancet* 2000; 355: 2076–7.

19. Saito T, Fujiuchi S, et al. Efficacy and safety of voriconazole in the treatment of chronic pulmonary aspergillosis: experience in Japan *Infection* 2012; 40: 661–7.
20. Shetty J, Giri N, et al. Invasive aspergillosis in human immunodeficiency virus-infected children. *Pediatr Infect Dis J* 1997; 16: 216–21.
21. Slavin MA, Chakrabarti A. Opportunistic fungal infections in the Asia-Pacific region. *Med Mycol* 2011; 50: 18–25.
22. Ulsakarya A. Aspergilloma. *N Eng J Med* 2002; 346: 256.
23. Wheat LJ. Rapid diagnosis of invasive aspergillosis by antigen detection. *Transpl Infect Dis* 2003; 5: 158–66.

# CHAPTER 20

# Mucormycosis

Mucormycosis refers to diseases caused by fungi of the phylum Glomeromycota and the subphyla Mucoromycotina and Entomophthoromycotina. The principal human pathogens among the Mucormycetes are encompassed by two orders – Mucorales and the Entomophthorales. The order Entomophthorales contains two pathogenic genera, *Conidiobolus* and *Basidiobolus*. In the order Mucorales, pathogenic genera include *Mucor*, *Rhizopus*, *Lichtheimia* (formerly *Absidia*), *Rhizomucor*, *Apophysomyces* and *Syncephalastrum* (Table 20.1).

## ORDER: MUCORALES

Mucorales are ubiquitous molds widely distributed in the environment (soil, plants, and decaying organic material). They are frequent pathogens of plants and contaminants of grains and foods such as fruit or bread. Airborne spores are thought to be the infectious particles responsible for disease, particularly in immunocompromised individuals, and this explains the most frequent body localizations (skin, sinuses,

Table 20.1. Common causative agents of mucormycosis

| Phylum | Subphylum | Order | Family | Genera |
|---|---|---|---|---|
| Glomeromycota | Mucoromycotina | Mucorales | Mucoraceae | • *Mucor*<br>• *Rhizopus*<br>• *Lichtheimia* (formerly *Absidia*)<br>• *Rhizomucor*<br>• *Apophysomyces*<br>• *Syncephalastrum* |
| | | | Cunninghamellaceae | • *Cunninghamella*<br>• *Saksenaea* |
| | Entomophthoromycotina | Entomophthorales | Entomophthoraceae<br>Basidiobolaceae | • *Conidiobolus*<br>• *Basidiobolus* |

and lungs). These molds are frequently found as laboratory contaminants and may cause nosocomial infections. The Mucorales are rapid growers and thermotolerant. Their asexual reproductive structures, sporangia borne on sporangiophores are large enough to be seen with unaided eye.

Hyphae of these fungi are coenocytic and mostly nonseptate, making them clearly distinguishable from those of other filamentous fungi. These fungi are responsible for a broad spectrum of infections, that are somewhat infrequent but often fatal. *Rhizopus* species are the frequent cause of mucormycosis, accounting for approximately half of the cases; with *R. arrhizus* the most common species, followed by *R. microsporus* var. *rhizopodiformis*, the second most frequently encountered species. *Mucor* species account for approximately 18% of reported cases, followed by *Cunninghamella bertholletiae*, *Apophysomyces elegans* (6%) and *Lichtheimia* about 5%.

## PATHOGENESIS

Most of the Mucormycetes (order Mucorales) have a wide geographic distribution in which they use a variety of substrates as nutrient sources. They are able to grow at temperatures greater than 37°C. They are found in decaying vegetables, foodstuffs, fruits, soil, animal excreta and other substrates high in sugar content. Mucormycosis is not contagious, the source of infection for man and animals is the environmental habitats mentioned above, and man's exposure to sporangiospores of these fungi must be frequent.

In general, members of the Mucorales cause the more severe forms of disease and the Entomophthorales cause more chronic disease of the nasal mucosa and subcutaneous tissue. Mucormycosis is rare in healthy individuals, unless trauma has provided a portal of entry for the fungus. Lesions usually remain localized around the initial site of the inoculation and respond well to local debridement and antifungal therapy.

Mucormycosis in debilitated patients is acute and fulminate fungal infection. The disease typically involves the rhinofaciocranial area, lungs, gastrointestinal tract, skin or less commonly other organs. **Predisposing factors** include diabetes, metabolic acidosis, hyperglycemia, corticosteroid therapy, immunosuppressive therapy for organ or bone marrow transplantation, neutropenia, trauma, HIV infection, and therapy with deferoxamine (an iron-chelating agent for treatment of iron overload). The latter is probably because Mucorales use this chelator as a siderophore to obtain more iron. One of the most important risk factors is diabetes mellitus, especially when ketoacidosis is present. The increased concentration of glucose stimulates rapid growth of Mucormycetes. It may lead to:

### 1. Rhinocerebral mucormycosis

This is the most serious and fulminating type of disease. It is usually associated with acute, uncontrolled diabetes mellitus or acidosis. Other predisposing factors include steroid-induced hyperglycemia, especially in patients with leukaemia and lymphoma, renal transplant recipients, and those receiving concomitant treatment with corticosteroids and azathioprine, and in patients with chronic alcoholism.

The infection begins in the nasal mucosa and extends to the palate, paranasal sinuses, orbit, face, and brain. Patient develops acute sinusitis mimicking bacterial sinusitis with fever, unilateral headache, nasal or sinus congestion or pain, and a serosanguineous nasal discharge. A direct examination of nasal discharge often reveals broad irregular hyphae. Other symptoms include orbital pain, diplopia, ophthalmoplegia, proptosis of the eye, lid edema, conjunctivitis, and ulceration of cornea.

Fungus has a predilection for invading blood vessels and nerves rather than muscles. This leads to infarction of the invaded areas and extension into the brain. Most human cases of rhinocerebral mucormycosis are caused by *R. arrhizus* (previously referred to as *R. orizae*).

### 2. Pulmonary mucormycosis

Pulmonary mucormycosis develops by inhalation of sporangiospores into the bronchioles and alveoli, leading to rapidly progressive bronchopneumonia, segmental or lobar consolidation, signs of cavitation and rarely pleural effusion. Haematogenous dissemination to other organs, particularly the brain, often occurs.

### 3. Gastrointestinal mucormycosis

This is acquired by ingestion of food contaminated with the fungal elements. Ulceration of gastric mucosa with thrombosis of associated vessels occurs. Invasive gastrointestinal mucormycosis has been reported in liver, renal and heart transplant patients, and in neonates. Lesions are most common in the stomach, colon, and ileum. Intestinal infections are usually fatal within 2–3 weeks as a result of bowel infarction, sepsis or haemorrhagic shock.

### 4. Disseminated mucormycosis

The Mucormycetes may become widely disseminated affecting lungs, kidneys, gastrointestinal tract, heart and brain. It is usually seen in neutropenic patients with pulmonary infection and less commonly from gastrointestinal tract, burns, or other cutaneous lesions.

### 5. Cutaneous mucormycosis

Cutaneous mucormycosis is usually caused by the traumatic implantation of fungal elements through the skin especially in patients with extensive burns, diabetes, or steroid-induced hyperglycemia. This leads to a chronic indolent ulcer. It may resolve spontaneously or extend into subcutaneous tissue and become rapidly progressive. Occasionally, the mold can be seen growing on the edge of the wound.

## LABORATORY DIAGNOSIS

### Clinical material

Sputum and needle biopsy from pulmonary lesions, bronchoalveolar lavage fluid, nasal discharges, scrapings and aspirates from sinuses in patients with rhinocerebral lesions, skin scrapings from cutaneous lesions, and biopsy tissue from patients with gastrointestinal and/or disseminated disease.

Mucorales have coenocytic hyphae that will often be damaged and become nonviable during the biopsy procedure (especially scrapings and aspirates), or by the chopping up or tissue grinding process in the laboratory. This is why these fungi which are clearly visible in direct microscopic or histopathologic mounts are often difficult to grow in culture from clinical specimens.

If on clinical and/or radiological evidence mucormycosis is suspected then try to avoid excessive tissue damage when collecting the specimen and in the laboratory the tissue should be gently teased apart and inoculate directly onto the isolation media. **Therefore, a positive direct microscopy, especially from a sterile site, should be considered significant, even if the laboratory is unable to culture the fungus.**

### *Direct microscopy*

The specimen should be observed with a microscope after mounting the material in a few drops of 10–20% potassium hydroxide (KOH) and gently heating the slide to clear the tissue. Broad (7–15 μm), nonseptate hyphae with non-parallel walls can be seen. Chlamydoconidia (15–30 μm in diameter) that may resemble yeast cells and distorted hyphae are often seen. Branching differs from that of *Aspergillus* spp. by the fact that it occurs frequently at a 90° angle to the main hyphae. In acute aspergillosis the hyphae are septate 3–5 μm in diameter with characteristic dichotomous branching. The hyphae have a tendency to branch repeatedly. The branches arise at an angle of 45°.

### *Histopathology*

Tissue sections should be stained with haematoxylin and eosin (H&E), Gomori methenamine silver (GMS) and periodic acid-Schiff (PAS) stains. The characteristic pathological changes in mucormycosis are suppuration and necrosis. Mucormycetes have a predilection for invasion of blood vessels, causing thrombosis and infarction. In tissues, the organisms appear as irregularly branched, nonseptate, very broad hyphae (7–15 μm in diameter). Unlike *Aspergillus* spp. mycelium, Mucormycetes hyphae are usually clearly visible in H&E-stained sections. On the other hand, the colouration by special fungus stains such as Gridley, PAS and in some cases GMS may be very poor (Figs. 20.1 and 20.2).

True septa are rarely seen in the hyphae but under low magnification, cross folds in the walls of the hyphae may resemble septa. Occasionally, sporangia with well-delineated columellae and sporangiospores may be seen in tissue sections of nasal and pulmonary

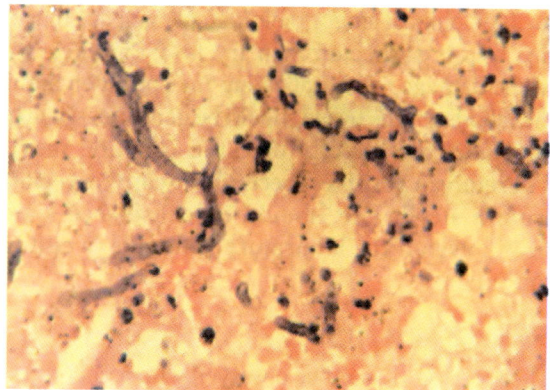

**Fig. 20.1.** Mucormycosis showing broad nonseptate hyphae in H&E staining (×400).

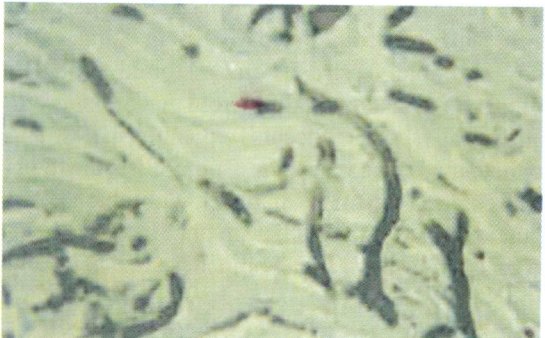

**Fig. 20.2.** Section stained by Gomori methenamine silver stain (×400) showing broad nonseptate hyphae.

tissue that are well-aerated. Mucorales do not sporulate in tissue unless there is an air interface. Cross-sections of large hyphae in tissue can superficially resemble yeast cells similar to that seen with *Aspergillus* infection. In tissues, aspergillosis can be easily differentiated from mucormycosis in its uniform dichotomous pattern of branching, the presence of many septa and its much easier detection by the special stains than the routine H&E stain.

### Culture

Members of the order Mucorales grow on most routine fungal culture media provided they do not contain cycloheximide. The use of antibacterial antibiotics such as chloramphenicol and gentamicin in primary isolation media is recommended to prevent bacterial contamination. Sabouraud dextrose agar (SDA) containing antibacterial antibiotics is used as primary isolation medium. Most mucoraceous species are fast growing and sporulate profusely.

Growth is rapid and usually visible after 24 hours of incubation at 25–37°C. Growth matures within 4 days. The colony quickly covers agar surface with dense growth that is cotton candy-like. Colonies are white at first and then gray or yellowish brown. Reverse is white.

Some genera produce root-like rhizoids connected by hyphae called stolons. Asexual reproductive structures are important characters for identification purposes. Spores are produced in globose sporangia which develop at the tips of a stalk, the sporangiophore. Most sporangiophores with sporangia are between 500 μm and 2 mm in length, large enough to be seen with the unaided eye. Sporangium has two compartments. The first compartment is the columella, a swollen extension of the sporangiophore that protrudes into the sporangium. The columella is separated from the second or spore-containing compartment by a membrane. During maturation the cytoplasm of the sporangium divides into hundreds of sporangiospores. When the sporangium is mature, the sporangium wall dissolves, releasing the sporangiospores.

Isolation from sputum of *Lichtheimia corymbifera*, and species of *Rhizopus* and *Mucor* must be interpreted with caution. Patients with bronchiectasis may cough up spores of all these fungi, as well as those of *Aspergillus fumigatus* for several days after exposure to them in a dusty environment. If there is no invasion of pulmonary tissue, the sputum is usually free of fungi after the patients have been hospitalized for a few days. Negative cultures can occur as often as 40% of the time. Repeated sampling is useful in cases of negative culture with positive histologic examination.

### Species identification

Species identification of the Mucorales can be carried out by microscopic examination of lactophenol cotton blue mounts.

### *Rhizopus spp.*

These show broad hyphae (6–15 μm in diameter) and have no or very few septa. Numerous stolons run among the mycelia, connecting groups of long sporangiophores that usually are unbranched. At the point where the stolons and sporangiophores meet, rootlike hyphae (rhizoids) are produced. The sporangiophores are long (up to 3 mm) and terminate with a dark, round sporangium (40–275 μm in diameter) containing a columella and many oval, colourless or brown sporangiospores (4–9 μm in diameter) (Fig. 20.3).

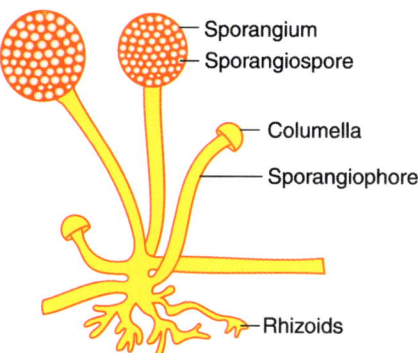

Fig. 20.3. *Rhizopus*.

After sporangiospore release, the apophyses and columella often collapse to form an umbrella-like structure. This genus is differentiated from *Mucor* spp. by presence of rhizoids, and usually unbranched sporangiophores. It is differentiated from *Lichtheimia* (*Absidia*) spp. by the sporangiophores that arise from the stolon in between the rhizoids, and small (20–120 μm in diameter) and slightly pear-shaped sporangia.

### Mucor spp.

Hyphae are wide (6–15 μm) and nonseptate. Sporangiophores arise randomly along aerial mycelium. They are erect, long and often branched without apophyses and with well-developed columellae. They bear terminal globose to spherical sporangiospore-filled sporangia (50–100 μm in diameter). Sporangial wall dissolves, scattering the round or slightly oblong sporangiospores (4–8 μm in diameter), revealing the columella and sometimes leaving a collarette (Fig. 20.4). Sporangiospores are hyaline, gray or brownish, globose to ellipsoidal, and smooth-walled. The genus *Mucor* can be differen-

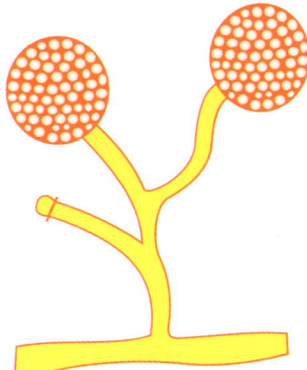

Fig. 20.4. *Mucor*.

tiated from *Lichtheimia*, *Rhizopus* and *Rhizomucor* by the absence of rhizoids.

### Lichtheimia (Absidia) corymbifera

Hyphae are wide (6–15 μm in diameter) and nonseptate. It possesses rhizoids and branched sporangiophores that arise from the stolon in between the rhizoids not opposite them. This feature separates the species of *Lichtheimia* from those of the genus *Rhizopus*, where sporangiophores arise opposite the rhizoids. The sporangiophores are up to 450 μm long and are branched. The sporangia are relatively small (20–90 μm in diameter) and slightly pear-shaped instead of spherical and are supported by a characteristic funnel-shaped apophysis. This distinguishes the genus *Lichtheimia* from the genera *Mucor* and *Rhizomucor*, which have large, globose sporangia without an apophysis. *A. corymbifera* is the only species of *Lichtheimia* known to cause disease in humans and animals (Fig. 20.5).

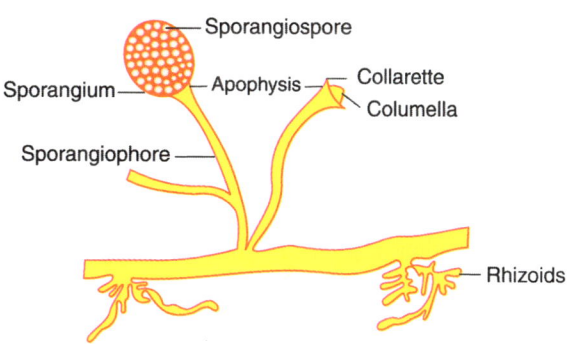

Fig. 20.5. *Lichtheimia*.

## SECTION 5 : Opportunistic Mycoses

### Rhizomucor spp.

These appear to be intermediate between *Rhizopus* and *Mucor* spp. Sporangia are round and are usually 40–100 µm in diameter. They possess a few primitive, short, irregularly branched rhizoids thus differentiating them from *Mucor* spp. They differ from *Rhizopus* spp. by having branched sporangiophores and by the location of rhizoids. Rhizoids may arise at the base of the sporangiophore or at the points between the sporangiophores (Fig. 20.6).

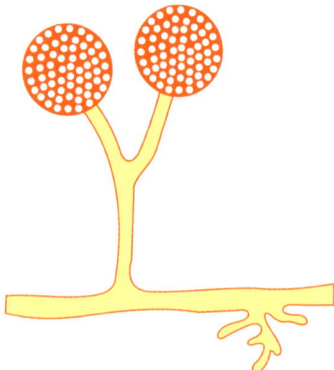

**Fig. 20.6.** *Rhizomucor.*

### Saksenaea vasiformis

On routine media the organism does not sporulate, it only forms broad, mostly nonseptate, branched, hyaline hyphae. For stimulation of sporulation grow the isolate on SDA plate at 25°C for 1 week. Aseptically cut out 1 cm$^2$ agar block permeated with the hyphal growth. Transfer the block to petri plate containing 20 ml of sterile distilled water and 0.2 ml of filter-sterilized 10% yeast extract. Seal the plate to prevent spillage. Incubate the block in water solution at 35–37°C. After 5 days of incubation, a thin film of growth appears over the surface of water. Make wet preparations with lactophenol cotton blue of portions of the film on days 5, 10 and 15 of incubation. Examine microscopically.

Sporangiophores (24–60 µm long) bear sporangia that are flask-shaped (50–150 µm long) having a swollen portion near the base and a long neck that broadens at the apex. Sporangiospores are elongate (3–4 µm long) and smooth. Rhizoids form near the base of sporangiophore and are dichotomously branched (Fig. 20.7), and darken with age.

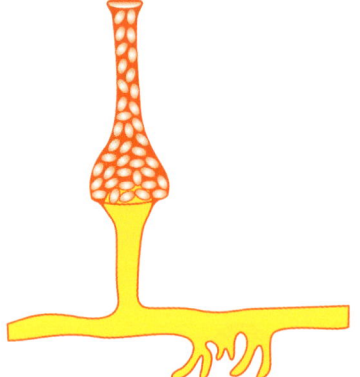

**Fig. 20.7.** *Saksenaea vasiformis.*

### Cunninghamella bertholletiae

It shows broad hyphae, almost nonseptate. Sporangiophores are long, branched and end in swollen vesicles (30–65 µm in diameter). Vesicles on lateral branches are smaller (14–35 µm in diameter). The vesicles are covered with spine-like denticles, each supporting a round to oval sporangiolum (5–8 × 6–14 µm). Each sporangiolum contains one spore (Fig. 20.8). Rhizoids may be seen. Zygospores and chlamydoconidia may also be formed.

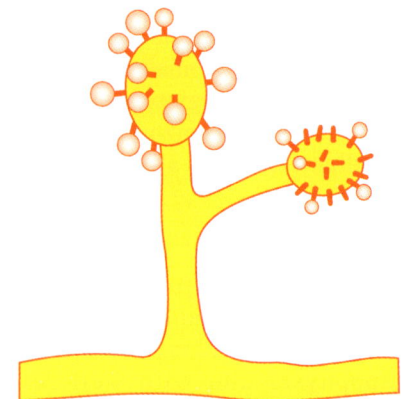

**Fig. 20.8.** *Cunninghamella bertholletiae.*

### Apophysomyces elegans

On routine culture media only broad, almost non-septate hyphae (4–8 µm in diameter) are seen. For stimulation of sporulation same method is used as in case of *Saksenaea vasiformis*. Sporangiophores are

164

unbranched, straight or curved, slightly tapering towards the apex. They are up to 530 μm long. Sporangiophores arise singly at right angles from the aerial hyphae and often have a septate basal segment resembling the 'foot cell' commonly seen in *Aspergillus* spp. The apex of the sporangiophore widens to form a funnel-shaped apophysis (11–40 μm in diameter at widest part) and hemispherical columella. Sporangia are small (20–55 μm in diameter) and typically pyriform in shape. Sporangiospores are smooth, mostly oblong (5 × 8 μm in length) and may appear pale brown in mass. Rhizoids are thin-walled and may be between the points of origin of the sporangiophores or opposite the sporangiophore (Fig. 20.9).

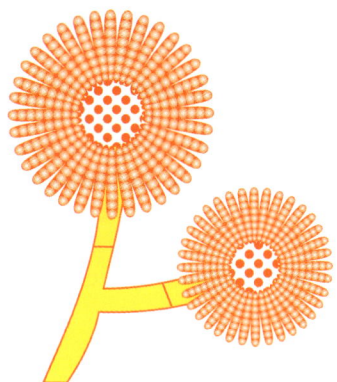

**Fig. 20.10.** *Syncephalastrum racemosum*.

- Antifungal drugs – only amphotericin B and posaconazole – have anti-*Mucor* activity. Early administration of lipid formulations of amphotericin B at high dose (3–5 mg/kg/day) is recommended.
- Reversal of risk factors – control of diabetes, reduction of steroid dose to minimum requirement, recovery of neutropenia after granulocyte transfusion.

## ORDER: ENTOMOPHTHORALES

Entomophthorales are classified into six families with 22 genera containing 132 species. However, *Basidiobolus ranarum*, *Conidiobolus coronatus*, and *C. incongruus* are the only species that are known to cause human disease. They cause entomophthoromycosis, which is chronic granulomatous subcutaneous, mucocutaneous and visceral infection.

In contrast to members of the order Mucorales, which cause acute, angioinvasive infections among immunocompromised patients with very high mortality, Entomophthorales cause chronic subcutaneous, mucocutaneous and visceral infections mainly in immunocompetent patients. These are prevalent in India, China and Thailand. Entomophthoromycosis has a much better prognosis than infections caused by Mucorales.

### Basidiobolus ranarum

*B. ranarum*, etiologic agent of entomophthoromycosis basidiobolae, occurs as a saprophyte in soil,

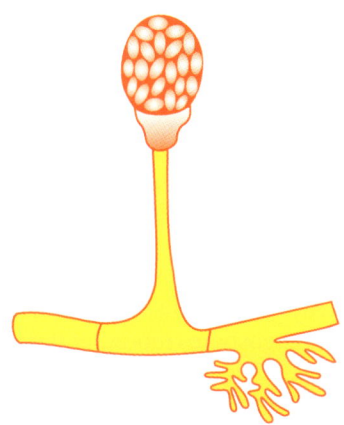

**Fig. 20.9.** *Apophysomyces elegans*.

### Syncephalastrum racemosum

Hyphae are broad (4–10 μm in diameter) and almost nonseptate. Sporangiospores are short and branched and terminate in a large round vesicle. On the vesicle are borne chains of round spores enclosed in fingerlike tubular sporangia (4–6 × 9–60 μm). Rhizoids are usually formed. Tubular sporangia and absence of phialides differentiate *S. racemosum* from *Aspergillus* (Fig. 20.10).

### Treatment

- Aggressive surgery wherever possible to minimize fungal load and to remove necrosed tissue so that antifungal drug may reach the site of fungal infection.

decaying fruit and vegetable matter, and in the intestinal contents of various insectivorous reptiles (lizards, chameleons), amphibian (toads), and mammals (bats, kangaroos, and wallabies). Infection due to *B. ranarum* is reported mainly in tropical areas of Asia (India, Indonesia and Myanmar), Africa (Uganda, Nigeria, Cameroon, Togo, Ivory Coast, Sudan, Senegal, Somalia and Kenya), South America (mainly Brazil), North America (Mexico) and Australia.

### Pathogenesis

The portal of entry of *B. ranarum* is believed to be the skin after insect bites, scratches, and minor cuts. It causes entomophthoromycosis basidiobolae, which is a chronic inflammatory or granulomatous disease generally restricted to limbs, chest, back, or buttocks. The lesions are huge, palpable, hard, non-ulcerating subcutaneous masses. Occasionally, it may cause gastrointestinal infections.

## Conidiobolus coronatus

*C. coronatus*, etiologic agent of entomophthoromycosis conidiobolae, is found as a saprophyte in soil, decaying vegetation, and in the gastrointestinal tract of lizards and toads. It has been reported from tropical portions of Africa (mostly Cameroon and Nigeria, but also Chad, Zaire, Kenya, Central African Republic, Guinea) and the Americas (Costa Rica, Caribbean islands, Columbia, Brazil).

### Pathogenesis

The spores are believed to enter the body by inhalation. It causes entomophthoromycosis conidiobolae, which is a chronic inflammatory or granulomatous disease usually restricted to the nasal mucosa. It can spread to adjacent subcutaneous tissue and cause disfigurement of the face. The disease is characterized by polyps or palpable subcutaneous masses. Rarely, it may cause deeply invasive, life-threatening infections.

### Laboratory diagnosis

#### KOH mount

A piece of biopsy tissue is mounted in 10% KOH on a glass slide, teased apart, and gently heated to dissolve the tissue prior to microscopic examination. It shows broad 5–15 µm wide, infrequently septate, thin-walled hyphae.

#### Histopathology

Tissue sections should be stained with H&E, PAS and GMS. H&E-stained sections are best to observe thin-walled hyphae surrounded by an eosinophilic sheath (**Splendore-Hoeppli material**).

#### Culture

Biopsy tissue should be inoculated onto SDA containing antibacterial antibiotics, but without cycloheximide. Both *Basidiobolus* and *Conidiobolus* grow rapidly. Growth matures within 5 days.

**Basidiobolus ranarum:** The colony is thin, flat, waxy, buff to gray. It becomes heaped up or radially folded, grayish brown. After several days the colony is covered with white aerial hyphae. Reverse is white.

Lactophenol cotton blue (LPCB) mount shows wide (8–20 µm in diameter) hyphae forming numerous round (20–50 µm in diameter), smooth, thick-walled intercalary zygospores that have two closely appressed beak-like appendages (Fig. 20.11A).

The zygospores are formed after the conjugation of two adjacent hyphal cells. Beak-like appendages attached to the zygospores represent the remnants of the conjugation tubes. The production of 'beaked' zygospores is diagnostic of the genus.

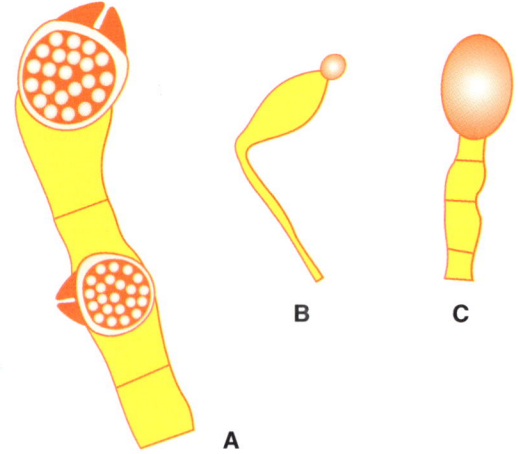

Fig. 20.11. *Basidiobolus ranarum*: (A) Zygospore, (B) Primary spore, (C) Secondary spore.

# Mucormycosis

Two types of asexual spores are formed – primary and secondary. Primary spores are globose, one-celled, solitary, and forcebly discharged from a sporophore. The sporophore has a distinct swollen area just below the spore, which actively participates in the discharge of the spore. Secondary spores are clavate, one-celled, have a knob-like adhesive tip and are passively released from a sporophore which is not swollen at its base. These spores can function as sporangia producing more sporangiophores.

**Conidiobolus coronatus:** Colonies grow rapidly and are flat, waxy, buff or gray, becoming radially folded. They become sparsely covered with short white aerial hyphae. Sides of culture tube or the lid of the petri dish soon become covered with conidia that were forcibly discharged by the conidiophores. The colour of the colony may become tan to brown with age.

LPCB mount shows hyphae which have few septa. Conidiophores are unbranched. They bear terminal conidia, which are spherical, 24–40 μm in diameter, multinucleate, single-celled and have a broad, tapering projection. A conidium may also develop a number of short extensions that give rise to a corona of secondary conidia. Conidia may also produce short, hairlike appendages (Fig. 20.12).

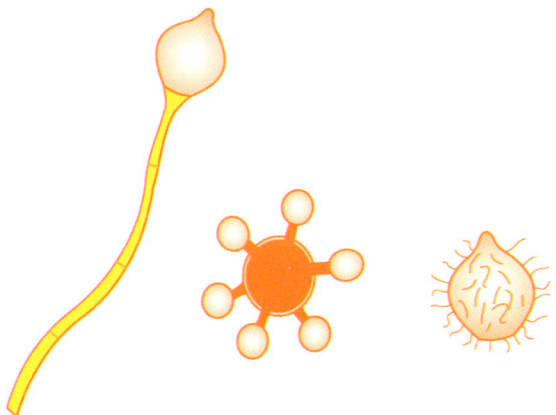

**Fig. 20.12.** *Conidiobolus coronatus.*

## Serological tests

Antibodies against both *Basidiobolus* and *Conidiobolus* spp. can be detected by immunodiffusion test.

## Treatment

The best management consists of aggressive surgical treatment combined with amphotericin B and control of predisposing factors when possible.

### Important Questions

1. Classify fungi causing mucormycosis. Discuss predisposing factors, pathogenesis and laboratory diagnosis of mucormycosis.
2. Discuss morphology and cultural characteristics of fungi causing mucormycosis.
3. Discuss briefly causative agents, pathogenesis and laboratory diagnosis of entomophthoromycosis.

### Multiple Choice Questions

1. Rhizoids are absent in:
   (a) *Lichtheimia.*
   (b) *Rhizopus.*
   (c) *Rhizomucor.*
   (d) *Mucor.*
2. The sporangia are supported by apophysis in:
   (a) *Lichtheimia.*
   (b) *Mucor.*
   (c) *Rhizomucor.*
   (d) All of the above.
3. Formation of numerous round, smooth, thick-walled intercalary zygospores that have two closely appressed beak-like appendages is diagnostic of:
   (a) *Conidiobolus coronatus.*
   (b) *Basidiobolus ranarum.*
   (c) *Apophysomyces elegans.*
   (d) *Cunninghamella bertholletiae.*
4. Which of the following fungi **does not** belong to order Mucorales?
   (a) *Mucor.*
   (b) *Lichtheimia.*
   (c) *Rhizopus.*
   (d) *Conidiobolus.*
5. Mucormycosis is caused by:
   (a) *Rhizopus arrhizus.*
   (b) *Basidiobolus ranarum.*
   (c) *Conidiobolus coronatus.*
   (d) All of the above.

## SECTION 5 : Opportunistic Mycoses

6. Hyphae of which of the following fungi are damaged and become nonviable during biopsy procedure or by tissue grinding process in the laboratory?
   (a) *Aspergillus fumigatus*.
   (b) *Penicillium marneffei*.
   (c) *Coccidioides immitis*.
   (d) Mucorales.

7. In which of the following fungi hyphae branch at an angle of 45°?
   (a) *Aspergillus* spp.
   (b) *Rhizopus* spp.
   (c) *Mucor* spp.
   (d) *Lichtheimia* spp.

8. In the tissue, aspergillosis can be differentiated from mucormycosis by:
   (a) uniform dichotomous pattern of branching of hyphae.
   (b) presence of many septa.
   (c) much easier detection by special stains than the routine H&E stain.
   (d) All of the above.

9. Which of the following statements best describes the growth of Mucorales?
   (a) Rapid grower.
   (b) Cannot grow at 37°C.
   (c) Requires enriched medium.
   (d) Slow grower.

10. Sporangiophores that are unbranched with rhizoids opposite the sporangiophores describes which Mucorales species?
    (a) *Cunninghamella bertholletiae*.
    (b) *Mucor circinelloides*.
    (c) *Lichtheimia corymbifera*.
    (d) *Rhizopus oryzae*.

11. The most common species isolated from a case of mucormycosis is:
    (a) *Cunninghamella bertholletiae*.
    (b) *Mucor* spp.
    (c) *Rhizomucor* spp.
    (d) *Rhizopus oryzae*.

12. In H&E staining thin-walled hyphae surrounded by eosinophilic sheath are seen in:
    (a) entomophthoromycosis.
    (b) hyalohyphomycosis.
    (c) aspergillosis.
    (d) penicilliosis.

### ANSWERS TO MCQs

1. (d), 2. (a), 3. (b), 4. (d), 5. (a), 6. (d), 7. (a), 8. (d), 9. (a), 10. (d), 11. (d), 12. (a).

### Further Reading

1. Abdel-Naser NB, Yousef N, et al. Invasive zygomycosis with a fatal outcome. *Arch Dermatol* 2005; 141: 1211–3.
2. Al Jarie A, Al-Mohsen I, et al. Pediatric gastrointestinal basidiobolomycosis. *Pediatr Infect Dis J* 2003; 22: 1007–14.
3. Benbow EW, Stodart RW. Systemic zygomycosis. *Postgraduate Med J* 1986; 62: 985–96.
4. Bittencourt AL, Marback R, Nossa LM. Mucocutaneous entomophthoromycosis acquired by conjunctival inoculation of the fungus. *Am J Trop Med Hyg* 2006; 75: 936–8.
5. Bouza E, Munoz P, Guinea J. Mucormycosis: an emerging disease? *Clin Microbiol Infect* 2006; 12 (Suppl. 7): 7–23.
6. Chayakulkeeree M, Ghannoum MA, Perfect JR. Zygomycosis: the re-emerging fungal infection. *Eur J Clin Microbiol Infect Dis* 2006; 25: 215–9.
7. Dammin TC. Orbital mucormycosis. *N Engl J Med* 2002; 347: 855–6.
8. Freifeld AG, Iwen PC. Zygomycosis. *Semin Respir Crit Care Med* 2004; 25: 221–31.
9. Godara SM, Kute VB, et al. Mucormycosis in renal transplant recipients: predictors and outcome. *Saudi J Kidney Dis Transpl* 2011; 22: 751–6.
10. Hammond SP, Bialek R, et al. Molecular methods to improve diagnosis and identification of mucormycosis. *J Clin Microbiol* 2011; 49: 2151–3.
11. Hernandez MJ, Landaeta W, et al. Subcutaneous zygomycosis due to *Conidiobolus incongruus*. *Int J Infect Dis* 2007; 11: 468–9.
12. Hoogendijk CF, van Heerden WF, et al. Rhino-orbitocerebral entomophthoromycosis. *Int J Oral Maxillofac Surg* 2006; 35: 277–80.

13. Kaufman CA. Zygomycosis: re-emergence of an old pathogen. *Clin Infect Dis* 2004; 39: 588–90.
14. Lanternier F, Sun HY, et al. Mucormycosis in organ and stem cell transplant recipients. *Clin Infect Dis* 2012; 54: 1629–36.
15. Prasad PA, Vaghan AM, Zaoutis TE. Trends in zygomycosis in children. *Mycoses* 2012; 55: 352–6.
16. Petrikkos G, Skiada A, et al. Epidemiology and clinical manifestations of mucormycosis. *Clin Infect Dis* 2012; 54 (Suppl 1): S23–S34.
17. Pyrgos V, Shoham S, Walsh TJ. Pulmonary zygomycosis. *Semin Respir Crit Care Med* 2008; 29: 111–20.
18. Sundaram C, Mahadevan A, et al. Cerebral zygomycosis. *Mocoses* 2005; 48: 396–407.
19. Zaoutis TE, Roilides E, et al. Zygomycosis in children: a systemic review and analysis of reported cases. *Pediatr Infect Dis J* 2007; 26: 723–7.

# CHAPTER 21

# Hyalohyphomycosis

The term hyalohyphomycosis is used for infections caused by molds that lack melanin in their cell walls, form colourless (hyaline), septate hyphae in host tissue and which do not have other specific, well-established names, such as aspergillosis. Hyphae are parallel-walled, typically showing irregular branching at both 45° and 90°. They measure 2–8 µm in diameter. Colony colour varies widely, but is never darkly pigmented. Presently, more than 20 genera and 70 species of fungi are the known causative agents of hyalohyphomycosis. Common causative agents are given in Table 21.1.

**Table 21.1.** Common causative agents of hyalohyphomycosis

| More common fungi | Less common fungi |
|---|---|
| • *Fusarium* spp.<br>• *Penicillium* spp.<br>• *Scedosporium* spp.<br>• *Paecilomyces* spp.<br>• *Acremonium* spp.<br>• *Scopulariopsis* spp. | • *Beauveria* spp.<br>• *Chaetoconidium* spp.<br>• *Chrysosporium* spp.<br>• *Myriodontium keratinophilum*<br>• *Neurospora sitophila*<br>• *Trichoderma* spp. |

## PATHOGENESIS

Hyalohyphomycetes or hyaline filamentous fungi are normally found as saprophytes in soil and vegetative matter and are opportunistic pathogens. They cause superficial, deep tissue, and disseminated infections. Deep infections may involve the lungs, sinuses, heart, liver, spleen, kidney, bones or central nervous system. These are commonly acquired through the respiratory tract, gastrointestinal tract (e.g., after major surgery), or blood vessels (e.g., catheter-related). Infection may remain localized in deep tissue and organs, or may disseminate haematogenously or via lymphatic system. Disseminated infections tend to occur among severely immunocompromised patients such as those undergoing transplantation and patients with acquired immunodeficiency syndrome. Following penetrating trauma localized infections may occur in otherwise healthy individuals.

The most common tissue responses are acute inflammation and necrosis with occasional granulomatous inflammation. Invasion of blood vessels with subsequent thrombosis and infarction also occurs.

## Fusarium spp.

*Fusarium* species are common fungi found worldwide in soil, in plant debris, and as important pathogens. These fungi produce potent mycotoxins (fumonisins, trichothecenes). In immune-normal persons it may cause nail infections, keratitis, and secondary infections in burn patients. In immunocompromised hosts it may cause haematogenously disseminated disease with skin lesions, invasive sinusitis, nail infections with paronychia, and pulmonary infection.

*Fusarium* mycosis is noncommunicable. Conidia are inhaled, ingested or acquired through a penetrating injury or burn. Aerosols from hospital water supply or other water source may be involved in transmission. Conidia may be introduced by walking barefoot and by local abrasions leading to nail infections and, rarely, tinea pedis.

*F. solani* is the most common species recovered from clinical specimens followed by *F. oxysporum*, *F. verticillioides* and *F. proliferatum*. *Fusarium* spp., after aspergillosis, are the second most common cause of invasive mold mycosis in haematologic malignancy and stem cell transplant patients.

## Acremonium spp.

*Acremonium* spp. are extremely common in man's environment, found in soil, decaying vegetation, and food stuffs. They have been identified as the pathogens in cases of mycetoma, keratomycosis, postoperative endophthalmitis and onychomycosis.

## Paecilomyces spp.

*Paecilomyces* spp. are widespread soil saprophytes. These have been associated with ocular mycosis, endocarditis, sinusitis, nephritis, cutaneous infection, and infection of the lacrimal sac. Unlike *Fusarium* the majority of infections caused by *Paecilomyces* spp. have occurred in immunocompetent patients.

## Scopulariopsis spp.

*Scopulariopsis* spp. cause infection of nails (usually toe nails) and are rarely associated with subcutaneous and invasive infection. They are also commonly encountered as contaminants.

## Penicillium spp.

*Penicillium* spp. are among the most common laboratory contaminants. However, they are known to cause corneal, cutaneous, external ear, respiratory and urinary tract infections, and endocarditis after insertion of valve prostheses. Disseminated disease may occur in severely immunocompromised patients.

When *Penicillium* is isolated from a patient, a diagnosis of penicilliosis can be confirmed only if the fungus has been demonstrated in tissue sections.

## LABORATORY DIAGNOSIS

Hyalohyphomycetes are commonly encountered as laboratory contaminants. Furthermore, isolation of fungus, particularly from respiratory tract, may simply represent colonization. Therefore, a positive culture from a nonsterile site, such as sputum, must be interpreted with caution. Histological detection of hyphae in normally sterile body fluids and/or tissue sections is essential for definitive diagnosis.

### Direct microscopy

Sputum, bronchial washings, aspirates, skin scrapings, skin biopsy, nail clippings, and corneal specimens should be examined using 10% KOH and Parker ink (1 : 1), Gram stain, or, preferably, a fluorescent chitin dye such as calcofluor white. Centrifuged deposit of body fluids and exudates should be examined microscopically.

### Histopathology

Tissue sections should be stained with haematoxylin and eosin (H&E), periodic acid-Schiff (PAS) and Gomori methenamine silver (GMS) stains. Hyalohyphomycetes are poorly stained with H&E. In histological sections various genera of hyaline molds, and agents of hyalohyphomycosis cannot be distinguished.

The hyphae of hyalohyphomycetes are usually irregular and haphazardly arranged. They measure 2–8 μm in diameter, and exhibit branching at both 45° and 90°. In tissue sections, hyalohyphomycetes can be differentiated from *Aspergillus* by pattern of branching at both 45° and 90°. All hyalohyphomycetes differ from Mucorales in forming hyphae that are narrower, and are regularly septate (Fig. 21.1). They differ from *Aspergillus*, Mucorales and Entomophorales in having the capacity to produce conidia and phialides within a closed lesion. Phialides usually appear as tapering structures along the sides or at the ends of the hyphae. The conidia commonly have a rounded apex and a flat basal scar when detached.

# SECTION 5: Opportunistic Mycoses

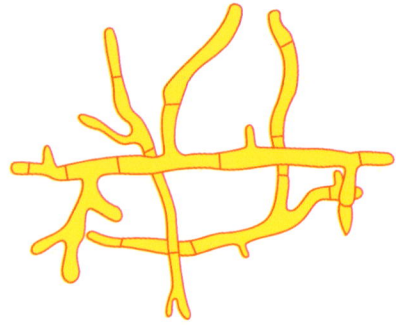

**Fig. 21.1.** Hyalohyphomycetes in tissues.

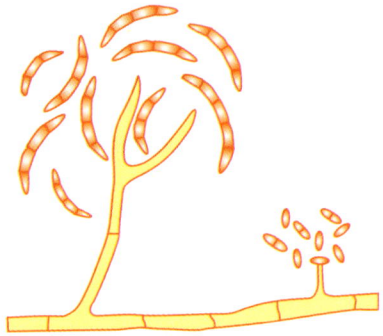

**Fig. 21.2.** *Fusarium* spp.

## Culture

Culture is almost always required for definitive identification of the causative agent of hyalohyphomycosis. All specimens (sputum, bronchial washings, aspirates, and biopsy tissue) should be cultured on Sabouraud dextrose agar (SDA). **Cycloheximide should not be added to SDA since many hyalohyphomycetes are sensitive to this compound.** Some organisms grow rather slowly, therefore, cultures should be incubated for 4–6 weeks, at 30°C. Definitive identification of the etiologic agents can be accomplished using macroscopic and microscopic morphology.

## *Fusarium* spp.

Colonies of majority of species of *Fusarium* grow rapidly. Growth matures within 4 days. Initially colonies are white and cottony, but often quickly develop a pink or violet centre with a lighter periphery. Reverse may be pale but can darken to purple, red, green, blue, or brown as culture matures. Lactophenol cotton blue mount shows septate hyphae. There are two types of conidiations:

1. Unbranched or branched conidiophores with phialides that produce large (2–6 × 14–80 µm) smooth sickle-shaped macroconidia with 3–5 transverse septa.
2. Long or short simple conidiophores bearing small (2–4 × 4–8 µm), smooth, oval microconidia. They are generally unicellular, although two- or three-celled varieties are occasionally observed. Microconidia are borne singly or in clusters (Fig. 21.2). Chlamydoconidia may be present in some species.

## *Scedosporium* spp.

Infections are caused by two species – *S. apiospermum* and *S. prolificans*. The latter is regarded as dematiaceous (darkly pigmented) fungus. It is classified as an agent of **phaeohyphomycosis**. *S. apiospermum* is the asexual state of teleomorph *Pseudallescheria boydii*, which is homothallic (sexual reproduction requiring only a single organism).

*S. apiospermum* causes sinusitis, pneumonia, and disseminated infections in immunocompromised hosts and mycetoma in immunocompetent patients. Pneumonia due to *S. apiospermum* is clinically indistinguishable from that due to *Aspergillus* spp. As with pulmonary aspergillosis, dissemination complicating *S. apiospermum* pneumonia often involves the central nervous system. Access to the brain can be haematogenous or spread from a sinus, or it can be due to trauma. Meningitis due to *Scedosporium* is rare and usually associated with immunosuppression.

On SDA the colonies of *S. apiospermum* grow rapidly (40 mm within 7–10 days). The sexual stage (*P. boydii*) is inhibited by cycloheximide but the asexual stage (*S. apiospermum*) is not inhibited. The surface of the colony has a spreading, white, cottony aerial mycelium which later turns gray or brown. The reverse is at first white but usually becomes gray or black.

Microscopically, the hyphae are septate (2–4 µm in diameter), with simple long or short conidiophores bearing conidia singly or in small groups. The conidia are unicellular, smooth and oval with the broader end towards the apex and appear cut off at the base. They measure 3–5 μm in diameter. They are initially colourless or pale but with age they become brown and thick-walled (Fig. 21.3A). In the sexual stage (the teleomorph *P. boydii*), large brown cleistothecia (fruiting bodies) 50–250 μm in diameter which contain asci and ascospores are produced (Fig. 21.3B). However, it is rare for clinical strains to produce these sexual structures, prolonged incubation may be required to induce their formation. The sexual stage may sometimes be induced by culturing on cornmeal agar or potato dextrose agar. Cleistothecia are most likely formed in the centre of the colony.

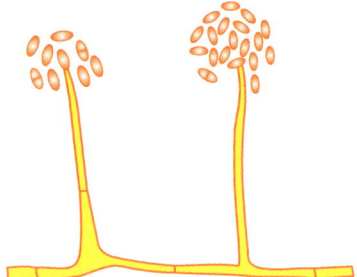

Fig. 21.4. *Acremonium* spp.

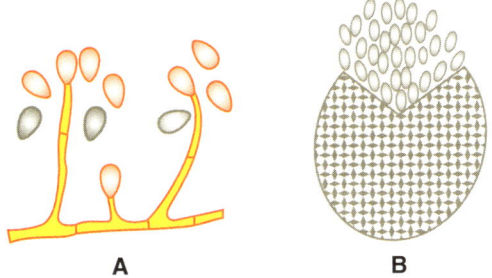

Fig. 21.3. *Scedosporium apiospermum*.

and taper to a long, slender tube. They bend away from the axis of the conidiophore and may appear singly along the hyphae. The conidia (2–4 × 2.5–5 μm) are elliptical or oblong (Fig. 21.5), representing **basipetal** conidiation in which each new conidium is formed directly from the tip of the phialide, pushing the previous conidium ahead of it. The older conidia at the tip are larger and more deeply staining.

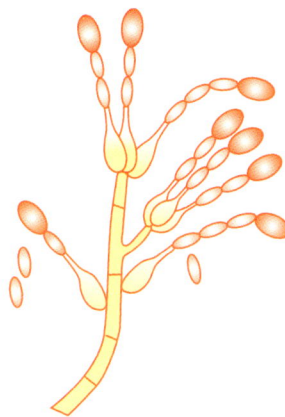

Fig. 21.5. *Paecilomyces* spp.

### Acremonium spp.

*Acremonium* spp. have moderate growth (generally slower than *Fusarium* spp.) on SDA without cycloheximide. The colonies are white-gray or rose in colour, with a velvety to cottony surface. Reverse is colourless, pale yellow, or pinkish. Microscopically, hyphae are septate. Phialides are erect, unbranched, tapering, and form directly on the fine, narrow hyphae, some of them have a septum at the base delimiting them from the hyphae. Conidia are oblong (2–3 × 4–8 μm) and usually one-celled but occasionally two-celled. The conidia form easily disrupted clusters at the tips of the phialides (Fig. 21.4).

### Paecilomyces spp.

*Paecilomyces* spp. grow rapidly (mature within 3 days) on SDA without cycloheximide. Colonies are at first floccose and white, becoming brownish or violet; the texture is woolly or powdery. Reverse is off-white, pinkish, yellow, or pale brown. Microscopically, it resembles *Penicillium* spp., but the phialides of *Paecilomyces* spp. are more elongated

### Scopulariopsis spp.

*Scopulariopsis* spp. produce rapidly growing colonies; mature within 5 days. The surface of the colonies is at first white and glabrous and then usually becomes powdery light brown with a light tan periphery. The reverse of the colony is usually tan with brownish centre. Microscopically, it shows septate hyphae. The conidiogenous cells (annellides) are produced from unbranched or branched "penicillus-like" conidiophores. Conidia are in chains with the youngest conidium at the base of the chain next to the tip of annellide. The conidia are rounded (4–9 μm in diameter), thick-walled, rough and spiny when mature, sometimes slightly pointed at the apex, and are cut off at the base, forming a short neck (Fig. 21.6). Sharp focus of the microscope objective may reveal a short rodlike connection between adjacent conidia. *Scopulariopsis* spp. can be distinguished from *Penicillium* spp. by their thick-walled, lemon-shaped annelloconidia, typically with truncate bases.

phores that have secondary branches known as metulae. On the metulae, arranged in whorls, are flask-shaped phialides that bear unbranched chains of smooth or rough, round conidia (2.5–5 μm in diameter). The entire structure forms characteristic "brush" appearance (Fig. 21.7).

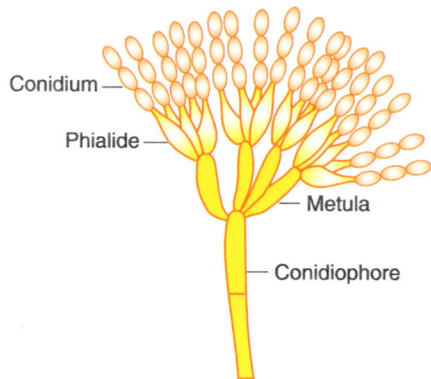

Fig. 21.7. *Penicillium* spp.

### *Beauveria bassiana*

*Beauveria bassiana* can cause keratitis following invasive procedures on the eye. It grows rapidly on SDA (growth matures within 4 days). Surface is white to cream, occasionally pinkish, fluffy to powdery. Reverse is white. Microscopically, hyphae are septate, narrow and delicate. Conidia-producing structures are flask-shaped, with a narrow zigzag terminal extension bearing a conidium at each bent point on a tiny denticle. Conidia are small (2–4 μm in diameter), and round to oval (Fig. 21.8).

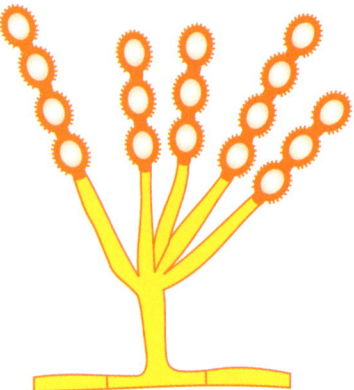

Fig. 21.6. *Scopulariopsis* spp.

### *Penicillium* spp.

There are more than 250 species of genus *Penicillium*. They occur as saprophytes in the soil and decomposing organic debris. However, some species are implicated in causing allergic fungal infections and mycotoxicosis. *P. marneffei* is an important pathogen encountered in immunocompromised patients (see Chapter 18). Non-*marneffei* spp. of genus *Penicillium* (*P. brevicompactum*, *P. chrysogenum*, *P. citrinum*, *P. commune*, *P. crustaceum*, *P. decumbens*, *P. dupontii*, *P. funiculosum*, *P. glaucum* and *P. purpurogenum*) may be occasionally seen as causative agents of hyalohyphomycosis among patients with underlying predisposing conditions.

*Penicillium* spp. show rapid growth (mature within 4 days) on SDA without cycloheximide. It usually shows no or poor growth at 37°C. Colony surface at first is white, then becomes very powdery and bluish green with a white border. Reverse is usually white, but may be red or brown.

Microscopically, hyphae are septate (1.5–5 μm in diameter) with branched or unbranched conidio-

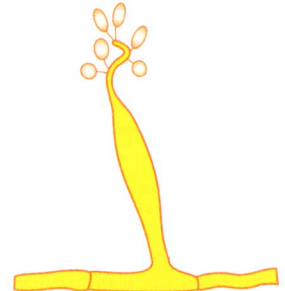

Fig. 21.8. *Beauveria bassiana*.

### *Chrysosporium* spp.

*Chrysosporium* spp. have been reported to cause disseminated disease and invasive sinusitis among immunocompromised hosts. In healthy individuals they may cause keratitis, pulmonary granulomas, endocarditis and osteomyelitis.

Growth is moderately rapid (matures within 6 days). Surface of the colony is cottony or powdery, flat or raised. It is usually white, yellow or tan but may be pink or slightly orange. Reverse is usually white, yellow, tan, or brown. Microscopically, it shows septate hyphae. Conidia may form directly on the hyphae or at the ends of simple or branched short or long conidiophores. Conidia are clavate (2–9 × 3–13 µm), with rounded apex and broad flattened base (Fig. 21.9).

Conidiophores are short and often branched at wide angles. Phialides are flask-shaped. Conidia are round (3–4 µm in diameter) or slightly oval (2–3 × 2.5–5 µm) and clustered together at the end of each phialide (Fig. 21.10).

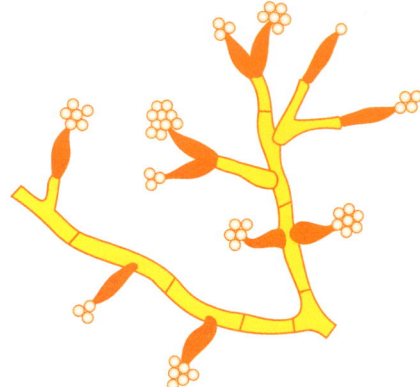

Fig. 21.10. *Trichoderma* spp.

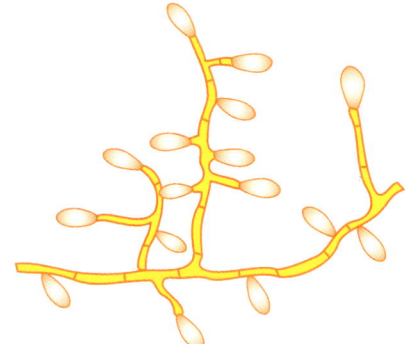

Fig. 21.9. *Chrysosporium* spp.

### Myriodontium keratinophilum

*Myriodontium keratinophilum* has been isolated from a patient with frontal sinusitis secondary to nasal polyps. The hyphae of *M. keratinophilum* in the sinus contents resemble those of *Aspergillus* but lack dichotomous branching. There was no evidence of tissue invasion by the fungus.

### Trichoderma spp.

*Trichoderma* spp. is commonly considered as a contaminant, but it has been reported to cause peritonitis in patients undergoing peritoneal dialysis and invasive infections in immunocompromised patients.

Growth is rapid (matures within 5 days). Colony is white fluff and later becomes compact and woolly. Eventually green patches are produced due to formation of conidia. Reverse is colourless or light tan to yellow. Microscopically, hyphae are septate.

### Treatment

1. Localized infection by *Fusarium* spp. is likely to benefit from surgical debridement. Keratitis can be treated with topical antifungal agents, and natamycin is the drug of choice. Disseminated infection requires systemic agents. Voriconazole has been used to effectively treat invasive *Fusarium* infection.
2. *Scedosporium apiospermum* is susceptible to itraconazole, voriconazole and posaconazole.
3. *Paecilomyces* is susceptible to triazoles (itraconazole, voriconazole and posaconazole).
4. *Acremonium* spp. are susceptible to amphotericin B, voriconazole and posaconazole.
5. Oral itraconazole and terbinafine, and topical natamycin may be used for the treatment of onychomycosis caused by *Scopulariopsis* spp. Invasive infections require surgical and medical treatment.

### Important Questions

1. Name causative agents of hyalohyphomycosis. Discuss pathogenesis and laboratory diagnosis of hyalohyphomycosis.
2. Discuss cultural characteristics of fungi causing hyalohyphomycosis.

# SECTION 5 : Opportunistic Mycoses

## Multiple Choice Questions

1. Which of the following fungi is **not** the causative agent of hyalohyphomycosis?
   (a) *Aspergillus* spp.
   (b) *Penicillium* spp.
   (c) *Fusarium* spp.
   (d) *Acremonium* spp.

2. Which of the following fungi invade/invades blood vessels?
   (a) *Rhizopus* spp.
   (b) *Mucor* spp.
   (c) *Penicillium* spp.
   (d) All of the above.

3. Which of the following fungi possess darkly pigmented hyphae?
   (a) *Cladosporium* spp.
   (b) *Aspergillus* spp.
   (c) *Penicillium* spp.
   (d) *Fusarium* spp.

4. Which of the following fungi produces conidia and phialides within a closed lesion?
   (a) *Aspergillus* spp.
   (b) *Rhizopus*.
   (c) Hyalohyphomycetes.
   (d) *Blastomyces dermatitidis*.

5. Which of the following fungi produces large, smooth sickle-shaped macroconidia?
   (a) *Fusarium* spp.
   (b) *Acremonium* spp.
   (c) *Paecilomyces* spp.
   (d) *Scopulariopsis* spp.

6. Which of the following fungi is the asexual state of teleomorph *Pseudallescheria boydii*?
   (a) *Scedosporium prolificans*.
   (b) *Scedosporium apiospermum*.
   (c) *Penicillium marneffei*.
   (d) *Beauveria bassiana*.

7. Which of the following morphological features is/are useful in identifying a mold as a *Fusarium* species?
   (a) Sickle-shaped multicelled macroconidia.
   (b) Acute angle branching hyphae.
   (c) Macroconidia formed on small denticles in a floret arrangement on apical swollen conidiophores.
   (d) Right angle branching hyphae.

8. Which *Fusarium* species is most commonly recovered from clinical specimens?
   (a) *F. oxysporum*.
   (b) *F. solani*.
   (c) *F. proliferatum*.
   (d) *F. verticillioides*.

9. Which *Fusarium* species is most commonly isolated from keratitis associated with contact lens use?
   (a) *F. oxysporum*.
   (b) *F. proliferatum*.
   (c) *F. solani*.
   (d) *F. verticillioides*.

10. Which statement best describes the growth of Mucorales species on laboratory media?
    (a) Cannot grow above 37°C.
    (b) Lid lifter.
    (c) Requires enriched medium.
    (d) Slow grower.

11. "Sporangiophores that are unbranched with rhizoids opposite the sporangiophores" describe which Mucorales species?
    (a) *Cunninghamella bertholletiae*.
    (b) *Mucor circinelloides*.
    (c) *Lichtheimia corymbifera*.
    (d) *Rhizopus oryzae*.

12. Columella is a:
    (a) branched hypha, root-like in appearance, which grows into substrate.
    (b) dome-like expansion at the apex of a sporangiophore, below a sporangium.
    (c) funnel-shaped swelling at the tip of a sporangiophore, below the sporangium.
    (d) suspensor cell supporting the zygospore.

13. Most common species isolated from mucormycosis is:
    (a) *Cunninghamella bertholletiae*.
    (b) *Mucor* spp.
    (c) *Rhizopus pusillus*.
    (d) *Rhizopus oryzae*.

## ANSWERS TO MCQs

1. (a), 2. (d), 3. (a), 4. (c), 5. (a), 6. (b), 7. (a), 8. (b), 9. (c), 10. (b), 11. (d), 12. (b), 13. (d).

**Further Reading**

1. Assaf C, Goerdt S, et al. Cutaneous hyalohyphomycosis. *Lancet* 2000; 356: 1185.
2. Bodey GP, Boktour M, et al. Skin lesions associated with *Fusarium* infection. *J Am Acad Dermatol* 2002; 47: 659–66.
3. Cortez KJ, Roilides E, et al. Infections caused by *Scedosporium* spp. *Clin Microbiol Rev* 2008; 21: 157–97.
4. Gardner JM, Nelson NM, Heffernan MP. Chronic cutaneous fusariosis. *Arch Dermatol* 2005; 141: 794–5.
5. Hay RJ. *Fusarium* infections of the skin. *Curr Opin Infect Dis* 2007; 20: 115–7.
6. Horre R, Jovanic B, et al. Fatal pulmonary scedosporiosis. *Mycoses* 2003; 46: 418–21.
7. Karaarslan A, Arikan S, et al. Skin infection caused by *Scedosporium apiospermum*. *Mycoses* 2003; 46: 524–6.
8. Nagano Y, Millar BC, et al. Emergence of *Scedosporium apiospermum* in patients with cystic fibrosis. *Arch Dis Child* 2007; 92: 607.
9. Nucci M, Anaissie E. Emerging fungi. *Infect Dis Clin N Am* 2006; 20: 563–79.
10. Posteraro P, Frances C, et al. Persistent subcutaneous *Scedosporium apiospermum* infection. *Eur J Dermatol* 2003; 13: 603–5.
11. Schinabeck MK, Ghannoum MA. Human hyalohyphomycosis: a review of human infections due to *Acremonium* spp., *Paecilomyces* spp., and *Scopulariopsis* spp. *J Chemother* 2003; 15 (Suppl. 2): 5–15.

# SECTION 6

# MISCELLANEOUS MYCOSES

**Chapter 22** Oculomycosis
**Chapter 23** Adiaspiromycosis
**Chapter 24** Rhinosporidiosis
**Chapter 25** Mycotoxicoses

# Oculomycosis

Oculomycosis is the fungal infection that occurs in the eye and its associated structures. Such infections are being increasingly recognized as important causes of morbidity and blindness. Cornea is the site most frequently affected causing keratomycosis. However, orbit, lids, lacrimal apparatus, conjunctiva, sclera, and intraocular structures may also be involved. Fungal infections of the eye and adnexa are divided into three broad categories:

A. Fungal (mycotic) keratitis
B. Fungal endophthalmitis
C. Fungal infections of ocular adnexa

## A. FUNGAL (MYCOTIC) KERATITIS

The cornea is the transparent avascular anterior-most structure of the eye, measuring 10–12 mm in diameter. It has a central thickness of about 0.5 mm. Like skin, it is the external anatomic barrier between the environment and deeper tissues. It is the ocular structure most frequently damaged by external trauma. The corneal surface is normally protected by the physical barrier of eyelids to foreign material, regular blink response, tight junctions between conjunctival and corneal epithelial cells, immune mediators (conjunctival mast cells, conjunctiva-associated lymphoid tissue which is responsible for local antigen processing), immunoactive substances in the tear film (IgA, lysozyme, β-lysine, lactoferrin, and tear-specific albumin), plasma cells, macrophages and T lymphocytes. Mycotic keratitis is relatively infrequent in the developed world but constitutes a large proportion of corneal infections in developing countries. In general, fungal infections of the cornea are more common in warmer climates.

Inflammatory processes involving the cornea, whether infectious or non-infectious, are termed "keratitis". Fungal keratitis is suppurative, usually ulcerative, fungal infection of cornea. Risk factors for fungal keratitis are corneal trauma with plant or organic material contaminated with fungi, immunocompromised state, and contact lens wear. The inflammatory response leads to cellular infiltration with destruction of the corneal collagen, thinning of the stroma and, in severe cases, perforation of the cornea with leakage of the aqueous humor and risk of intraocular extension, i.e., endophthalmitis. The inflammatory reaction and tissue destruction in fungal keratitis are caused by antigenic fungal cellular components, mycotoxins, and fungal proteases assisting in deeper stromal invasion.

### Causative agents

The fungi causing fungal keratitis are opportunistic organisms and colonize when natural defences of eye are abrogated by corneal trauma, use of topical corticosteroids or any other predisposing factors. Most of these are saprophytic fungi and are rarely associated with true infections among healthy individuals. Fungi causing keratitis are given in Table 22.1.

**Table 22.1.** Fungi causing keratitis

**A. Hyaline filamentous fungi**
- *Fusarium solani*
- *F. dimerum*
- *F. oxysporum*
- *F. nivale*
- *Aspergillus fumigatus*
- *A. flavus*
- *A. terreus*
- *Paecilomyces farinosus*
- *P. lilacinus*
- *Acremonium* spp.
- *Penicillium* spp.
- *Scedosporium apiospermum* (*Pseudallescheria boydii*)

**B. Dematiaceous fungi**
- *Curvularia* spp.
- *Bipolaris* spp.
- *Exophiala* spp.
- *Exserohilum* spp.
- *Fonsecaea* spp.
- *Lecythophora* spp.
- *Phialophora* spp.
- *Lasiodiplodia* spp.

**C. Yeast and yeast-like fungi**
- *Candida albicans*
- *C. parapsilosis*
- *C. tropicalis*
- *Cryptococcus neoformans*

**Hyaline filamentous fungi are the principal causes of mycotic keratitis in most parts of the world.** Filamentous fungal keratitis occurs most commonly in healthy young men engaged in agricultural work or outdoor occupations. *Fusarium* spp. are the most frequently encountered etiologic agents of keratitis, particularly in tropical or sub-tropical regions.

Fungi of the genus *Aspergillus* abound in the environment, thriving on various substrates, including corn, decaying vegetation, and soil. These fungi are also found commonly in hospital air. They are important causes of keratitis following occupational trauma or surgery in both tropical and temperate zones of the world. *A. fumigatus* is the most commonly isolated species, followed by *A. flavus* and *A. terreus*. Species of *Paecilomyces* are found worldwide in soil and decaying vegetation. They may also contaminate sterile solutions. Keratitis may develop following surgical procedures.

*Scedosporium apiospermum* is found in soil, sewage and polluted water. It may lead to keratitis. *Acremonium* spp. are ubiquitous, being found in abundance in the soil and air. These may also lead to keratitis.

Dematiaceous fungi are common soil and plant saprophytes. They are reported to be responsible for 10–15% of all fungal keratitis and are the third most frequently encountered fungi following *Fusarium* and *Aspergillus*.

Keratitis due to yeasts and yeast-like fungi is most frequently caused by *Candida albicans*. Less frequent causes include *C. parapsilosis*, *C. tropicalis* and *Cryptococcus neoformans*.

### Clinical features

Patient develops ocular pain, redness, diminished vision, photophobia and discharge. The eyelids may be erythematous and oedematous. The slit-lamp examination reveals breach in corneal epithelium and in Bowman's membrane. Later corneal findings may include an immune ring that can form focally in the corneal stroma around the infection, satellite lesions, and an endothelial plaque. In advanced fungal keratitis the cornea becomes white, resembling bacterial keratitis, and corneal perforation through necrosis and ulceration may ensue. Sometimes, endophthalmitis may result in later stage of infection due to perforation of corneal ulcer.

### Laboratory diagnosis

For the diagnosis of fungal keratitis, corneal material (such as scrapings or biopsy material) is the specimen of choice. It is collected by using a platinum spatula, surgical blades or calcium alginate swabs. Debride material from the base and edges of the ulcerated part of the cornea. This should be done several times to obtain as much material as possible. Cotton-tipped swabs do not seem to be useful means of debriding the necrotic corneal slough. Calcium alginate swabs (premoistened with tryptone soy broth), when used for debridement, may facilitate recovery of fungi in culture. If corneal scrapings do not yield positive results, a corneal biopsy may help in the diagnosis since a greater quantum of tissue can be obtained from a greater depth of the cornea.

### Direct examination

Examination of a wet preparation (using 10% KOH), a smear stained by the Gram stain or Giemsa stain and a smear stained by special fungal stains, such as Gomori methenamine silver (GMS), periodic acid-Schiff (PAS) and calcofluor white, reveal septate hyphae, yeast cells, pseudohyphae and/or true hyphae. It may not be possible to identify the fungal genus involved. However, presence of conidial structures in corneal material may aid in the differentiation of genera of hyaline filamentous fungi, such as *Acremonium*, *Fusarium* and *Paecilomyces*. The inflammatory reaction seen in mycotic keratitis is less severe than bacterial keratitis and usually consists of lymphocytes and plasma cells. There may be coagulative necrosis of the corneal stroma with "satellite microabscesses".

### Fungal culture

A diagnosis of mycotic keratitis is confirmed by isolation of fungi from corneal scrapes or biopsies which are inoculated onto the surface of two sets of SDA by making rows of 'C' streaks (two rows for each scraping). One set each of the inoculated media is incubated at 25°C and 37°C respectively. Only growth on the 'C' streaks are considered significant rather than laboratory contaminant. Antibacterial compounds, such as chloramphenicol (40 µg/ml) or a penicillin-streptomycin combination, are usually incorporated in the media to suppress bacterial growth, but **cycloheximide must never be used since it may suppress most ocular fungal pathogens**.

Although, ocular fungal pathogens are usually recovered in culture within 3–4 days, culture media need to be incubated for 4–6 weeks. A fungal strain is considered significant if it is recovered in culture from corneal material more than once. The mycelial fungal isolates are identified by their colony characteristics, microscopic morphology in lactophenol cotton blue mount and by slide culture. The yeast isolates are identified by sugar fermentation and assimilation test, formation of germ tubes, production of chlamydoconidia on cornmeal agar, and urease test.

### Histopathology

Corneal material for histopathology is obtained as a biopsy or button following penetrating keratoplasty. Sections are stained by haematoxylin and eosin (H&E), GMS and PAS stains. With H&E stain, evoked tissue response can be seen but species of *Fusarium* or *Candida* may not be stained at all. While fungi can be easily detected in sections of corneal tissue stained by GMS or PAS stains, little else can be visualized. However, a section stained by GMS can be counterstained by H&E to simultaneously demonstrate a mycotic agent and the evoked tissue response. Filamentous fungi are usually found deep in, and arranged parallel to, the corneal stromal lamellae.

The purulent inflammatory cellular reaction consists mostly of lymphocytes and plasma cells, with variable involvement of polymorphonuclear leucocytes. It is usually less intense in fungal than in bacterial keratitis.

## B. FUNGAL ENDOPHTHALMITIS

Endophthalmitis is a panophthalmic infectious or inflammatory process caused by either exogenous or endogenous microbial contamination of intraocular tissues. **Exogenous endophthalmitis** is usually associated with penetrating injury to the eye. It can also result from contamination of the internal eye by surgical instruments, fluids, and foreign materials introduced into the eye during surgery. The patients are otherwise healthy hence do not have any underlying immunodeficiency. It may also occur in patients receiving contaminated intravenous fluids.

**Endogenous endophthalmitis** is principally the result of haematologic spread of microorganisms from a distant focus of infection. It occurs most often in immunocompromised patients, e.g., organ transplant recipients and HIV-infected patients.

Endophthalmitis may also occur as a result of pre-existing scleritis or keratitis and mucormycosis of the surrounding soft tissue. Intravenous drug abusers are at a great risk to develop fungal endophthalmitis, probably because they may use contaminated drugs, syringes, needles or cotton.

### Causative agents

Fungi causing endophthalmitis are given in Table 22.2.

---
**Table 22.2.** Fungi causing endophthalmitis
---
- *Candida* spp.
- *Aspergillus* spp.
- *Fusarium* spp.
- *Cryptococcus neoformans*
- *Penicillium* spp.
- *Coccidioides immitis*
- *Blastomyces dermatitidis*
- *Histoplasma capsulatum*
- *Sporothrix schenckii*
- *Acremonium* spp.
---

*Candida* spp. are the most common cause of fungal endophthalmitis. *C. albicans* is the most frequently isolated species although other non-*albicans* species, including *C. parapsilosis*, *C. krusei* and *C. tropicalis* have also been implicated. *Candida* endophthalmitis has been reported in association with gastrointestinal surgery, corticosteroid therapy, lymphomas, and diabetes.

*Aspergillus* spp. are the second most common fungal cause of endophthalmitis with *A. flavus* the most frequently encountered species. Other *Aspergillus* spp. include *A. fumigatus*, *A. niger*, *A. terreus*, *A. glaucus* and *A. nidulans*. *Aspergillus* demonstrates tropism for vascular tissue with angio-invasion of the hyphae observed in pathologic specimens. *Aspergillus* endophthalmitis is most common in organ transplant recipients, neutropenic patients, patients receiving chemotherapeutic agents or corticosteroids, and those undergoing valvular cardiac surgery.

### Clinical features

Patient with fungal endophthalmitis develops redness, pain and diminished or blurred vision in the involved eye. Occasionally, hypopyon may be visible which is whitish layer of inflammatory cells and debris in the inferior anterior chamber. Patient with fungal endophthalmitis develops chorioretinitis, chorioretinal fungal mass penetrating through the inner limiting membrane of the retina into vitreous cavity, and retinal detachment.

### Laboratory diagnosis

Pass 27 or 30 gauge needle through the peripheral cornea at the limbus into the anterior chamber and withdraw 0.1 ml of aqueous fluid. Fungal endophthalmitis can be confirmed by direct microscopic demonstration of fungal hyphae or yeast cells in 10% KOH wet mounts, or smears stained by calcofluor white and the Gram method. In addition, Gram and Giemsa stains should be performed routinely on clinical samples.

Aqueous fluid is plated on blood agar, chocolate agar, Sabouraud dextrose agar, thioglycollate broth, and anaerobic medium. Direct inoculation of aqueous fluid on the culture media immediately after collection is recommended.

Polymerase chain reaction can provide rapid identification of the infecting organism in aqueous fluid.

## C. FUNGAL INFECTION OF OCULAR ADNEXA

Fungi may cause infection of eyelids, conjunctiva and lacrimal sac.

### Mycotic infection of eyelids

Infections of eyelids are caused most frequently by bacteria (particularly *Staphylococcus* spp.). However, fungi may also cause superficial or deep eyelid lesions. Fungi causing infection of the eyelids are given in Table 22.3.

---
**Table 22.3.** Fungi causing infection of eyelids
---
- *Sporothrix schenckii*
- *Blastomyces dermatitidis*
- *Paracoccidioides brasiliensis*
- *Cryptococcus neoformans*
- *Candida* spp.
- *Malassezia* spp.
- *Microsporum* spp.
- *Trichophyton* spp.
- *Rhinosporidium seeberi*
---

- *Sporothrix schenckii*, *Blastomyces dermatitidis* and *Paracoccidioides brasiliensis* may cause chronic ulcerative lesions of the eyelids.
- *Cryptococcus neoformans* may cause necrotizing fasciitis of eyelids and periorbital area. An eyelid nodule and ulcerative lesions have been reported to constitute a sentinel lesion of disseminated cryptococcosis in a patient with AIDS.
- *Candida* spp. may cause chronic severe ulcerative blepharitis. Ulceration begins at the base of an eyelash; small granulomata appear at its edge, and vesicles and pustules may also be present.
- *Malassezia* spp. may cause seborrheic blepharitis and pityriasis versicolor, a chronic and mild skin infection sometimes found around the eyebrows and eyelids.
- *Microsporum* and *Trichophyton* cause erythematous scaly papules that slowly enlarge and result in hair breaking at the levels of the skin surface.
- Rhinosporidiosis of the lid margins is a rare occurrence.

## Mycotic conjunctivitis

Normally, fungi are transient inhabitants of the normal conjunctival sac. But the unrestricted use of antibacterials and corticosteroids may predispose to fungal infection. *Candida* spp. cause simple acute or subacute superficial epithelial conjunctivitis. *Malassezia* spp. cause catarrhal conjunctivitis.

*Sporothrix schenckii* may cause nodular conjunctivitis and local lymphadenopathy. *Blastomyces dermatitidis*, *Coccidioides immitis* and *Paracoccidioides brasiliensis* cause follicular conjunctivitis. *Aspergillus niger* causes chronic conjunctivitis with black conjunctival secretions. Fungi causing conjunctivitis are given in Table 22.4.

## Mycotic dacryocystitis

Dacryocystitis is an infection of the lacrimal sac. It generally arises due to the stasis accompanying obstruction of nasolacrimal duct. Mycotic dacryocystitis is caused by *Acremonium* spp., *Aspergillus* spp., *Candida* spp., *Paecilomyces* spp., *Rhinosporidium seeberi*, dermatophytes, and *Sporothrix schenckii*. *Acremonium* spp. and *Sporothrix schenckii* cause chronic suppurative dacryocystitis with pre-

**Table 22.4.** Fungi causing conjunctivitis

| Fungi | Manifestations |
|---|---|
| *Candida* spp. | Simple acute or subacute superficial epithelial conjunctivitis |
| *Malassezia* spp. | Catarrhal conjunctivitis |
| *Sporothrix schenckii* | Nodular conjunctivitis and local lymphadenopathy |
| *Blastomyces dermatitidis*, *Coccidioides immitis* and *Paracoccidioides brasiliensis* | Follicular conjunctivitis |
| *Aspergillus niger* | Chronic conjunctivitis with black conjunctival secretions |

auricular and submaxillary lymphadenitis. *Aspergillus* spp., *Candida* spp., *Paecilomyces* spp., *Rhinosporidium seeberi*, and dermatophytes cause chronic granulomatous dacryocystitis.

Patient develops erythema, induration, and sensation of pressure in the medial canthus; pressure over the area usually results in a purulent discharge through the lower punctum. Eye may be red and the eyelids edematous. Patient may develop acute pain in the lower forehead and tenderness in the medial canthus.

### Treatment

Natamycin 5% suspension administered topically is used for fungal keratitis. Topical natamycin with oral itraconazole or oral ketoconazole is used for *Aspergillus* keratitis. For *Candida* and cryptococcal keratitis amphotericin B 0.15% solution is used. Natamycin alone or in combination with topical clotrimazole or topical miconazole is effective in keratitis caused by dematiaceous fungi. Systemic therapy with ketoconazole (400 mg/day) or itraconazole (400 mg/day) is given in severe cases.

 **Important Questions**

1. Classify fungi causing keratitis. Discuss predisposing factors, clinical features and laboratory diagnosis of fungal keratitis.
2. Name fungi causing endophthalmitis. Discuss pathogenesis, clinical features and laboratory diagnosis of fungal endophthalmitis.

# SECTION 6 : Miscellaneous Mycoses

3. Write short notes on:
   (a) Mycotic infection of eyelids
   (b) Mycotic conjunctivitis
   (c) Mycotic dacryocystitis.

## Multiple Choice Questions

1. The most frequently encountered etiologic agents of keratitis are:
   (a) *Fusarium* spp. and *Aspergillus* spp.
   (b) *Penicillium* spp. and *Acremonium* spp.
   (c) *Curvularia* spp. and *Exophilia* spp.
   (d) *Candida albicans* and *Candida parapsilosis*.

2. Which of the following fungi are the most common cause of fungal endophthalmitis?
   (a) *Candida* spp.
   (b) *Aspergillus* spp.
   (c) *Fusarium* spp.
   (d) *Acremonium* spp.

## ANSWERS TO MCQs

1. (a), 2. (a).

## Further Reading

1. Ahearn DG, Zhang S, et al. *Fusarium* keratitis and contact lens wear: facts and speculations. *Med Mycol* 2008; 46: 397–410.
2. Alfonso EC, Cantu-Dibildox J, et al. Insurgence of *Fusarium* keratitis associated with contact lens wear. *Arch Ophthalmol* 2006; 124: 941–7.
3. Andreola C, Ribeiro MP, et al. Multifocal choroiditis in disseminated *Cryptococcus neoformans* infection. *Am J Ophthalmol* 2006; 142: 346–8.
4. Bhansali A, Sharma A, et al. Mucor. endophthalmitis. *Acta Ophthalmol Scand* 2001; 79: 88–90.
5. Bradley JC, George JG, et al. *Aspergillus terreus* endophthalmitis. *Scand J Infect Dis* 2005; 37: 529–31.
6. Bradley JC, Hirsch BA, et al. *Pseudoallescheria boydii* keratitis. *Scand J Infect Dis* 2006; 38: 1101–3.
7. Burgess EH, Moro Vieira LF. Endogenous endophthalmitis. *N Engl J Med* 2007; 357: 163.
8. Cohen EJ. *Fusarium* keratitis associated with soft contact lens wear. *Arch Ophthalmol* 2006; 124: 1183–4.
9. Figueroa MS, Fortum J, et al. Endogenous endophthalmitis caused by *Scedosporium apiospermum* treated with voriconazole. *Retina* 2004; 24: 319–20.
10. Gaudio PA, Gopinathan U, et al. Polymerase chain reaction based detection of fungi in infected corneas. *Br J Ophthalmol* 2002; 86: 755–60.
11. Gupta PN, Ichhpujani RL, Bhatia R, Arora DR, Chugh TD. Effect of pre-treatment with dexamethasone on corneal pathogenicity of *Candida albicans*. *J Commun Dis* 1983; 15: 200–4.
12. Jain A, Egbert P, et al. Endogenous *Scedosporium apiospermum* endophthalmitis. *Arch Ophthalmol* 2007; 125: 1286–9.
13. Kiratli H, Uzun O, et al. *Scedosporium apiospermum* chorioretinitis. *Acta Ophthalmol Scand* 2001; 79: 540–2.
14. Kirszrot J, Rubin PA. Invasive fungal infections of the orbit. *Int Ophthalmol Clin* 2007; 47: 117–32.
15. Kumar M, Mishra NK, Shukla PK. Sensitive and rapid polymerase chain reaction based diagnosis of mycotic keratitis through single-stranded conformation polymorphism. *Am J Ophthalmol* 2005; 140: 851–7.
16. Saha R, Das S. *Bipolaris* keratomycosis. *Mycoses* 2005; 48: 453–5.
17. Shukla PK, Kumar M, Keshava GB. Mycotic keratitis: an overview of diagnosis and therapy. *Mycoses* 2008; 51: 183–99.
18. Srinivasan M. Fungal keratitis. *Curr Opin Ophthalmol* 2004; 15: 321–7.
19. Thomas PA. Fungal infections of the cornea. *Eye* 2003; 17: 852–62.
20. Wang MX, Shen DJ, et al. Recurrent fungal keratitis and endophthalmitis. *Cornea* 2000; 19: 558–60.

# CHAPTER 23

# Adiaspiromycosis

Adiaspiromycosis is a pulmonary mycosis of man and animals. The disease name is based on the cells found in tissues which have been termed adiaspores (adiaconidia). Many species of burrowing animals including rodents, small carnivores, insectivores, marsupials, and edentates throughout the world have been found to be infected. In humans, it is often self-limited, benign and asymptomatic, with rare cases progressing to fatal outcome. Adiaspiromycosis is caused by three species of the genus *Emmonsia* – *E. parva*, *E. crescens* and *E. pasteuriana*. Genetic studies place them in the family Ajellomycetaceae. Human adiaspiromycosis has been reported from Central and South America, Europe, USA and North Africa.

## Pathogenesis

Occurrence of adiaspiromycosis in burrowing rodents, the pulmonary alveolar position of the fungi, and experimental infections, indicate that *Emmonsia* spp. are soil inhabiting fungi, and that contaminated soil is the source of infection. Humans, as in animals, acquire infection by inhalation of dust-borne conidia of causative saprophytic soil fungus of the genus *Emmonsia*. Adiaconidia are formed *in vivo* when inhaled conidia, which initially measure about 4 µm in diameter, enlarge to form thick-walled spherule-like cells reaching 15–300 µm in diameter. The size of the adiaconidia varies with the species involved, with those of *E. crescens* being larger than those of *E. parva* and *E. pasteuriana*.

Adiaconidia of *Emmonsia* spp. resemble the spherules produced by *Coccidioides immitis* but adiaconidia do not form internal spores (endoconidia), nor do they further replicate. Each inhaled conidium grows *in vivo* to its ultimate enormous size at the site of implantation in an alveolus or a bronchiole without any type of germination, reproduction, and it eventually dies and may become calcified in this site. The large fungal cell which develops *in vivo* is called **adiaconidium**, a name derived from Greek roots which signify the remarkable growth in size of the fungus without multiplication.

Adiaspiromycosis is a pulmonary disease seen mainly in rodents and small animals living in soil; only occasionally in humans. This mycosis is characterized by the *in vivo* enlargement without multiplication of inhaled conidia. The mycosis is usually self-limited, benign and localized, but may be more severe; disseminated infection has been reported in patients with AIDS. A heavy or repeated exposure may result in acute pulmonary disease with bilateral granulomatous lesions. Patients are either asymptomatic or present with non-productive cough, dyspnea on exertion, low grade fever, and less often haemoptysis.

### Laboratory diagnosis

The diagnosis of adiaspiromycosis rests upon radiological and histopathological findings by demonstration of adiaconidia in various stages of development.

### Histopathology

In biopsy specimens the **adiaconidia of *E. crescens*** are generally found within granulomas, with each granuloma containing one or occasionally two adiaconidia. They are oval or globose, measure 200–400 µm in diameter with thick (20–70 µm thick) cell wall. The narrow outer layer of the adiaconidial wall is eosinophilic; a thin middle layer of the wall has irregular perforations that may appear as unstained spots; the inner layer of the wall is broad, hyaline, and composed predominantly of chitin. The walls can be readily stained with haematoxylin and eosin, and stain extremely well with Gomori methenamine silver, periodic acid-Schiff and Gridley stains. The interior of the conidium usually appears empty but small (1–3 µm in diameter), refractile, eosinophilic hyaline globules may be seen along the inner surface of the wall. There is no evidence of replication or endosporulation. Adiaconidia may be surrounded by a few macrophages and lymphocytes or by a granulomatous inflammatory reaction composed of epithelioid cells, macrophages, lymphocytes, plasma cells, neutrophils and fibrous tissue. Multinucleated giant cells may be seen in some granulomas.

**Adiaconidia of *E. parva*** are oval or globose, 10–40 µm in diameter with thin wall (2–4 µm). *E. pasteuriana* has small and large yeast cells; small cells are oval to pyriform (2–4 µm), often intracellular; and occasionally larger thick-walled (8–15 µm); all with narrow-based buds. Adiaspiromycosis should be carefully differentiated from spherules of *Coccidioides immitis* or nonbudding yeast cells of *Blastomyces dermatitidis*. Spherules of *C. immitis* are smaller (30–60 µm), have walls about 2 µm thick and contain endoconidia 2–5 µm in diameter.

### Culture

*Emmonsia* spp. grow well on Sabouraud dextrose agar without cycloheximide, but conidiation is enhanced on media such as potato dextrose agar. *Emmonsia* spp. form small, colourless, glabrous colony which later produce white aerial hyphae. At 20–25°C colonies reach a diameter of about 5 cm in 2 weeks. Microscopically, *Emmonsia* spp. appear similar to each other. Lactophenol cotton blue mount shows narrow (1–2.5 µm wide) septate and branching hyphae forming solitary sessile conidia or at the ends of narrow, often slightly swollen stalks that arise at right angles to the vegetative hyphae. Conidia are round or almost so (2–4.5 µm in diameter) and are smooth to slightly roughened (Fig. 23.1).

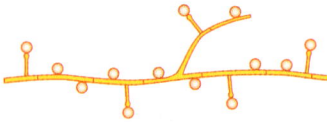

**Fig. 23.1.** Microscopic morphology of *Emmonsia* spp.

When the hyphae and conidia are incubated at their maximum temperature on enriched medium, the hyphae become distorted and usually disintegrate while the conidia swell to become round, thick-walled adiaconidia. The adiaconidia of *E. crescens* are produced at 37°C and measure 20–140 µm in diameter. The adiaconidia of *E. parva* are best produced at 40°C and range from 10–25 µm in diameter. When grown on enriched media such as brain heart infusion agar at 37°C, *E. pasteuriana* converts to a yeast phase consisting of oval to lemon-shaped, small (2–4 µm) yeast-like cells having narrow-based buds but conversion is incomplete and hyphal forms are present. Adiaconidia are produced on phytone-yeast-extract agar. Blood supplementation does not enhance adiaconidia production. Adiaconidia *in vivo* are larger and have thicker cell wall.

### Immunodiagnosis

Delayed type hypersensitivity reaction to antigens of *E. crescens* and precipitating antibodies in sera can be demonstrated in patients with adiaspiromycosis. Immunological crossreactivity has been demonstrated between *Emmonsia* spp. and

*B. dermatitidis* and *Histoplasma capsulatum* but not with *C. immitis*.

## Treatment

For the treatment of adiaspiromycosis itraconazole with prednisone may be used. Amphotericin B alone or in combination with flucytosine or prednisolone may also be used.

### Important Questions

Discuss pathogenesis and laboratory diagnosis of adiaspiromycosis.

### Multiple Choice Questions

1. Which of the following causes adiaspiromycosis?
   (a) *Rhinosporidium seeberi*.
   (b) *Emmonsia parva*.
   (c) *Coccidioides immitis*.
   (d) *Blastomyces dermatitidis*.

2. Which of the following statements is **incorrect** in case of adiaspiromycosis?
   (a) Adiaconidia do not form internal conidia.
   (b) Adiaconidia do not replicate.
   (c) Adiaspiromycosis is usually limited to lungs.
   (d) The causative fungus of adiaspiromycosis does not grow in laboratory culture media.

3. What is the name of the mycosis in which the inhaled conidium only enlarges and never germinates or reproduces in the host tissue?
   (a) Pneumocystosis.
   (b) Lobomycosis.
   (c) Adiaspiromycosis.
   (d) None of the above.

4. Adiaconidium is:
   (a) a conidium that enlarges but does not replicate.
   (b) a spherule.
   (c) a sporangium.
   (d) the sexual stage of *Emmonsia crescens*.

### ANSWERS TO MCQs

1. (b), 2. (d), 3. (c), 4. (a).

### Further Reading

1. dos Santos VM, Fatureto MC, et al. Pulmonary adiaspiromycosis: report of two cases. *Rev Soc Bras Med Trop* 2000; 33: 483–8.
2. Echevarria E, Cano EL, Restrepo A. Disseminated adiaspiromycosis in a patient with AIDS. *J Med Vet Mycol* 1993; 31: 91–7.
3. England DM, Hochholzer L. Adiaspiromycosis: an unusual fungal infection of the lung: report of 11 cases. *Am J Surg Pathol* 1993; 17: 876–86.
4. Hubalek Z, Burda H, et al. Emmonsiosis of subterranean rodents (*Bathyergidae*, *Spalacidae*) in Africa and Israel. *Med Mycol* 2005; 43: 691–7.
5. Stebbins WG, Krishul A, et al. Cutaneous adiaspiromycosis: a distinct dermatologic entity associated with *Chrysosporium* species. *J Am Acad Dermatol* 2004; 51 (Suppl. 5): S185–9.
6. Sun Y, Bhuiya T, et al. Fine needle aspiration of pulmonary adiaspiromycosis: a case report. *Acta Cytol* 2007; 51: 217–21.
7. Turner D, Burke M, et al. Pulmonary adiaspiromycosis in a patient with acquired immunodeficiency syndrome. *Eur J Clin Microbiol Infect Dis* 1999; 18: 893–5.
8. Wellinghausen N, Kern WV, et al. Chronic granulomatous lung infection caused by the dimorphic fungus *Emmonsia* spp. *Int J Med Microbiol* 2003; 293: 441–5.

# CHAPTER 24

# Rhinosporidiosis

Rhinosporidiosis is primarily an infection of mucous membranes, leading to a chronic granulomatous disease characterized by the development of pedunculated or sessile, red, spongy, friable, polypoid, granulomatous growths in the nose, conjunctiva and occasionally in ears, larynx, bronchus, penile urethra, vagina, rectum and skin. It was thought to be caused by a fungus, *Rhinosporidium seeberi*, but all attempts at isolation from clinical material failed. On the basis of modern molecular based studies, it is now considered to be a **hydrophilic protistan** hence called pseudofungal organism.

Taxonomically, it is now included, along with some fish and amphibian pathogens, in a new clade – **Mesomycetozoa**, a clade of fish parasites that form a branch of the evolutionary tree near the animal-fungal divergence. It is known to infect not only humans but a large variety of domestic and wild animals in all the continents except Australia. More than 90% of cases have been reported from India, Sri Lanka and South America. In India, sporadic cases occur all over but endemic foci exist in parts of Orissa, Andhra Pradesh, Kerala, Chennai and Raipur (Chhattisgarh). Very rarely, there is haematogenous spread with metastatic lesions in the lungs, brain and bones.

***Rhinosporidium seeberi* has not been cultured and animal inoculation is also not successful.**

Nothing definite is known about the mode of transmission of infection. However, it has been suggested that the organism is transmitted in dust or water. It is believed that fish may be the natural hosts of *R. seeberi*. Infection is more common in:

- Persons bathing in muddy stagnant pools of water.
- Those who dive into streams to collect sand from riverbeds.
- Paddy cultivators.
- In dry areas, after dust storm and eye injuries.

It is believed that *R. seeberi* gains entrance to the infected tissues by trauma. Anterior urethral rhinosporidiosis in Muslim males has been attributed to infection conveyed by pieces of stone or brick probably contaminated by soil-borne *R. seeberi* applied to absorb the last drops of urine. Trauma from *R. seeberi* contaminated pieces of stone or brick used for mopping up residual drops of urine is claimed to be responsible for anterior urethral rhinosporidiosis in males.

Deposits of water from a reservoir in Sri Lanka in which many rhinosporidial patients had bathed, showed bodies on periodic acid-Schiff (PAS)-stained smears, that were comparable in size and shape with rhinosporidial endoconidia.

Rhinosporidiosis is an infective disease in the sense that the tissue lesions are always associated with the presence of pathogen. No evidence has been adduced that it is also an infectious disease, as no transmission has ever been documented of cross-infection between members of the same family or between animals and humans. In addition to numerous cases in humans, rhinosporidiosis has also been documented as having occurred in several species of farm, domestic and wild animals – cattle, buffaloes, dogs, cats, goats, horses, mules, several species of ducks, swans, geese and water fowl.

Rhinosporidial infection spreads locally, regionally, and to distant, anatomically unrelated sites. Spillage of endoconidia from polyps after trauma or surgery is thought to be followed by auto-inoculation in the adjacent epithelium. Development of subcutaneous granulomata in the limbs, without breach of the overlying skin, could be attributed to haematogenous dissemination, from a subclinical, upper respiratory focus of infection.

Infected humans and animals have usually been associated with wet environments prior to infection. *R. seeberi* was, therefore, placed within the hydrophilic pathogens. However, the finding of human rhinosporidiosis in dry areas after sandstorms suggests that *R. seeberi* may develop resistant conidia in dry environments. These conidia could remain viable in aquatic as well as in dry ecologic niches for long periods of time, acting as infectious particles for susceptible hosts.

## PATHOGENESIS

Rhinosporidiosis in upper respiratory sites is thought to be initiated by the implantation of endoconidia from the aquatic habitat into the respiratory mucosa, added by abrasions caused, for instance, by sand particles in river sand workers who dive into the water or by vigorous cleaning of the anterior nares with the fingers. Autoinoculation of the mucosa by endoconidia released from sporangia or after surgery may lead to satellite polyps in the adjacent regions. Polyps on the skin may result from implantation of endoconidia by scratching with contaminated fingers or through haematogenous dissemination from respiratory sites.

No clear evidence of transmission between humans, even between those living in close contact, has been recorded. Ocular rhinosporidiosis, as it occurs in dry regions in the Middle Eastern countries, is believed to have been due to the dust-borne pathogen. Dust storms have been suggested as the possible vehicle although ocular disease has been recorded in wet regions as well. There is no evidence that humans can acquire the disease from animals. Both humans and animals probably acquire the pathogen from the common source of ground waters. Trauma acts as a predisposing factor for acquisition of rhinosporidiosis.

*R. seeberi*, as in the other mesomycetozoans, develops sporangia (cysts) with endoconidia. The endoconidia are subsequently released from mature sporangia in the infected host tissues and to the environment. Susceptible hosts may then acquire the infection after traumatic implantation of the resistant conidia. However, experimental infection in animals has so far been unsuccessful.

Painless obstructive polypoidal masses that easily bleed are commonly found in the eye, nostrils, pharynx, nasopharynx, and less frequently in other anatomic areas. Unusual cases involving internal organs occur sporadically. About 15% of cases of rhinosporidiosis are ocular in location, in the bulbar and palpebral conjunctiva. Rhinosporidiosis of the lacrimal sac and nasolacrimal duct has also been documented. Other sites of solitary polyps include the external urethral meatus especially in males. *The absence of rhinosporidiosis in the sexual partners of these patients is the evidence that the disease is neither infectious nor contagious.*

Dissemination to the limbs, trunk and viscera has been described in a few cases. Characteristically, rhinosporidial lesions in the nasal passages are polypoidal, granular, red in colour due to pronounced vascularity, with a surface containing yellowish pin head-sized spots which represent underlying mature sporangia. Nasopharyngeal polyps are often multilobed with a variegated appearance, with typical strawberry like regions and other areas which have relatively less vascular lobes with smooth surfaces.

Polyps on the skin, and in respiratory sites, could be sessile or pedunculated and non-infiltrating into deeper tissues. This feature makes the radical excision of pedunculate polyps possible with minimal spillage of endoconidia and uncommon recurrence, while excision of sessile polyps might be incomplete, with contamination of adjacent mucosa by endoconidia leading to recurrence. Polyps in respiratory sites are usually covered with mucus in which numerous endoconidia may be detected in stained smears. Growths on the skin may undergo ulceration and secondary infection, and then mimic malignant tumours.

Disseminated rhinosporidiosis is relatively rare, and presents with masses of varying size on face, trunk, limbs, and in the viscera including the liver, spleen, brain, and kidneys. The disease is not life-threatening, but it can cause breathing difficulties when the polyps obstruct the nose or laryngeal passages. Rhinorrhea and bleeding are common with polyps located in the nose.

## THE ORGANISM AND ITS LIFE CYCLE

In infected tissue *R. seeberi* develops a complex life cycle. It starts with the enlargement of non-flagellated 5–20 µm in diameter endoconidia released from mature sporangia through programmed pore formation. The endoconidia enlarge to become immature 40–60 µm diameter sporangia with refractile eosinophilic walls approximately (2–3 µm thick) and no endoconidia. These forms evolve to become mature sporangia with a thick wall (about 5 µm) and hundreds of endoconidia. The mature sporangia may reach 100–500 µm in diameter, a feature that contrasts with the smaller (30–100 µm) spherical phenotypes of *Coccidioides immitis* (Table 24.1).

**Table 24.1.** Differences between sporangia of *R. seeberi* and spherules of *C. immitis*

| Character | Sporangia of *R. seeberi* | Spherules of *C. immitis* |
|---|---|---|
| Size | 100–500 µm | 30–100 µm or more in diameter |
| Size of endoconidia | 5–20 µm | 2–4 µm |
| Staining with mucicarmine | + | – |

## LABORATORY DIAGNOSIS

The definitive diagnosis of rhinosporidiosis depends on the histopathological examination of biopsied or resected tissues. The infected tissue shows hyperplasia with a chronic granulomatous inflammatory response. Lymphocytes, plasma cells, macrophages, giant cells and, rarely eosinophils are usually found around the spherical phenotypes of *R. seeberi*. **Large numbers of sporangia at different stages of development are a main feature of the histopathologic tissue sections.** Active macrophages are also seen with engulfed endoconidia. However, sufficient numbers of endoconidia evade elimination to become immature and mature sporangia.

*R. seeberi* can be identified in haematoxylin and eosin stained sections, but sometimes one may need special stains such as Gomori methenamine silver (GMS) and periodic acid-Schiff (PAS) stains to demonstrate the causative agent. Sporangia can be seen with the naked eye as small white dots. The mature sporangium measures 100–500 µm in diameter and contains hundreds of endoconidia 5–20 µm in diameter (Table 24.1 and Fig. 24.1)

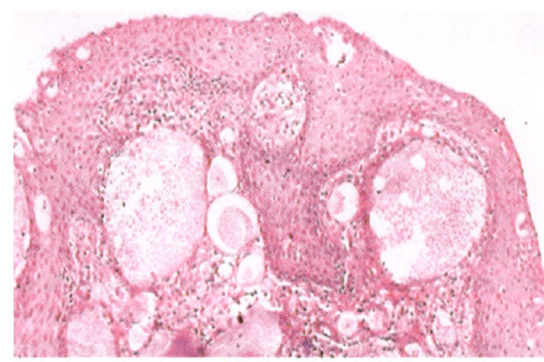

**Fig. 24.1.** Rhinosporidiosis showing sporangia and endoconidia (H&E stain, ×400).

Rhinosporidiosis should be differentiated from coccidioidomycosis in which *Coccidioides immitis* has mature stages which consist of large, thick-walled bodies which are smaller than the sporangia of *R. seeberi*, but which also contain endoconidia which are also smaller than those of *R. seeberi* (Table 24.1).

## CYTODIAGNOSIS

Cytodiagnosis is a useful method in diagnosis on aspirates from nonulcerated lumps in extra respiratory sites. Smears of the endoconidia-laden mucoid covering on the surfaces of polyps in the respiratory passages and from ulcerated polyps elsewhere in the body, and washings of sinuses and bronchi are stained with suitable stains such as GMS, Papanicolaou's, PAS and Meyer's mucicarmine. These reveal diagnostic features, especially the endoconidia.

## Wet mount

Wet mount preparations from clinical specimens from cases of rhinosporidiosis usually show the presence of mature and immature spherical sporangia with numerous endoconidia.

## TREATMENT

Surgical removal resulting in complete eradication of the disease is the treatment of choice.

## Important Questions

Discuss morphology, life cycle, pathogenesis and laboratory diagnosis of *Rhinosporidium seeberi*.

## Multiple Choice Questions

1. *Rhinosporidium seeberi* is a:
   (a) fungus.
   (b) algus.
   (c) protozoan.
   (d) hydrophilic protisan.
2. *Rhinosporidium seeberi* can be cultured on:
   (a) Sabouraud dextrose agar.
   (b) brain heart infusion agar.
   (c) blood agar.
   (d) None of the above.
3. Rhinosporidiosis is:
   (a) an infective disease.
   (b) an infectious disease.
   (c) a contagious disease.
   (d) All of the above.

## ANSWERS TO MCQs

1. (d), 2. (d), 3. (a).

## Further Reading

1. Ahluwalia KB. Causative agent of rhinosporidiosis. *J Clin Microbiol* 2001; 39: 413–5.
2. Ali A, Flieder D, et al. Rhinosporidiosis: an unusual affliction. *Arch Pathol Lab Med* 2001; 125: 1392–3.
3. Arseculeratne SN. Recent advances in rhinosporidiosis and *Rhinosporidium seeberi*. *Indian J Med Microbiol* 2002; 20: 119–131.
4. Arseculeratne SN. Rhinosporidiosis: What is the cause? *Curr Opin Infect Dis* 2005; 18: 113–8.
5. Chakraborty S, Chakraborti A, et al. Orbital rhinosporidiosis. *J Indian Med Assoc* 2005; 103: 383–4.
6. de Silva NR, Huegel H, et al. Cell-mediated immune responses (CMIR) in human rhinosporidiosis. *Mycopathologia* 2001; 152: 59–68.
7. Echejoh GO, Manasseh AN, et al. Nasal rhinosporidiosis. *J Natl Med Assoc* 2008; 100: 713–5.
8. Fredricks DN, Jolley JA, et al. *Rhinosporidium seeberi*: a human pathogen from a noval group of aquatic protistan parasites. *Emerg Infect Dis* 2000; 6: 273–82.
9. Ghorpade A. Giant cutaneous rhinosporidiosis. *J Eur Acad Dermatol Venereol* 2006; 16: 190–2.
10. Kumar BV, Osmani M, Mudhar HS. Rhinosporidiosis: an unusual presentation. *Int Ophthalmol* 2005; 26: 243–5.
11. Laxmisha C, Thappa DM. Subcutaneous swellings due to rhinosporidiosis. *J Dermatol* 2005; 32: 150–2.
12. Loh KS, Chong SM, et al. Rhinosporidiosis: differential diagnosis of a large nasal mass. *Otolaryngol Head Neck Surg* 2001; 124: 121–2.
13. Mendoza L, Herr RA, Ajello L. Causative agent of rhinosporidiosis. *J Clin Microbiol* 2001; 39: 413–5.
14. Mohanty RC, Khalkho J, Sahu A. Diagnosis of disseminated rhinosporidiosis by fine needle aspiration cytology. *Acta Cytol* 2006; 50: 234.
15. Pathak D, Neelaiah S. Disseminated cutaneous rhinosporidiosis: diagnosis by fine needle aspiration cytology. *Acta Cytol* 2006; 50: 111–2.

# CHAPTER 25

# Mycotoxicoses

Mycotoxicosis is poisoning by ingestion of toxins of fungal origin (mycotoxins) in foods which have been altered or damaged by the growth of toxin-producing molds. Some yeasts and basidiomycetes (mushrooms) have the capacity to form mycotoxins.

Not all toxic compounds produced by fungi are classified as mycotoxins; for example, compounds mainly toxic to bacteria are termed antibiotics, while those toxic to plants are called phytotoxins. There are more than 100 toxigenic fungi and more than 300 compounds toxic to vertebrates in low concentrations, which are currently recognized as mycotoxins. These toxins can cause acute or chronic intoxication and damage. The mycotoxins are secondary metabolites and their effects are not dependent on fungal infection or viability. Among the commodities, maize and groundnut are the most frequently contaminated feeds.

Mycotoxins form in hyphae, may be incorporated into conidia during conidiogenesis, or may be expelled into the environment. These substances are thought to be produced by fungi as ecologic survival aids designed to reduce competition for nutrients and living space by other fungi and organisms such as bacteria, insects and arachnids. Depending on the mycotoxin, various effects on protein, DNA, RNA synthesis or disruption of cell membranes are produced, resulting in either impaired cellular function or death.

## MODE OF ACQUISITION OF MYCOTOXINS

Humans and animals may acquire mycotoxins by eating contaminated food like cereals and grains, by skin contact and subsequent absorption of the mycotoxins, or by inhalation of mycotoxins or fungal elements (conidia or hyphal fragments) containing mycotoxins. Of these, consumption of contaminated food like cereals and grains is the most common. Contamination of cereals and grains may result from pre-harvest growth of mycotoxin-producing fungi on the grain, or fungal growth during storage. A few mycotoxins can be absorbed through the skin or mucous membranes. These may be used as **bioweapons**. Not all strains of a given species of a fungus are capable of mycotoxin production. Mycotoxin-producing species of fungi belong to genera *Aspergillus*, *Fusarium* and *Penicillium*.

Mycotoxicoses may manifest as acute or chronic disease, ranging from rapid death to tumour formation. Mycotoxicoses are more common in undeveloped countries where methods of food handling and storage are inadequate. Some mycotoxins are dermonecrotic, and cutaneous or mucosal contact with mold-infected substrates may result in disease. Likewise, inhalation of spore-borne toxins also contributes an important form of exposure. Mycotoxicoses are not communicable from person to person. Those fungi, such as *Aspergillus fumigatus*, which are both important opportunistic pathogens and are capable of producing gliotoxins, generally, do not produce the toxin in significant amounts during the course of human disease to have an effect on the disease process. **Whereas an opportunistic fungus must be able to grow at human body temperature (37°C) to cause disease, the optimum temperature for biosynthesis of most mycotoxins is much lower (20°C–30°C).**

Mycotoxins produced by various species of fungi are aflatoxins, ergot alkaloids, ochratoxins, fumonisins, gliotoxin, zearalenone, trichothecenes and citrinin.

## Aflatoxins

Aflatoxins are difuranocoumarin derivatives, of which there are over a dozen, with types $B_1$, $B_2$, $G_1$, $G_2$ being the major types. Type $B_1$ is the main aflatoxin produced. Types $B_1$, $B_2$ and $G_1$, $G_2$ exhibit blue and green fluorescence when irradiated under ultraviolet light on thin layer chromatography plates respectively. Aflatoxins are produced by *Aspergillus* spp., primarily *A. flavus, A. parasiticus A. nomius*, and *A. niger*.

*A. flavus* is a common contaminant of agricultural products among which are corn, figs, cottonseeds, peanuts, certain tree nuts, and tobacco. Milk, eggs and meat products are sometimes contaminated because of the animal consumption of aflatoxin-contaminated feed. However, the commodities with the highest risk of aflatoxin contamination are corn, peanuts, and cottonseed. Corn is probably the commodity of greatest worldwide concern, because it is grown in climates that are likely to have perennial contamination with aflatoxins and corn is the staple food of many countries. Contamination of crops can occur in the fields before harvest, especially in times of drought, or during storage, depending upon the moisture content of the substrate and the relative humidity of the storage conditions.

Aflatoxin is associated with both toxicity and carcinogenicity in human and animal populations. **Acute toxicity** is caused when large doses of aflatoxin are ingested. Humans are exposed to aflatoxins by consuming foods contaminated with products of fungal growth. Acute toxicosis from aflatoxins has been associated with contaminated grains, particularly maize. It may lead to **acute hepatitis** with centrilobular necrosis and steatosis. **Kwashiorkor** is a childhood disease that has manifestations of severe protein deficiency, hepatic steatosis, and ascites. The disease has been associated geographically with the seasonal occurrence of aflatoxins in food. Aflatoxins have been detected in the livers of children who died with the disease.

**Chronic toxicity** is due to long-term exposure to moderate to low aflatoxin concentration. Relationship between aflatoxin $B_1$ and **hepatocellular carcinoma** (HCC) is an example of chronic aflatoxicosis. It is believed that aflatoxin $B_1$ is involved in the pathogenesis of some cases of HCC, and it has been classified as a **Group 1 carcinogen by the International Agency for Research on Cancer**.

## Ergot alkaloids

Ergot alkaloids are compounds produced as a toxic mixture of alkaloids in the sclerotia (fruiting structure) of species of *Claviceps*. These fungi grow on rye and related plants, and produce alkaloids. The ingestion of ergot sclerotia from infected cereals, commonly in the form of bread produced from contaminated flour, cause ergotism. Human poisoning due to the consumption of rye bread made from ergot-infected grain was common in Europe in the Middle Ages. It was known as Saint Anthony's fire. *Claviceps* includes 50 known species, mostly in the tropical regions.

There are two forms of ergotism – gangrenous, affecting blood supply to extremities, and convulsive, affecting the central nervous system. Modern methods of grain cleaning have significantly reduced ergotism as a human disease, however, it is still an important veterinary problem. Ergot alkaloids have been used pharmaceutically.

## Ochratoxins

Ochratoxins are a group of mycotoxins produced by some *Aspergillus* and *Penicillium* spp. Ochratoxin A is the most prevalent and relevant fungal toxin of this group, while ochratoxins B and C are of lesser importance. Ochratoxin A is a dihydroisocoumarin produced by *Aspergillus ochraceus* and at least seven other *Aspergillus* species, including *A. niger* and *A. carbonarius*. *Penicillium verrucosum*, found on some grains and corn, also produces this mycotoxin.

Ochratoxin A has been detected in a variety of grains such as barley, oats, rye, and wheat and other commodities such as coffee beans, cocoa, various nuts, spices, and wines and beer. It is fat soluble and poorly excreted, and, as such, finds its way into food animals (particularly pork) through feeds, from which it can be consumed by humans. Human exposure can also occur through consumption of contaminated food products, particularly contaminated grain products as well as coffee, wine grapes and dried grapes. It acts by disrupting phenylalanine metabolism.

Ochratoxins are nephrotoxic, hepatotoxic, immunosuppressant, teratogenic, and a carcinogen in all experimental animals tested so far. **Ochratoxin A is potentially carcinogenic to humans** (Group 2B).

## Fumonisins

Fumonisins are a group of at least 15 chemically related toxic fungal metabolites (mycotoxins) produced by members of genus *Fusarium*, with *F. verticillioides* probably the most important, but other species such as *F. proliferatum* may also produce fumonisins. *Fusarium* spp. may colonise cereals, especially maize, in the field. Fumonisins have been found in maize and maize products worldwide. Therefore, they are of concern from a food safety point of view.

Biochemically, these mycotoxins consist of a 20 carbon aliphatic backbone with two ester-linked hydrophilic side chains, and the compound bears resemblance to sphingosine. This resemblance appears to play a role in inhibiting sphingolipid metabolism in animals. Fumonisins are known to cause adverse health effects in livestock and other animals and are considered to be potentially toxic to humans.

In humans, fumonisins may induce **neural tube defect**. These are defects of the brain and spinal cord in the embryo resulting from failure of the neural tube to close. **Fumonisins have been noted to have a possible link with esophageal cancer**. There is the co-occurrence of a high incidence of *F. verticillioides* contamination of grain and a high incidence of esophageal cancer in areas of South Africa, China and Italy. Fumonisins may also cause acute mycotoxicosis (food poisoning) by consumption of food products contaminated by fungi. This leads to diarrhoea and abdominal pain.

## Gliotoxin

Gliotoxin is an epipolythiodioxopiperazine. It is produced by *Aspergillus fumigatus*, *Trichoderma virens*, *Penicillium* spp., and *Candida albicans*. The cytotoxic activity of gliotoxin is generally mediated by direct inactivation of essential protein thiols and by inhibition of the respiratory burst in neutrophils by disrupting NADPH oxidase assembly, thereby facilitating *in vivo* fungal dissemination.

Gliotoxin possesses immunosuppressive properties as it may suppress and cause apoptosis in certain types of cells of the immune system, including neutrophils, eosinophils, granulocytes, macrophages, and thymocytes. It may be a virulence factor in infections caused by *A. fumigatus* and *C. albicans*. *In vivo* it displays antiinflammatory activity. It acts by blocking thiol groups in the cell membranes.

## Zearalenone

Zearalenone, also known as F-2 mycotoxin, is a nonsteroidal oestrogen or phytoestrogen. It is produced by *Fusarium graminearum* and several other *Fusarium* species, all of which are found in abundance in association with grains. These species are known to colonise cereals and tend to develop particularly during cool, wet growing and harvest seasons. It may be produced in maize, wheat, barley, rice and other cereals.

Zearalenone is the most common of the mycotoxins associated with *Fusarium* and it has been stated that up to approximately one quarter of corn consumed by humans contains this mycotoxin. Its structure resembles 17β estradiol. It is capable of binding to mammalian steroid receptors and has demonstrated **estrogenic effects**. Pigs are particularly sensitive to its action, and consumption in contaminated feed results in hyperoestrogenic syndrome that may include both **infertility and teratogenic effects**. Decreased fertility, abnormal estrus cycle, swollen vulvas, vaginitis, reduced milk production and mammary gland enlargement are most common findings reported in cattle and swine. To date epidemiologic studies have not confirmed any demonstrable adverse effects in humans.

## Trichothecenes

Trichothecenes are a very large family of chemically related mycotoxins produced by various species of *Fusarium, Trichoderma, Myrothecium, Phomopsis, Trichothecium*, and *Stachybotrys*. The most important structural features causing the biological activities of trichothecenes are the 12,13-epoxy ring, the presence of hydroxyl or acetyl groups at appropriate positions on the trichothecene nucleus and the structure and position of the side chain. They act by inhibiting protein synthesis, although different trichothecenes act at different stages in the process.

The most important trichothecene mycotoxin is deoxynivalenol (DON), a common contaminant of wheat, barley, oats, rye and maize. DON is also called vomitoxin. Humans consuming flour made from wheat contaminated with DON often develop nausea, fever, headache, and vomiting. Another trichothecene mycotoxin known as T-2 toxin may contaminate small grains. **T-2 toxin has been implicated as part of the alleged chemical warfare agent 'yellow rain' in Southeast Asia. T-2 toxin causes fatal disease of humans known as alimentary toxic aleukia (ATA).** Symptoms of ATA in humans include vomiting, diarrhoea, complete degeneration of bone marrow, and eventually death.

## Citrinin

Citrinin is a simple, low-molecular-weight compound that crystallizes as lemon-coloured needles. It is produced by *Penicillium citrinum, P. expansum, P. viridicatum, P. camemberti, Aspergillus niveus, A. oryzae, A. terreus* and *Monascus* spp. It has been associated with Japanese yellow rice disease. It has also been found in various other grains, peanuts, and fruits. Citrinin has demonstrated nephrotoxic effects on all animal species tested. It has been shown to inhibit dehydrogenase activity in rats' kidneys, liver, and brain. Its relevance to human health is unknown.

## BIOTERRORISM

There is concern about the possible use of mycotoxins in bioterrorism:

- Choice of aflatoxin as a weapon of mass destruction is odd at best, since the effects (liver cancer) of aflatoxicosis are too long-term to be effective during war.
- Trichothecenes are much more suited for warfare than aflatoxins because they act immediately upon contact and several milligrams can be lethal.

### Treatment

Treatment of mycotoxicosis is mostly symptomatic.

### Important Questions

1. Name and discuss various mycotoxins.
2. Write short notes on:
   (a) Mycotoxins associated with human cancer
   (b) Aflatoxins
   (c) Ergot alkaloids
   (d) Ochratoxins
   (e) Gliotoxin
   (f) Zearalenone
   (g) Trichothecenes.
   (h) Citrinin.

### Multiple Choice Questions

1. Which of the following commodities are most frequently contaminated with mycotoxins?
   (a) Wheat.
   (b) Gram.
   (c) Groundnut.
   (d) Cashewnut.
2. Humans and animals may acquire mycotoxins by:
   (a) eating contaminated food like cereals and grains.
   (b) skin contact and subsequent absorption of mycotoxins.
   (c) inhalation of mycotoxins or fungal elements containing mycotoxins.
   (d) All of the above.
3. Mycotoxin-producing species of fungi belong to genus/genera:

## SECTION 6 : Miscellaneous Mycoses

   (a) *Aspergillus*.
   (b) *Fusarium*.
   (c) *Penicillium*.
   (d) All of the above.
4. Which of the following mycotoxins may cause hepatocellular carcinoma?
   (a) Fumonisins.
   (b) Gliotoxin.
   (c) Zearalenone.
   (d) Aflatoxin $B_1$.
5. Which of the following mycotoxins causes alimentary toxic aleukia?
   (a) Trichothecenes.
   (b) Zearalenone.
   (c) Gliotoxin.
   (d) Fumonisins.
6. Which of the following toxins has/have been used in biological warfare?
   (a) Botulinum toxin.
   (b) Trichothecenes.
   (c) Ricin.
   (d) All of the above.
7. Which of the following mycotoxins have a possible link with esophageal cancer?
   (a) Fumonisins.
   (b) Aflatoxin $B_1$.
   (c) Zearalenone.
   (d) Gliotoxin.
8. Which of the following mycotoxins has/have possible link with human cancer?

   (a) Aflatoxin $B_1$.
   (b) Ochratoxins.
   (c) Fumonisins.
   (d) All of the above.

### ANSWERS TO MCQs

1. (c), 2. (d), 3. (d), 4. (d), 5. (a), 6. (d), 7. (a), 8. (d).

###  Further Reading

1. Bennett JW, Klich M. Mycotoxins. *Clin Microbiol Rev* 2003; 16: 497–516.
2. Burton JR Jr, Ryan C, Shaw-Stiffel TA. Liver transplantation in mushroom poisoning. *J Clin Gastroenterol* 2002; 35: 276–80.
3. Fox M, Gray G, et al. Detection of *Aspergillus fumigatus* mycotoxins: immunogen synthesis and immunoassay development. *J Microbiol Methods* 2004; 56: 221–30.
4. Hori K, Fukui H, Fujimori T. Haemorrhagic enteritis due to poisonous mushrooms. *Int J Surg Pathol* 2008; 16: 62.
5. Mas A. Mushrooms, amatoxins and the liver. *J Hepatol* 2005; 42: 166–9.
6. Pit JI. Toxigenic fungi and mycotoxins. *Br Med Bull* 2000; 56: 184–92.
7. Richard JL. Some major mycotoxins and their mycotoxicoses – an overview. *Int J Food Microbiol* 2007; 119: 3–10.
8. Saviuc P, Danel V. New syndromes in mushroom poisoning. *Toxicol Rev* 2006; 25: 199–209.

# SECTION 7

# APPENDICES

**Appendix A** Culture Media
**Appendix B** Laboratory Procedures
**Appendix C** Staining Methods
**Appendix D** Glossary
**Appendix E** Overview of Medical Mycology

# APPENDIX A

# Culture Media

Media for isolation of pathogenic fungi are designed to be inhibitory to bacteria and in certain cases selective against other fungi as well. Following culture media are commonly used in the mycology laboratory.

## FOR PRIMARY ISOLATION OF FUNGI

### 1. Sabouraud dextrose agar (SDA)

**Original formula:**

| | |
|---|---|
| Dextrose | 40 g |
| Peptone | 10 g |
| Agar | 15 g |
| Distilled water | 1000 ml |

Dissolve the ingredients by boiling and adjust pH at 5.6. Dispense in tubes, and autoclave at 121°C for 10 minutes. Allow tubes to cool in slanted position. Store in refrigerator.

### 2. Emmons' modification of Sabouraud dextrose agar or neutral Sabouraud dextrose agar

| | |
|---|---|
| Dextrose | 20 g |
| Peptone | 10 g |
| Agar | 17 g |
| Distilled water | 1000 ml |

Dissolve the ingredients by boiling and adjust pH at 6.9. Dispense in tubes, and autoclave at 121°C for 10 minutes. Allow tubes to cool in slanted position. Store in refrigerator.

### 3. Sabouraud-cycloheximide-chloramphenicol agar

| | |
|---|---|
| Dextrose | 20 g |
| Peptone | 10 g |
| Agar | 20 g |
| Chloramphenicol | 40 mg |
| Cycloheximide | 500 mg |
| Distilled water | 1000 ml |

After dextrose, peptone and agar are dissolved, heat to boiling, add 40 mg of chloramphenicol which has been suspended in 10 ml of 95% alcohol and quickly remove from heat. Add 500 mg cycloheximide, which has been dissolved in 10 ml of acetone. Dispense in tubes, and autoclave at 121°C for 10 minutes. Allow tubes to cool in slanted position. Store in refrigerator.

This medium is useful for isolation of fungi from contaminated specimens. **Chloramphenicol** inhibits bacterial contaminants. **However, it partially inhibits** *Nocardia* **and actinomycetes.**

**Cycloheximide** reduces the rate of growth of many saprophytic fungi. It is toxic for *Cryptococcus* *neoformans*, *Candida* spp. and other yeasts. It also inhibits growth of the yeast forms of some dimorphic fungi when they are incubated at 37°C.

## NUTRITIONALLY DEFICIENT MEDIA

### 1. Cornmeal agar

| | |
|---|---|
| Cornmeal | 40 g |
| Agar | 20 g |
| Tween 80 (polysorbate 80) | 10 ml |
| Distilled water | 1000 ml |

Mix cornmeal well with 500 ml of water; heat to 65°C for 1 hour. Filter through gauze and then paper until clear; restore to original volume. Adjust to pH 6.6–6.8; add agar dissolved in 500 ml of water. Add Tween 80, autoclave at 121°C for 15 minutes. Dispense into petri plates.

Cornmeal agar is low in nutrients. It suppresses vegetative growth while stimulating sporulation of many fungi. It is used in distinguishing the different genera of yeasts and various species of *Candida*. It is also useful in slide culture. If 10 g of dextrose is added to the medium in place of the Tween 80, the medium can be used to differentiate *Trichophyton mentagrophytes* from *T. rubrum* on the basis of pigment production. On this medium the latter produces red pigment while the former is negative.

### 2. Rice-Tween 80 agar

| | |
|---|---|
| Cream of rice | 10 g |
| Tween 80 | 10 ml |
| Agar | 10 g |
| Distilled water | 1000 ml |

To 1 litre of boiling distilled water add 10 g cream of rice and continue boiling for 30 seconds. Filter through cotton and restore volume. Add 10 g agar and dissolve with heat. Add 10 ml Tween 80. Autoclave at 121°C for 15 minutes. Pour into a cylinder and leave overnight in a water bath at 60°C. Decant clear portion, refilter through cotton, dispense in flasks and autoclave at 121°C for 15 minutes. Pour in petri plates.

Rice-Tween 80 agar is used for the production of chlamydoconidia by *Candida albicans* faster as compared to cornmeal agar.

## ENRICHED MEDIA

### 1. Brain heart infusion (BHI) agar

| | |
|---|---|
| Brain heart infusion | 8 g |
| Peptic digest of animal tissue | 5 g |
| Pancreatic digest of casein | 16 g |
| Sodium chloride | 5 g |
| Dextrose | 2 g |
| Disodium phosphate | 2.5 g |
| Agar | 13.5 g |
| Distilled water | 1000 ml |

Dissolve ingredients by boiling and dispense into screw-cap tubes and autoclave at 121°C for 15 minutes. Chloramphenicol 40 mg is often added to inhibit bacteria, and sheep blood is added to further enrich the medium and enhance the growth of fastidious pathogenic fungi. BHI agar is recommended for the cultivation of fastidious pathogenic fungi, such as *Histoplasma capsulatum* and *Blastomyces dermatitidis*.

### 2. Histoplasma mold to yeast form conversion medium

| | |
|---|---|
| Brain heart infusion agar base | 5.2 g |
| Glutamine | 1 ml |
| Sheep blood | 5 ml |
| Distilled water | 100 ml |

Prepare brain heart infusion agar base. Autoclave at 121°C for 15 minutes. Cool it to 50°C and add glutamine and sheep blood. Dispense in test tubes. Slant the test tubes.

### 3. Blood agar

The medium is prepared by adding 5% sterile sheep blood to sterile nutrient agar that has been melted and cooled to 50°C. This is used for isolation of *Histoplasma capsulatum*, *Blastomyces dermatitidis* and *Cryptococcus* spp.

# Culture Media

## SELECTIVE AND DIFFERENTIAL MEDIA

### 1. Bird seed agar or niger seed agar

Bird seed agar is a selective and differential medium used for primary isolation of *Cryptococcus* spp. The colonies of *Cryptococcus* spp. on this medium are dark brown to black in colour because phenoloxidase produced by these organisms breaks down the substrate (*Guizotia abyssinica* seeds or niger seed) to melanin, which is deposited in the yeast cell wall. This imparts a dark brown to black pigmentation of the colonies.

| | |
|---|---|
| *Guizotia abyssinica* (niger seed or bird seed) | 50 g |
| Distilled water | 1000 ml |

Boil for 30 minutes. Filter through gauze and add the following:

| | |
|---|---|
| $KH_2PO_4$ | 1 g |
| Creatinine | 1 g |
| Agar | 15 g |

(Glucose, 1 g is added in the formulation for identification of *Candida dubliniensis*, but it inhibits pigment production by *Cryptococcus neoformans*. Chloramphenicol, 1 g may be added in the formulation for pigment production and isolation of *C. neoformans*.)

Mix well. Autoclave at 121°C for 15 minutes. Pour into tubes and cool in slanted position.

### Test procedure

#### A. For pigment production by *C. neoformans*

Inoculate with suspected *Cryptococcus* spp. and incubate at 25–30°C for 7 days. Only *C. neoformans* varieties *neoformans* and *gattii* produce phenoloxidase which break down the substrate resulting in the production of melanin and the development of dark brown to black colonies. Colonies of other yeasts are cream in colour.

#### B. For differentiation of *Candida dubliniensis* versus *C. albicans*

Inoculate a plate of this medium with a 48-hour-old colony. Incubate at 30°C for 3–5 days. Examine macroscopic morphology of colonies. Colonies of *C. dubliniensis* are rough and may have hyphal fringe. On the other hand, colonies of *C. albicans* are smooth.

### 2. Dermatophyte test medium (DTM)

| | |
|---|---|
| Phyton | 10 g |
| Dextrose | 10 g |
| Agar | 20 g |
| Phenol red solution | 40 ml |
| 0.8 M HCl | 6 ml |
| Cycloheximide | 0.5 g |
| Gentamicin sulphate | 0.1 g |
| Chlortetracycline HCl | 0.1 g |
| Distilled water | 1000 ml |

Dissolve phyton, dextrose, and agar by boiling them in water. While stirring, add 40 ml of phenol red solution (0.5 g of phenol red dissolved in 15 ml of 0.1 N NaOH made up to 100 ml with distilled water). While stirring, add 0.8 M HCl. Dissolve cycloheximide in 2 ml of acetone, and add to hot medium while stirring. Dissolve gentamicin sulphate in 2 ml of distilled water, and add to the medium while stirring. Autoclave at 12 lb/in$^2$ for 10 minutes and cool to approximately 47°C. Dissolve chlortetracycline in 25 ml of sterile distilled water in sterile container, and add to medium while stirring. Dispense into sterile 30-ml screw-cap tubes; slant and cool. The final pH of the medium is 5.4–5.6, and the medium should be yellow in colour. Store in refrigerator at 4°C.

The dermatophyte test medium is used for presumptive diagnosis of dermatophytes. They change the colour of the medium from yellow to red due to liberation of alkaline metabolites within 14 days. Care must be taken in specimen collection and interpretation of results, as many contaminants and other fungi increase the number of false-positive changes in colour. DTM cannot be used to study pigment production because of the intense red colour of the indicator.

### 3. Urea agar (Christensen medium)

| | |
|---|---|
| Peptone | 1 g |
| Dipotassium hydrogen phosphate ($K_2HPO_4$) | 2 g |
| Sodium chloride (NaCl) | 5 g |

| | |
|---|---|
| Phenol red | |
| (1 in 500 aqueous solution) | 6 ml |
| Agar | 20 g |
| Distilled water | 1 litre |
| Glucose, 10% solution, sterile | 10 ml |
| Urea, 20% solution, sterile | 100 ml |

Sterilize the glucose and urea solutions by filtration. Prepare the basal medium without glucose and urea. Adjust to pH 6.8–6.9 and sterilize by autoclaving in a flask at 121°C for 30 minutes. Cool to about 50°C, add glucose and urea and tube the medium as deep slopes.

This medium detects the ability of an organism to produce urease enzyme. In the presence of suitable substrates, urease splits urea producing ammonia. It raises pH of the medium and phenol red indicator changes amber colour to pinkish red.

Urease-positive fungi are *Trichophyton mentagrophytes*, *Trichosporon* spp., *Cryptococcus neoformans* and *Rhodotorula*. Urease-negative fungi are *Trichophyton rubrum*, *Geotrichum candidum*, *Candida* and *Saccharomyces*,

## ASSIMILATION MEDIA FOR YEASTS

Assimilation is the utilization of carbon (or nitrogen) source by a microorganism in the presence of oxygen. A positive reaction is indicated by the presence of growth or a pH shift in the medium. **Since all yeasts assimilate glucose, it acts as a positive control.**

### 1. Carbon assimilation medium

| | |
|---|---|
| Yeast nitrogen base | 6.7 g |
| Appropriate pure carbohydrate | 5 g |
| Distilled water | 100 ml |

Heat to dissolve. Sterilize by Seitz or membrane filtration. Add 0.5 ml of the solution to 4.5 ml of sterile distilled water in screw-cap tubes. Store in refrigerator. These may be used for one month.

### 2. Nitrate assimilation medium

| | |
|---|---|
| Yeast carbon base | 11.7 g |
| Potassium nitrate | 0.78 g |
| Distilled water | 100 ml |

Warm gently to dissolve. Sterilize by Seitz or membrane filtration. Add 0.5 ml of medium to 4.5 ml of sterile distilled water in screw-cap tubes. Store in refrigerator. These may be used for one month.

### Test procedures

Make a suspension of the yeast in sterile distilled water. This suspension should not exceed the turbidity of McFarland No. 1 standard. Add 0.1–0.2 ml of the yeast suspension to each tube of medium. Include a tube of yeast nitrogen base without any carbon source, and a tube of yeast carbon base without potassium nitrate, as controls for carryover. Incubate tubes at the yeast's optimal temperature. Examine cultures over a period of 7–14 days for dense turbidity caused by growth. The negative-control tubes without a carbon or nitrogen source should show no growth.

## AUXANOGRAPHIC PLATE METHOD

### 1. Carbon assimilation tests

| | |
|---|---|
| Yeast nitrogen base | 0.67 g |
| Noble or washed agar | 20 g |
| Distilled water | 1000 ml |

Dispense in 20-ml quantities into 18 × 150 mm screw-cap tubes. Autoclave at 121°C for 15 minutes. Allow to harden as butts. Store in refrigerator.

### Test procedure

- Melt a tube of nitrogen base medium in a boiling-water bath. Allow to cool to 47–48°C.
- With a sterile cotton-tipped applicator, make a heavy suspension of a 24- to 72-hour yeast culture in 4 ml of sterile distilled water. The density of the suspension should be equal to that of a McFarland No. 4 or 5 standard.
- Pour the yeast suspension into the tube of molten yeast nitrogen base agar. Mix thoroughly by inverting tube several times.
- Pour the yeast-agar mixture into a sterile 15 × 150 mm petri plate. Allow to solidify at room temperature.
- Place carbohydrate-containing disks, evenly spaced, on the plate.

- Incubate at 30°C for 18–24 hours and then examine for growth around each disk. Growth around a disk indicates that the yeast assimilates that sugar.

## 2. Nitrate assimilation tests
### Medium

| | |
|---|---|
| Yeast carbon base | 12 g |
| Noble or washed agar | 20 g |
| Distilled water | 1000 ml |

Tube in 20-ml aliquots and autoclave at 121°C for 15 minutes. Store in refrigerator.

### Peptone solution for positive control

| | |
|---|---|
| Peptone | 10 g |
| Distilled water | 100 ml |

Sterilize by filtration store in refrigerator

### Test procedure
- Melt a tube of yeast carbon base medium in a boiling-water bath. Allow to cool to 47–48°C.
- Make an aqueous solution suspension of the yeast to a density equal to a McFarland No. 1 standard.
- Add 0.1 ml of yeast suspension to the tube of medium. Mix thoroughly.
- Pour the yeast-agar mixture into a sterile petri plate. Allow to solidify at room temperature.
- Place approximately 1 mg of potassium nitrate crystals on agar surface away from the centre of the plate.
- Place about 0.1 ml of peptone solution (positive control) on agar surface opposite potassium nitrate site.
- Incubate at 30°C for 48–96 hours.

For test to be valid growth must occur in the peptone area. If growth is seen in the "peptone area", examine for growth in the potassium nitrate area (growth indicates assimilation of potassium nitrate).

# APPENDIX B

# Laboratory Procedures

## COLLECTION AND PREPARATION OF SPECIMEN

Isolation and identification of fungi from clinical specimens are not likely to be accomplished unless the specimen is properly collected and sent immediately to the laboratory. All specimens should be transported in sterile containers and processed as soon as possible.

### General rules for collection and transportation of specimen

- Apply strict aseptic techniques throughout the procedure.
- Wash hands before and after the collection.
- Prevent contamination of the specimen with externally present organisms or normal flora of the body.
- Collect the specimen from the actual infection site.
- Collect adequate quantity for the desired tests.
- Collect the specimen aseptically in a sterile and appropriate container.
- Close the container tightly so that its contents do not leak during transportation.
- Ensure that the outside of the specimen container is clean and uncontaminated.
- Label the container appropriately and complete the requisition form.
- Immediately transport the specimen to the laboratory.
- *If a specific fungus is suspected by the physician, the laboratory should be notified, as special media and culture procedures may be needed, and the information will be helpful for the safety of laboratory personnel.*

### Criteria for rejection of specimens

- Missing or inadequate identifications.
- Incomplete forms.
- Leaking container or blood stained containers.
- Specimens collected in an inappropriate container.
- Haemolysed blood sample.
- Insufficient quantity.
- Dried-up specimen.
- Contamination suspected.
- Inappropriate transport or storage.

### Blood for fungal culture

Blood for fungal cultures must be collected aseptically and inoculated into broth or tubes containing polyanetholsulphonate in a final concentration of 0.03–0.05%. The incorporation of saponin to lyse the blood cells is also desirable. Recovery of fungi increases with the volume of blood tested and since fungal sepsis may be intermittent, at least two blood samples should be separately collected and cultured.

Biphasic blood culture medium consisting of broth with an agar slant is significantly better than broth alone. Conventional broth cultures may require 20–30 days before becoming positive and should be subcultured at regular intervals regardless of gross appearance.

## Blood for serological tests

For serological tests collect about 5 ml of blood to ensure there will be enough serum for all the tests that may be required. Immediately transfer the blood from the syringe into a dry stoppered sterile tube or bottle (without anticoagulant) and allow to clot. When the serum has separated, pipette it off into a sterile tube.

## Bone marrow

Decontaminate the skin, overlying the site from where specimen is to be collected, with spirit and tincture iodine. Aspirate 1 ml or more of bone marrow by sterile percutaneous aspiration with bone marrow aspiration needle. Collect in a sterile screw-cap tube. Immediately transport to the laboratory.

Alternatively, the specimen may be collected in a heparinized syringe and inoculated onto appropriate fungal media at the bedside. The specimen should also be smeared and stained with Giemsa or Wright stain if the presence of *Histoplasma capsulatum* is the possibility.

## Cerebrospinal fluid (CSF)

Cerebrospinal fluid must be collected by an experienced physician. Rigorous aseptic precautions must be observed to prevent the introduction of infection into the central nervous system. The fluid is usually collected from the arachnoid space.

A sterile wide-bore needle is inserted between fourth and fifth lumber vertebrae and the CSF is allowed to drip into a sterile dry container. Only 3–5 ml of fluid should be collected, because the removal of a larger volume may lead to headache. Immediately deliver the sample with a request form to the laboratory. The fluid should be handled with special care because a lumber puncture is required to collect the specimen.

CSF should be centrifuged at 2000 $g$ for 10 minutes. The supernatant should not be decanted unless a portion is needed for cryptococcal antigen testing. With a sterile pipette, the sediment is removed and used to inoculate the medium and prepare smears for microscopic examination. Any remaining sediment is resuspended, and the medium is reinoculated with fairly large amounts of the whole specimen. Filtration of CSF through a 0.45-μm pore-size membrane filter, followed by culture of the filter is sometimes preferred method.

## Sputum

Sputum should be collected as a first early-morning sample in a wide-mouthed container, which is preferably disposable, made up of transparent thin plastic, unbreakable and leak-proof.

- Ask the patient to rinse the mouth with plain water and then inhale deeply 2–3 times, cough up deeply and spit in the sputum container by bringing it close to the mouth.
- Make sure the sputum sample is of good quality and not just the saliva. A good quality sputum sample is thick, purulent and sufficient in amount (2–3 ml).
- Flecks containing pus, blood or caseous material should be sought and used in culture and smears.
- Twenty four-hour specimens are not satisfactory, as they easily become overgrown with bacteria and saprophytic fungi.
- Sputum decontaminated for culturing acid-fast bacilli is not acceptable because the sodium hydroxide in the procedure destroys a large number of fungi. A mucolytic agent without sodium hydroxide may be used with very viscous specimens.

## Stool

Specimens of stool are rarely worth culturing for fungi. Growth of a large amount of yeast has possible significance. If fungal infection of the gastrointestinal tract is suspected, biopsy specimens of tissue are usually required for diagnosis.

## Urine

Midstream urine sample is collected after giving proper instructions to the patient.

Clean the genitalia properly. In case of male, retract the prepuce, clean it with sterile normal saline and collect a "clean-catch" mid stream urine sample in a sterile container. In case of female, wash perineum and periurethral area with soap and water. Separate apart labia with fingers of one hand and collect a "clean-catch" mid stream urine sample in a sterile container.

Upon reaching the laboratory, the urine is centrifuged at 2000 $g$ for 10 minutes. The supernatant is decanted, and approximately 0.5 ml of the sediment is placed on each medium to be used. The clinical presentation of the patient must be given prime consideration in the determination of the significance of *Candida* spp. in urine. It should be kept in mind that yeast in urine may be a sign of dissemination in severely immunocompromised patients.

## Fluids

Fluids (e.g., pleural, peritoneal, or joint fluids) are collected with heparin to prevent clotting. The fluid is centrifuged at 2000 $g$ for 10 minutes. Any clotted material should be minced with a sterile scalpel and combined with the concentrated material. At least 0.3 ml of inoculum is placed onto each medium.

## Tissues

Tissues should be minced with a scalpel or ground with a mortar and pestle or tissue grinder. A small amount of sterile saline or broth may be added to facilitate grinding. *If infection with Mucorales is suspected, the tissue should be minced, not ground or homogenized, as these procedures destroy the hyphae and decrease the viability of the organisms.*

## Cutaneous specimens

### Skin

Specimens of skin are taken from an area previously cleansed with 70% alcohol. The active, peripheral edge of a lesion is scraped with a scalpel or the end of a microscope slide.

### Nails

Nail samples should be collected by taking clippings from any discoloured, dystrophic or brittle parts of the nail and, importantly, by scraping material from underneath the nail.

### Scalp and hair

Fungi causing infection of scalp and hair are best isolated by culturing the basal portion of the infected hair. Hairs infected with some dermatophytes fluoresce under UV light. Hairs that are fluorescent, distorted or fractured should be cultured.

Skin scrapings, hair stubs, and nail clippings or scrapings are collected into folded paper square for transport to the laboratory. The use of paper allows the specimen to dry out, which helps reduce bacterial contamination and provides conditions under which specimen can be stored for 12 months or more without appreciable loss of viability of the fungus.

## Exudates, pus, and drainage

Specimens of exudates, pus and drainage should be examined for granules by using a dissecting microscope. A portion of the specimen is teased apart gently, crushed between two glass slides, and examined microscopically. The remainder is washed several times in sterile distilled water, crushed with a sterile glass rod and inoculated onto appropriate media. If no granules are present, the specimen is examined microscopically for hyphae and other fungal elements and directly inoculated onto isolation medium.

# METHODS FOR DIRECT MICROSCOPIC EXAMINATION OF SPECIMENS

## Potassium hydroxide (KOH) preparation

A 10–20% solution of KOH is useful for detecting fungal elements in skin, hair, nails, and tissue. In this procedure, KOH is mixed in equal proportions with the specimen on a slide and the specimen material is teased with two inoculating needles. A coverslip is placed over it and heated gently. Preparation with KOH clears the tissue and cellular debris from all types of clinical specimens without damaging the fungal cells.

This clearing process requires only 5–10 minutes after which one can observe the fungal morphology as well as the pigment of the fungal cell wall under a phase-contrast or bright-field microscope using low-power followed by high-power objectives. **Reaction of KOH with pus, sputum, and skin may produce artifacts that superficially resemble hyphae or budding forms of fungi.** Therefore, experience is required in interpreting the results. Moreover, crystals can form on standing so that reading of the smear becomes difficult.

With KOH preparation, a definitive diagnosis of blastomycosis, paracoccidioidomycosis, coccidioidomycosis, mycetoma, phaeohyphomycosis, lobomycosis and rhinosporidiosis can be made. Tentative diagnosis can be derived from the presence of fungal elements compatible to the etiologic agents of aspergillosis, mucormycosis, dermatophytosis, candidiasis, sporotrichosis, or cryptococcosis. To confirm such a diagnosis, however, culture proof is necessary.

### KOH with calcofluor white

**Calcofluor white is an excellent fluorescent stain for detection of fungi in specimens.** It can be combined with KOH if clearing is required. A drop of 0.1% calcofluor white solution (fluorescent reagent) can be added to the KOH preparation prior to placing coverslip over it. Calcofluor white binds to polysaccharide present in the chitin of the fungus or to cellulose. Fungal elements fluoresce apple-green or blue-white, depending on the combination of filters used. The actual fungal structure must be seen before a positive preparation is reported.

### India ink

**India ink preparations may be used for detecting encapsulated yeast *Cryptococcus neoformans* in cerebrospinal fluid (CSF).** A drop of India ink is mixed with a drop of centrifuged deposit of CSF, and the preparation is examined under high power. With this negative stain, budding yeast surrounded by a large clear area against a dark background is presumptive evidence of *C. neoformans*. White blood cells and other artifacts may resemble encapsulated organisms; therefore, careful examination is necessary.

# APPENDIX C

# Staining Methods

## Gomori methenamine silver (GMS) stain

### Fixation
- Formalin 10%

### Technique
- Paraffin or frozen sections

### Solutions required
- 10% chromic acid
- 5% silver nitrate
- 3% methenamine
- 5% borax (sodium borate)
- 1% gold chloride
- 1% sodium metasulphite
- 5% sodium thiosulphate

### Preparation of stains

#### Methenamine-silver nitrate working solution

| | |
|---|---|
| 3% methenamine | 40 ml |
| 5% silver nitrate | 2 ml |
| 5% borax | 3 ml |
| Distilled water | 35 ml |

This solution must be freshly prepared before use. Other solutions may be reused up to 1 month.

#### Light green stock solution

| | |
|---|---|
| Light green, SF yellow | 0.2 g |
| Distilled water | 100 ml |
| Glacial acetic acid | 0.2 ml |

Solution is stable for 1 year

#### Working light green solution

| | |
|---|---|
| Stock light green solution | 10 ml |
| Distilled water | 40 ml |

Solution is stable for 1 month

### Staining procedure

1. Deparaffinize sections through 2 changes of xylene, absolute and 95% alcohols to distilled water. Other slides must be fixed by heating or submerging in alcohol. Positive control slides must be included each time the staining procedure is performed.
2. Oxidize in 10% chromic acid solution for 1 hour.
3. Wash in running tap water for 5 seconds.
4. Rinse in 1% sodium metasulphite for 1 minute to remove any residual chromic acid.
5. Wash in running tap water for 5–10 minutes.
6. Wash with 3 or 4 changes of distilled water.
7. Place in working methenamine-silver nitrate solution in oven at 58–60°C for 30–60 minutes until section turns yellowish-brown. Use paraffin-coated forceps to remove slide from this solution. Dip slide in distilled water and check for adequate

silver impregnation with microscope. Fungi should be dark brown in colour at this stage.
8. Rinse in 6 changes of distilled water.
9. Tone in 1% gold chloride solution for 2–5 minutes.
10. Rinse in distilled water.
11. Remove unreduced silver with 5% sodium thiosulphate solution for 2–5 minutes.
12. Wash thoroughly in tap water.
13. Counterstain with working light green for 30–45 seconds.
14. Dehydrate with 2 changes of 95% alcohol, absolute alcohol, clear with 2–3 changes of xylene. Place a drop of mounting medium on slide, and cover with coverslip.

## Results

- Fungi: Sharply delineated in black.
- Mucin: Taupe to dark gray.
- Inner parts of mycelia and hyphae: Old rose.
- Background: Pale green.

Methenamine silver nitrate is the most useful for screening clinical specimens. It provides better contrast and often stains fungal elements that may not be revealed by other procedures. Fungi are sharply delineated in black against a pale background. The inner parts of hyphae are charcoal gray. Certain bacteria (including *Nocardia* spp.) as well as some tissue elements also take the stain. Therefore, all that is gray or black is not necessarily a fungus.

## Mayer's mucicarmine stain for mucin and *Cryptococcus*

Meyer's mucicarmine stain is useful for differentiating *Cryptococcus neoformans* from other fungi of similar size and shape when found in samples of tissue. The mucopolysaccharide in the capsular material of the fungus stains red, whereas the other tissue elements stain yellow.

## Fixation

- Any well fixed tissue.

## Technique

- Six micrometer paraffin sections.

## Solutions

### Weigert's iron haematoxylin

**Solution A**
| | |
|---|---|
| Haematoxylin | 1 g |
| Alcohol 95% | 100 ml |

**Solution B**
| | |
|---|---|
| Ferric chloride, 29% aqueous solution | 4 ml |
| Distilled water | 95 ml |
| Hydrochloric acid, concentrated | 1 ml |

**Working solution**
Equal parts of solution A and B.
Prepare fresh.

### Metanil yellow solution

| | |
|---|---|
| Metanil yellow | 0.25 g |
| Distilled water | 100 ml |
| Glacial acetic acid | 0.25 ml |

### Mucicarmine stain

| | |
|---|---|
| Carmine | 1 g |
| Aluminium chloride, anhydrous | 0.5 g |
| Distilled water | 2 ml |

Mix stain in small test tube. Heat over small flame for 2 minutes. Liquid becomes almost black and syrupy. Dilute with 100 ml of 50% alcohol and let it stand for 24 hours. Filter. Dilute 1 to 4 with tap water for use.

### Staining procedure

1. Xylene, absolute and 95% alcohols to distilled water. Remove mercury precipitate through iodine and hypo solutions, if necessary.
2. Stain for 7 minutes in working solution of Weigert's haematoxylin.
3. Wash in tap water for 5–10 minutes.
4. Place in diluted mucicarmine solution for 30–60 minutes or longer.
5. Rinse quickly in distilled water.
6. Stain in metanil yellow solution for 1 minute.
7. Rinse quickly in distilled water.
8. Rinse quickly in 95% alcohol.
9. Dehydrate in 2 changes of absolute alcohol, clear with 2 to 3 changes of xylene and mount in Permount.

### Results
- Mucin: Red
- Nuclei: Black
- Other tissue elements: Yellow

### Periodic acid-Schiff (PAS) staining

#### Fixation
- 10% formalin

#### Technique
- Six micrometer paraffin sections.

#### Solutions

##### Schiff's leucofuchsin solution
Dissolve 1 g basic fuchsin in 200 ml hot distilled water. Bring to boiling point. Cool to 50°C. Filter and add 20 ml normal hydrochloric acid. Cool further and add 1 g anhydrous sodium metasulphite. Keep in dark for 48 hours until solution becomes straw coloured. Store in refrigerator.

##### 0.5% periodic acid solution

| | |
|---|---|
| Periodic acid crystals | 0.5 g |
| Distilled water | 100 ml |

##### 0.2% light green counterstain

| | |
|---|---|
| Light green crystal | 0.2 g |
| Distilled water | 100 ml |
| Glacial acetic acid | 0.2 ml |

#### Staining procedure
1. Bring sections to water (xylene → absolute alcohol → 95% alcohol → distilled water).
2. Oxidize with periodic acid solution for 5 minutes.
3. Rinse in distilled water.
4. Place in Schiff's leucofuchsin for 15 minutes.
5. Place in running tap water for 10 minutes for pink colour to develop.
6. Stain with light green counterstain for a few seconds.
7. Dehydrate in alcohol, clear in xylene and mount in synthetic resin medium.

#### Result
- Fungi: Red
- Nuclei: Blue
- Background: Pale green.

### Giemsa stain

Giemsa stain is used for the detection of intracellular yeast forms of *Histoplasma capsulatum* in bone marrow and buffy coat specimens. The fungus is usually seen as a small oval yeast cells that stain blue and have a hyaline halo that represents poorly staining cell wall. The stain can also be used to visualize the trophozoites of *Pneumocystis jirovecii*.

1. Place slide in 100% methanol for 1 minute (to fix smear).
2. Drain off methanol.
3. Flood slide with Giemsa stain (freshly diluted 1 : 10 with distilled water) for 5 minutes.
4. Wash with water, dry in air and mount.

#### Results
Nuclei: Purple
Cell cytoplasm: Blue to mauve
Red blood cells: Pink

### Gridley's fungus stain

#### Fixation
Any well fixed tissue.

#### Technique
Six micrometer paraffin sections.

#### Solutions

##### Chromic acid solutions

| | |
|---|---|
| Chromic acid | 4 g |
| Distilled water | 100 ml |

##### Coleman's Feulgen reagent
Bring 200 ml of distilled water to boil, remove from flame and add 1 g basic fuchsin. When fuchsin is dissolved, cool and filter. Add 2 g sodium meta-sulphite and 10 ml of normal hydrochloric acid. Let it bleach for 24 hours, and then add 0.5 g activated carbon, shake for about 1 minute and filter through coarse paper. The filtrate should be colourless. Store in refrigerator.

## Normal hydrochloric acid

Hydrochloric acid 83.5 ml
Distilled water 916.5 ml

## Sodium metasulphite solution

Sodium metasulphite 10 g
Distilled water 10 ml

## Sulphurous rinse

Sodium metasulphite, 10% solution 6 ml
Normal hydrochloric acid 5 ml
Distilled water 100 ml

## Aldehyde-fuchsin solution

Basic fuchsin 1 g
Alcohol, 70% 200 ml
Paraldehyde 2 ml
Hydrochloric acid, concentrated 2 ml

Let it stand at room temperature for 3 days until solution turns deep blue. Keep in refrigerator. Filter and warm to room temperature before using.

## Metanil yellow solution

Metanil yellow 0.25 g
Distilled water 100 ml
Glacial acetic acid 2 drops

## Staining procedure

1. Bring sections to distilled water (xylene → absolute and 95% alcohols → distilled water).
2. Place in 4% chromic acid for one hour (oxidizer).
3. Wash in running tap water for 5 minutes.
4. Place in Coleman's Feulgen reagent for 15 minutes.
5. Rinse in 3 changes of sulphurous acid rinse.
6. Wash for 15 minutes in running tap water.
7. Place slides in aldehyde-fuchsin solution for 15–30 minutes.
8. Rinse off excess stain with 95% alcohol.
9. Rinse in tap water.
10. Counterstain lightly with metanil yellow solution for 1 minute.
11. Rinse in tap water.
12. Dehydrate through 95% and absolute alcohols.
13. Clear in xylene and mount in Permount.

## Result

- Fungi, elastic tissue and mucin: Deep rose to purple.
- Background: Yellow.

## Alcian blue staining

Alcian blue and Meyer's mucicarmine stain are mucopolysaccharide stains. These are useful for visualizing the polysaccharide capsule produced by *Cryptococcus neoformans* in histological sections of tissue.

## Fixation

- Neutral 10% formalin.

## Technique

- Six micrometer paraffin sections.

## Solutions

### 3% acetic acid solution

Glacial acetic acid 3 ml
Distilled water 97 ml

### Alcian blue solution

Alcian blue 1 g
Acetic acid, 3% solution 100 ml

Adjust the pH to 2.5. Filter and add a few crystals of thymol.

### Kernechtrot solution

Kernechtrot 0.1 g
Aluminium sulphate, 5% solution 100 ml

Dissolve by aid of heat. Cool, filter, and add a few crystals of thymol.

### Hyaluronidase solution

Dissolve 1 vial (150 TR units) hyaluronidase with 1 ml saline.

## Staining procedure

1. Deparaffinize sections through 2 changes of xylene, absolute and 95% alcohols.
2. Wash in tap water. Rinse in distilled water.
3. Mordant in 3% acetic acid solution for 3 minutes.
4. Stain in Alcian blue solution for 30 minutes.
5. Wash in running tap water for 1 minute.

6. Rinse in distilled water.
7. Counterstain in kernechtrot for 5 minutes.
8. Wash in running tap water for 1 minute.
9. Dehydrate with 2 changes of 95% alcohol, absolute alcohol, clear with 2–3 changes of xylene and mount in Permount.

### Results

- Acid mucopolysaccharide: Blue
- Nuclei: Pink

## Haematoxylin and eosin (H&E) staining

1. Bring sections to distilled water.
2. Stain with Ehrlich's haematoxylin for 8 minutes.
3. Tip off stain and wash thoroughly with water.
4. Differentiate with 1% acid alcohol for 15 seconds.
5. Wash well in water and blue for 3–5 minutes.
6. Counterstain with 1% aqueous eosin for 2 minutes.
7. Wash in tap water.
8. Wash in 95% alcohol for a few seconds.
9. Dehydrate with absolute alcohol.
10. Clear the section in xylene.
11. Mount in DPX.

### Result

1. Tissue response can be demonstrated better than with any special stain.
2. Innate colour of the fungal elements whether phaeoid (pigmented) or hyaline, can be determined.
3. Haematoxylin stains nuclei of most yeast-like cells.
4. Some fungi, e.g., the aspergilli and Mucorales are haematoxylinophilic and readily delineated with H&E.

## Gram staining

Yeast cells and pseudohyphae generally stain Gram-positive and hyphae (septate and nonseptate) stain Gram-negative.

### Reagents

(a) **Crystal violet alcohol solution**

| | |
|---|---|
| Crystal violet, 85% dye content | 2 g |
| Ethyl alcohol, 95% | 10 ml |

Dissolve the dye in alcohol. Add 100 ml distilled water.

(b) **Ammonium oxalate solution**

| | |
|---|---|
| Ammonium oxalate | 4 g |
| Distilled water | 400 ml |

Dissolve ammonium oxalate in water.

Mix the crystal violet alcohol solution (a) with the ammonium oxalate solution (b).

### Gram iodine solution

| | |
|---|---|
| Iodine | 1 g |
| Potassium iodide | 2 g |

Dissolve iodine and potassium iodide completely in 5 ml of distilled water.

Add 240 ml distilled water and 60 ml sodium bicarbonate (5% aqueous solution).

Mix well; store in amber glass bottle.

### Counterstain

| | |
|---|---|
| Safranin O | 1 g |
| Ethyl alcohol, 95% | 40 ml |

Dissolve the dye in alcohol. Add 400 ml distilled water. Mix well.

### Staining procedure

1. Fix the smear by passing it over a flame.
2. Place crystal violet solution on the slide for 20 seconds.
3. Wash gently with tap water.
4. Apply Gram iodine solution to the slide for 20 seconds.
5. Wash gently with tap water.
6. Decolourize quickly in solution of equal parts of acetone and 95% ethanol.
7. Wash gently with tap water.
8. Counterstain with safranin for 10 seconds.
9. Wash with tap water, air dry and blot dry.

## Acid-fast modified Kinyoun stain for *Nocardia* spp.

### Reagents

*Kinyoun carbol fuchsin*

| | |
|---|---|
| Basic-fuchsin | 4 g |
| Phenol | 8 ml |

# Staining Methods

| | |
|---|---|
| Alcohol, 95% | 20 ml |
| Distilled water | 100 ml |

Dissolve the dye in the alcohol, and then add water and phenol.

## 1% aqueous $H_2SO_4$

| | |
|---|---|
| Concentrated $H_2SO_4$ | 1 ml |
| Distilled water | 99 ml |

Add acid to water, not vice versa.

## Counterstain

| | |
|---|---|
| Methylene blue | 2.5 g |
| Ethanol, 95% | 100 ml |
| or | |
| Brilliant green | 0.5 g |
| Distilled water | 100 ml |

## Staining procedure

1. Make a smear and fix over flame.
2. Flood slide with Kinyoun carbol fuchsin for 5 minutes.
3. Pour off excess stain.
4. Flood slide with 50% alcohol and immediately wash with tap water.
5. Decolorize with 1% aqueous sulphuric acid.
6. Wash with tap water.
7. Counterstain with methylene blue or brilliant green for 1 minute.
8. Rinse with water, dry, and examine under oil-immersion objective.

## Results

The filaments of *Nocardia* spp. usually appear at least partially acid-fast with this staining procedure. Acid-fast organisms stain pink to red.

## Lactophenol cotton blue stain

Lactophenol cotton blue (LPCB) consists of phenol, lactic acid, glycerol, and aniline (cotton) blue dye. It is used as both a mounting fluid and a stain. Lactic acid acts as a clearing agent and aids in preserving the fungal structure, phenol acts as a killing agent, glycerol prevents drying, and cotton blue gives colour to the structures.

| | |
|---|---|
| Lactic acid | 20 ml |
| Phenol crystals | 20 g |
| Glycerol | 40 ml |
| Distilled water | 20 ml |
| Cotton blue | 0.05 g |

Dissolve phenol in the lactic acid, glycerol, and distilled water by gently heating. Add cotton blue. Mix well.

There are several methods for microscopic examination of a fungus culture.

### A. Tease mount

1. Place a drop of LPCB on a clean glass slide.
2. With a bent dissecting needle, remove a small portion of the colony from the agar surface and place it in the drop of LPCB.
3. With 2 dissecting needles gently tease apart the mycelial mass of the colony on the slide, cover with coverslip, and observe under the microscope with low-power and high-dry magnifications.

Teasing the colony often disrupts the delicate fruiting structures of the filamentous molds, making it difficult in some instances to observe the characteristic spore arrangements or hyphal attachments necessary for a definitive identification. In such cases, a cellophane tape mount or slide culture may be required.

### B. Cellophane tape mount

1. Press the sticky side of a 4 cm strip of clear cellophane tape gently but firmly to the surface of the fungal colony and then pull the tape gently away. A portion of aerial mycelium will adhere to the tape. This operation should always be performed under a biologic safety hood. Fingers should not come in contact with the mold, therefore, gloves should be worn.
2. Place a small drop of LPCB on a glass slide.
3. Stick one end of the tape to the surface of the slide adjacent to the drop of stain.
4. Stretch the tape over the stain, gently lowering it, so that the mycelium becomes permeated with stain.
5. Examine under microscope.

This method is usually successful in retaining the original positions of the characteristic fungal structures but has the drawback of requiring the organism to be grown on plated medium.

## Slide culture

It is the best method for observing the actual structure of a fungus. It is indicated when teased mount of LPCB is inconclusive.

1. Cover the inside bottom of a 100 mm diameter sterile petri plate with a piece of filter paper.
2. Place a bent glass rod over the filter paper.
3. Place a clean, flamed glass microscope slide on the glass rod.
4. Put a piece of 1 square cm block of cornmeal agar or potato dextrose agar on the slide.
5. Inoculate the fungal strain under identification at four sides of agar block.
6. Place a flamed coverslip over the block and apply slight pressure to ensure adherence.
7. Place approximately 1.5 ml of sterile water on the filter paper to prevent drying of agar and incubate at room temperature.
8. Examine periodically for growth, and add sterile water if the medium begins to dry out. The fungus ordinarily grows on the surface of the slide and also on the undersurface of the coverslip. The closed petri plate can be placed on the microscope stage, and the slide culture can be examined with the low-power objective.
9. When growth appears, carefully remove the coverslip and place it on a drop of LPCB on a second slide.
10. With a needle or applicator stick, gently flip the agar block of the original slide into a container of antifungal disinfectant. Place a drop of LPCB on the slide, and place a new coverslip over it.
11. Both microscopic preparations from steps 9 and 10 can be sealed around the edges with nail polish for further study or as teaching aids. The mycelia which adhere to glass surface usually show characteristic microscopic appearance, which may be lost if teasing needles are used as it happens in routine LPCB mounts.

## Germ tube test for the presumptive identification of *Candida albicans*

**About 90% of yeasts isolated from human material are *Candida albicans*** and a rapid method of identification is available. The ability of this species to produce a germ tube in serum is shared only with *C. dubliniensis*. For the 'germ tube' test, lightly touch a single colony with a loop or Pasteur pipette; remove excess inoculum and then emulsify the yeast cells in 0.5 ml of sheep, horse or human serum in a small test tube with a loose cotton-wool plug. The optimum inoculum is $10^5$–$10^6$ cells per ml. An increased concentration of inoculum causes a significant decrease in the percentage of cells forming germ tubes. Incubate at 35–37°C for no longer than 3 hours. Place 1 drop of the yeast-serum mixture on a slide. Place a coverslip over the drop and examine microscopically for germ tube production. A known strain of *C. albicans* should be tested with each new batch of serum.

Germ tubes are the beginnings of true hyphae and appear as filaments that are not constricted at their points of origin on the parent cell. If the filaments are constricted and septate at their points of origin, they are pseudohyphae, not germ tubes (Fig. 15.6).

# APPENDIX D

# Glossary

**Acrogenous.** Conidia developing at the tip of a conidiophore.

**Acropetal.** A chain of conidia growing at the tip; having the youngest conidium at the apex of the chain.

**Acropleurogenous.** Conidia developing at the tip and along the sides.

**Adiaconidium.** A fungus conidium which when introduced into an animal or incubated *in vitro* at elevated temperatures, increases greatly in size without eventual reproduction or replication.

**Aerial hyphae/mycelium.** Hyphae growing above the colony surface, for example, on an agar base.

**Aflatoxin.** Toxin produced by the *Aspergillus flavus* group. The acronym 'aflatoxin' is derived from *Aspergillus flavus* toxin.

**Aleuriconidium.** Thick walled terminal or lateral conidium attached by a wide base to the conidiophore and released by fracture of the wall below the conidium.

**Anamorph.** An asexual or imperfect state of fungus.

**Angioinvasive.** Tending to invade the walls of blood vessels.

**Annellide.** A cell that produces and extrudes conidia; the tip tapers, lengthens, and acquires a ring of cell wall material as each conidium is released.

**Annelloconidium.** A conidium arising from an annellide.

**Annellophore.** The conidiophore or stalk supporting an annellide.

**Antheridium.** The male gametangium.

**Anthropophilic.** A dermatophyte that preferentially or exclusively infects humans, i.e., humans are its natural hosts.

**Antler hyphae.** Repeatedly branching hyphal tip resembling an antler.

**Apophysis.** Swelling of a sporangiophore immediately below the columella.

**Arthroconidium.** A conidium formed by septation of a hypha. The resulting conidium may be rectangular or barrel-shaped and thick or thin-walled, depending on the genus.

**Ascospore.** A sexual spore produced in a saclike structure known as an ascus.

**Ascocarp.** A fruiting body which bears asci and ascospores.

**Ascus.** A round or elongate sacklike structure usually containing two to eight haploid sexual ascospores. Asci are often formed within a fruiting body, such as cleistothecium or perithecium.

**Assimilation.** The ability of a fungus to use a specific carbon or nitrogen source for growth; assimilation is read by the presence or absence of growth.

**Asteroid body.** An eosinophilic antigen-antibody complex deposited *in vivo* surrounding *Sporothrix schenckii* yeast forms in tissue.

**Ballistospore.** A spore that, at maturity, is actively ejected, as in the Entomophthorales.

**Basidiospore.** A haploid sexual spore borne on a basidium.

**Basidiocarp.** Fruiting body seen in Basidiomycetes which contains basidia.

**Basidium.** The structure which bears basidiospores.

**Basipetal.** Growing in the direction of base, with the apical cell the oldest.

**Biseriate.** The phialide supported by a metula in genera *Aspergillus* and *Penicillium* as opposed to a uniseriate phialide, which forms directly on the vesicle.

**Blastic.** A mode of conidiogenesis best described as "budding".

**Blastoconidium.** A conidium formed by budding along a hypha, pseudohypha or single cell, as in the yeasts.

**Budding.** A process of asexual reproduction in which the fungal cell develops a smaller outgrowth from the parent cell. This is characteristic of yeast and yeast-like fungi.

**Capsule.** A colourless, transparent, mucopolysaccharide on the wall of a cell or spore. It is seen in *Cryptococcus* and *Rhodotorula* spp.

**Chlamydoconidium (syn: Chlamydospore).** A thick-walled, rounded, intercalary or terminal conidium containing stored food enabling it to assist in survival. It may be located at the end of the hypha (terminal) or inserted along the hypha (intercalary), singly or in chains. It is greater in diameter than the hypha on which it is borne.

**Clamp connection.** A short hypha which bypasses a hyphal septum and is attached to the two cells adjacent to the septum.

**Clavate.** Club-shaped.

**Cleistothecium.** A large, fairly round, closed multicellular fruiting body (ascoma) in which asci and ascospores are formed and held until the structure ruptures.

**Coenocytic.** Having many nuclei and few or no septa (cross-walls); nonseptate.

**Collarette.** Cup- or funnel-shaped remnant of cell wall present at the tip of phialide through which conidia are produced.

**Columella.** Enlarged, dome-shaped tip of sporangiophore extending into sporangium. Often the sporangium bursts, leaving the columella bare and readily visible upon microscopic examination.

**Conidiogenous cell.** The cell that produces the conidia.

**Conidiophore.** A specialized hypha which bears conidia.

**Conidium.** An asexual propagule that forms on the side or the end of hypha or conidiophore. It may consist of one or more cells, and the size, shape, and arrangement in groups are generally characteristic of the organism. It is always borne externally, i.e., not enclosed within a saclike structure such as a sporangium. If a fungus produces two types of conidia, those that are small and usually single-celled are referred to as *microconidia*, whereas the larger *macroconidia* are usually segmented into two or more cells.

**Cryptococcoma.** Cyst-like granuloma containing cryptococci, particularly common in the cerebral cortex but also found in the lung and elsewhere.

**Dematiaceous.** Pigmented fungi that have brown- or black-coloured cell walls in their conidia, mycelia and sclerotic bodies. This is due to melanotic pigment in the cell walls. They form brown to black colonies on culture.

**Denticle.** Small, narrow, projection bearing a conidium.

**Dermatomycosis.** A fungal disease of the skin, hair, or nails caused by nondermatophytic molds and yeasts.

**Dermatophyte.** A pathogenic fungus of the genera *Microsporum*, *Trichophyton*, or *Epidermophyton* causing a cutaneous infection of the stratum corneum, the hair, or nails.

**Dichotomous.** A type of branching in which the two branches are equal in diameter to the hypha from which they originated.

**Dimorphic.** Having two morphological forms (hyphal and yeast) produced by fungi such as *Histoplasma capsulatum*. It is due to temperature-

# Glossary

dependent changes in the organism on artificial culture media, i.e., fungi having mold phase when cultured at 25–30°C and a yeast phase when cultured at 35–37°C.

**Downy.** Colonies covered with short, fine hyphae.

**Dysgonic.** Growing with difficulty on artificial culture media.

**Echinulate.** Covered with small spines.

**Ectothrix.** Forming a sheath of arthroconidia outside the hair.

**Endothrix.** Arthroconidia within the hair shaft without a conspicuous external sheath of arthroconidia.

**Favic chandeliers.** Hyphae terminating in broad, irregular, antler-like branches. It is characteristic of *Trichophyton schoenleinii*.

**Floccose.** Cottony.

**Foot cell.** Base of the conidiophore. Here it merges with the hypha, giving the impression of a foot, typically seen in *Aspergillus* spp.

**Fusiform.** Spindle-shaped, i.e., wider in the middle and tapering towards both ends.

**Fragmentation.** Breaking of the hyphae into pieces (arthroconidia) which are capable of forming new organisms.

**Geophilic.** Those dermatophytes which are soil-inhabiting.

**Germ tube.** A tubelike outgrowth from a yeast, conidium or spore. It is the beginning of a true hypha.

**Glabrous.** Smooth; without aerial hyphae.

**Globose.** Round.

**Halophilic.** Requiring a salty environment.

**Halotolerant.** Tolerant of a salty environment.

**Heterothalic.** A fungus that is only capable of sexual reproduction after the fusion of two genetically dissimilar nuclei from two different thalli or strains of compatible mating types.

**Hilum.** Scar of attachment where the conidium was formerly attached to the conidiophore and/or another conidium.

**Homothalic.** A fungus that does not require two distinct thalli or strains for sexual reproduction.

**Hyaline.** Clear, transparent, colourless.

**Hyalohyphomycosis.** Infections caused by molds that lack melanin in their cell walls, form colourless (hyaline), septate hyphae in host tissue and which do not have established names such as aspergillosis.

**Hypha.** A filamentous structure of a fungus. It may be septate or nonseptate. Many hyphae together constitute the mycelium.

**Hyphomycete.** An asexual fungus possessing colourless (hyaline) or darkly pigmented (dematiaceous) mycelium.

**Id (Dermatophytid).** A cutaneous vesicular eruption, usually distinct from the site of a dermatophyte infection, but related to it. Ids are thought to result from interaction between circulating antigen and antibodies. Although usually vesicular, they may be papular or eczematous. They are sterile lesions and are most often seen in inflammatory dermatophytosis.

**Infectious propagules.** Particles capable of communicating infection; in mycology, spores, conidia or, exceptionally, hyphal fragments.

**Intercalary.** Formed between cells of a hypha, not at its ends.

**Isthmus.** A narrow neck or pore between mother and daughter yeast cells.

**Karyogamy.** Fusion of two nuclei.

**Keratinases.** Proteinases capable of digesting hair, nails, and skin scales.

**Keratinophilic.** Capable of digesting and using keratin, such as fungi causing cutaneous mycoses, the dermatophytes.

**Lenticular.** Having the shape of a double convex lens.

**Macroconidium.** The larger of two types of conidia in those fungi that produce both large and small conidia. It may be single-celled but usually is multi-celled.

**Metulae.** Secondary branches of conidiophore that support the phialide in genera such as *Aspergillus* and *Penicillium*.

**Microconidium.** The smaller of two types of conidia in those fungi which produce both large and small conidia. It is usually single-celled.

**Mold.** A filamentous fungus.

**Moniliform** (*monilia:* necklace). Hyphae with swellings at regular intervals. Beaded and joined together like a string of beads or pearls; that is regularly constricted and composed of globose cells.

**Monomorphic.** Growth exclusively in a single form, either as a mold or as a yeast.

**Morphogenesis.** Development or change in the form of an organism, for example, mold to yeast or yeast to mold dimorphism.

**Muriform.** An enlarged fungal cell with cross-walls produced both vertically and horizontally.

**Mycelium.** The mass of intertwined hyphae making up the colony of a fungus.

**Mycetoma.** Chronic granulomatous infection usually of exposed parts of the body especially feet and hands. It is classically characterized by tumefactions, deformities and draining sinuses discharging fungal or bacterial grains or granules (triad of symptoms).

**Mycology.** The study of fungi and their biologies.

**Mycosis** (pl. mycoses). Infection caused by a fungus.

**Nodular body.** Knot-like structure formed by intertwined hyphae. It is produced by some species of dermatophytes.

**Nonseptate (syn. coenocytic).** Lacking septa (cross-walls) between cells.

**Obclavate.** Club-shaped and thickened at the outer end.

**Obovoid.** An inverted egg-shaped conidium with the broad end up and narrow end down.

**Onychomycosis.** Fungal infection of the nail caused by any fungus (a dermatophyte or other fungus).

**Oogonium.** The female cell of Oomycetes.

**Ostiole.** A mouth or opening in an ascocarp or pycnidium through which conidia escape.

**Pectinate.** Resembling a comb.

**Penicillate.** Brush-like pattern of conidiophores and metulae. It is seen in *Penicillium* and *Scopulariopsis* species.

**Penicillus.** A brush-like asexual sporing head characteristic of the genus *Penicillium*.

**Perfect state.** The part of life cycle in which spores are formed after nuclear fusion (sexual reproduction).

**Perithecium.** A flask-shaped ascocarp usually having a small rounded opening (ostiole). It contains asci and ascospores.

**Phaeohyphomycosis.** Diseases caused by melanized fungi in which the hyphal or yeast-like tissue forms appear darkly pigmented. Excluded are agents of chromoblastomycosis which have a distinct tissue form.

**Phaeoid.** Darkly pigmented.

**Phialide.** A cell that produces and extrudes succession of conidia. It is usually flask-, vase-, or tenpin-shaped.

**Phialoconidium.** Conidium that is produced by flask-shaped conidiogenous cell called phialide. It is seen in *Phialophora* species.

**Pleomorphic.** Condition in which more than one form of sporulation occurs as seen in *Fonsecaea pedrosoi*.

**Pleurogenous.** Borne on the sides of a conidiophore or hypha.

**Propagule.** A reproductive unit that is capable of propagation.

**Pseudohypha.** A fragile chain of cells formed by budding and have elongated without detaching from adjacent cells. It differs from true hypha by being constricted at the septa, forming branches that arise at the septa, and having terminal cells smaller than the other cells.

**Pycnidium.** A spherical or flask-shaped asexual fruiting body containing conidia. It usually has an opening (osteole).

**Pyriform.** Pear-shaped.

**Racquet hypha.** A hypha with one enlarged (club-shaped) end. The enlarged end of one cell is attached to the smaller end of the adjacent cell.

**Rhizoid.** Rootlike, branched hypha growing into the medium.

**Ringworm.** A communicable skin disease affecting the outer layer of the epidermis, the stratum corneum, which may invade the hair and nails, caused by dermatophytes. The classic appearance of the skin lesion is circular with an active border, inflammation, scaling, and pruritis.

# Glossary

**Rugose.** Ridged, wrinkled, or roughened surface.

**Saprobe/Saprophyte.** An organism which uses dead organic matter as a source of nutrients.

**Sclerotic body.** Rounded, thick-walled, brown cell with a diameter of 5–12 µm. It has horizontal and/or vertical septations. It reproduces by equatorial splitting and not by budding.

**Septate hypha.** Hypha having cross-walls.

**Septum.** A cross-wall.

**Sessile.** A conidium arising directly from the surface of a hypha.

**Sexual state.** Life cycle in which the organism reproduces by the union of two nuclei. It is also known as *perfect state*.

**Spherule.** Large, round, thick-walled structure containing endoconidia. It is seen in *Coccidioides immitis*.

**Spinose.** Covered with small spines.

**Spiral hypha.** Hypha forming coiled or corkscrew-like turns.

**Splendore-Hoeppli material.** Eosinophilic material formed by antibodies or antigen-antibody complexes. It is found surrounding yeast cells of *Sporothrix schenckii*, grains of actinomycetoma, botryomycosis and actinomycosis, hyphae of Entomophthorales, *Schistosoma* eggs and microfilariae.

**Sporangiophore.** A specialized hyphal branch or stalk bearing a sporangium.

**Sporangium.** A closed saclike structure which produces asexual endoconidia by cleavage.

**Spore.** Propagule that develops by asexual means within a sporangium (sporangiospore or endoconidia), or by sexual reproduction (ascospores, basidiospores or zygospores).

**Sterigmata.** A small pointed structure arising from a hypha or cell and supporting a spore.

**Stolon.** A horizontal hypha, or runner that grows along the surface of the medium. It often bears rhizoids that penetrate the medium and sporangiophores that ascend into air.

**Subclavate.** Somewhat club-shaped.

**Syngamy.** Fusion of gametes in fertilization.

**Synonym.** Another name for a species or taxonomic group.

**Taxonomy.** Science of systematic classification of organisms.

**Teleomorph.** Sexual reproductive or perfect stage of fungus.

**Thallus.** The vegetative body of a fungus.

**Tuberculate.** Covered with finger-like outgrowths as seen in macroconidia of *Histoplasma capsulatum*.

**Umbonate.** Colony raised in the centre.

**Uncinate.** With tip bent to form hook.

**Uniseriate.** Phialides arising directly from the vesicle as in *Aspergillus fumigatus*.

**Vasiform.** Vase-shaped.

**Velvety.** Low aerial mycelia.

**Verrucose.** Furrowed colony.

**Verticillate.** Branches arranged in whorls.

**Vesicle.** Enlarged structure at the end of conidiophore or sporangiophore bearing metulae and/or phialides which, in turn, bear conidia, e.g., *Aspergillus* spp.

**Virulence.** Degree of the disease-producing ability of a microorganism.

**Yeast and yeast-like.** Unicellular organisms that reproduce by budding. If buds (blastoconidia) elongate and remain attached to the parent cell, they form chains known as pseudohyphae. Some organisms, e.g., *Candida albicans* also produce true hyphae, while others form no hyphal elements.

**Zoophilic.** Growing preferentially on lower animals rather than man.

# APPENDIX E

# Overview of Medical Mycology

*Fungal infections in the patients with immunodeficiency virus infection*

- Candidiasis
- Cryptococcosis
- Histoplasmosis
- Coccidioidomycosis
- Penicilliosis marneffei
- Aspergillosis

*Invasive fungal pathogens in cancer patients*

- *Candida* spp.
- *Aspergillus* spp.
- *Fusarium* spp.
- Mucorales
- *Scedosporium* spp.
- *Cryptococcus neoformans*
- *Pneumocystis jirovecii*

*Fungal infections in the organ transplant recipients*

- Blastomycosis
- Coccidioidomycosis
- Histoplasmosis
- Aspergillosis

*Invasive fungal infections in paediatric patients*

**Opportunistic yeasts**

- **Candida albicans**
- Non-***Candida albicans*** **spp., in particular *C. parapsilosis***
- *Cryptococcus neoformans*
- *Trichosporon beigelii*
- *Malassezia* spp.

**Opportunistic molds**

- ***Aspergillus* spp.**
- *Fusarium* spp.
- Mucorales
- *Acremonium* spp.
- *Pacilomyces* spp.
- *Trichoderma* spp.

**Dematiaceous molds**

- *Pseudallescheria boydii*
- *Alternaria* spp.
- *Curvularia* spp.
- *Bipolaris* spp.
- *Wangiella* spp.

**Endemic dimorphic molds**

- *Histoplasma capsulatum*
- *Coccidioides immitis*
- *Blastomyces dermatitidis*
- *Sporothrix schenckii*
- *Paracoccidioides brasiliensis*
- *Penicillium marneffei*

### Oral fungal infections
- Candidiasis
- Aspergillosis
- Mucormycosis
- Cryptococcosis
- Histoplasmosis
- Blastomycosis
- Coccidioidomycosis
- Paracoccidioidomycosis

### Cutaneous mycoses
- Dermatophytosis
- Candidiasis
- Pityriasis versicolor
- Black piedra
- White piedra

### Subcutaneous mycoses
- Mycetoma
- Chromoblastomycosis
- Sporotrichosis
- Rhinosporidiosis
- Entomophthoromycosis
- Phaeohyphomycosis
- Lobomycosis

### Fungi causing infections of bone and joint
- *Blastomyces dermatitidis*
- *Coccidioides immitis*
- *Cryptococcus neoformans*
- *Candida* spp.
- *Histoplasma capsulatum*

### Fungal infections of genitourinary tract
- Vaginal candidiasis
- Lower urinary tract candidiasis
- Renal candidiasis

### Fungal infections of respiratory tract
- Aspergillosis
- Mucormycosis
- *Fusarium* infections
- *Scedosporium apiospermum* infections
- Histoplasmosis
- Coccidioidomycosis
- Blastomycosis
- Paracoccidioidomycosis
- Penicilliosis marneffei

### Fungal infections of central nervous system
- Aspergillosis
- Candidiasis
- Blastomycosis
- Coccidioidomycosis
- Cryptococcosis
- Histoplasmosis
- Sporotrichosis
- Mucormycosis
- *Scedosporium apiospermum* infection
- *Cladophialophora bantiana* infection

### Haematogenously disseminated fungi
- *Candida* spp.
- *Aspergillus* spp.
- Mucorales
- *Histoplasma capsulatum*
- *Coccidioides* spp.
- *Blastomyces dermatitidis*
- *Sporothrix schenckii*
- *Paracoccidioides brasiliensis*
- *Penicillium marneffei*
- *Cryptococcus neoformans*
- *Fusarium* spp.
- *Trichosporon* spp.
- *Scedosporium* spp.

### Biosafety level 2 practices are recommended for handling and processing mold cultures of:
- *Blastomyces dermatitidis*
- *Histoplasma capsulatum*
- *Cryptococcus neoformans*
- *Penicillium marneffei*
- *Sporothrix schenckii*
- *Bipolaris* spp.
- *Cladophialophora bantiana*
- *Wangiella dermatitidis*
- *Exserohilum* spp.
- *Fonsecaea pedrosoi*
- *Ochraconis gallopava*
- *Scedosporium prolificans*

### Biosafety level 3 practices are recommended for handling and processing mold cultures of:
- *Coccidioides immitis*

# Index

## A

Absidia, 159
Acid-fast modified Kinyoun stain for *Nocardia* spp., 214
Acid-fast staining, 20
Acquired resistance, 35
*Acremonium* spp., 66
*Actinomadura madurae*, 67
*Actinomadura pelletieri*, 68
*Actinomyces*, 62
*Actinomyces israelii*, 62
Actinomycetomas
    Diagnostic characteristics of grains, 70
Acute atrophic candidiasis, 125
Acute pseudomembranous candidiasis, 124
Adiaconidium, 187
Adiaspiromycosis, 187
    Laboratory diagnosis, 188
    Pathogenesis, 187
    Treatment, 189
Aerial mycelium, 5
Aflatoxins, 195
Alcian blue staining, 213
Allergic fungal sinusitis, 83
*Alternaria* spp., 82
Alveolitis, 150
Antheridium, 11
Antifungal agents
    Mechanisms of resistance, 35
Azole resistance, 35
    Acquired, 35
    Intrinsic, 35
    Nonazole resistance, 36
Antifungal drugs, Classification
    Systemic, 28
    Allylamines, 32
        Terbinafine, 32
    Antibiotics, 28
        Amphotericin B, 28
        Griseofulvin, 29
    Antimetabolite, 32
        Flucytosine, 32
    Azoles, 29, 33
        Clotrimazole, 33
        Econazole, 33
        Fluconazole, 30
        Itraconazole, 30
        Ketoconazole, 30
        Miconazole, 33
        Oxiconazol, 33
        Posaconazole, 30
        Voriconazole, 30
    Echinocandins, 31
    Topical, 32
    Allylamines, 33
        Amorolfine, 34
        Butenafine, 33
        Naftifine, 34
    Benzoic acid, 34
    Ciclopirox olamine, 34
    Polyene antibiotics, 33
        Hamycin, 33
        Natamycin, 33
        Nystatin, 33
    Salicylic acid, 34
    Sodium thiosulphate, 34
    Tolnaftate, 34
    Undecylenic acid, 34
Antifungal drugs for the treatment of superficial and systemic mycoses, 35
*Apophysomyces*, 159
*Apophysomyces elegans*, 165
Arthroconidia, 7
Arthroderma, 47
Ascocarps, 10
Ascogonium, 11
Ascomycota, 10
    Life cycle, 11
Aspergilloma, 150
Aspergillosis
    Laboratory diagnosis, 152
        Culture, 154
            *Aspergillus flavus*, 154, 155
            *Aspergillus fumigatus*, 154, 155
            *Aspergillus nidulans*, 155
            *Aspergillus niger*, 155
            *Aspergillus terreus*, 155
    Pathogenesis, 150
        Acute invasive pulmonary aspergillosis, 151
        Allergic bronchopulmonary aspergillosis, 150

# Index

Cerebral aspergillosis, 152
Cutaneous aspergillosis, 152
Endocarditis, 152
Intracavitary aspergilloma (fungus ball), 151
Keratitis, 152
Otomycosis, 152
Paranasal *Aspergillus* granuloma, 151
Treatment, 156
*Aspergillus*, 150, 194
*Aspergillus niger*, 155
*Aspergillus terreus*, 155

## B

Basic fungal morphology, 5
*Basidiobolus*, 159
*Basidiobolus ranarum*, 165, 166
  Pathogenesis, 166
Basidiomycota, 12
  Life cycle, 13
Basidiospores, 12
Bird seed agar, 22
Blastoconidia, 7
*Blastomyces dermatitidis*, 103
  Phases, 106
Blastomycosis, 103
  Clinical types, 104
    Cutaneous blastomycosis, 104, 105
    Disseminated extrapulmonary blastomycosis, 104
    Pulmonary blastomycosis, 104
  Laboratory diagnosis, 105
  Oral manifestations, 105
  Pathogenesis, 104
  Treatment, 106
Blood agar, 22
Botryomycosis, 69
Brain heart infusion agar, 22

## C

Candida, 121
  Deep infections, 125
    Bone and joint *Candida* infection, 126
    Candidiasis of cardiovascular system, 126
    Candidiasis of gastrointestinal tract, 125

Candidiasis of respiratory system, 126
Candidiasis of liver, spleen and other organs, 126
Central nervous system candidiasis, 126
Ocular *Candida* infection, 126
Renal and urinary tract candidiasis, 125, 126
Superficial infections, 123
  Cutaneous infections, 123
  Mucosal infections, 124
  Nail infections, 124
*Candida* infection
  Laboratory diagnosis, 127
  Treatment, 131
*Candida albicans*, 121
*Candida dubliniensis*, 121, 122
*Candida glabrata*, 121, 122
*Candida guilliermondii*, 121, 122
*Candida kefyr*, 121, 122
*Candida krusei*, 121, 122
*Candida lusitaniae*, 121, 122
*Candida parapsilosis*, 121, 122
*Candida tropicalis*, 121, 122
*Candidal intertrigo*, 123
Candidemia, 127
Candidiasis
  Clinical features, 123
  Clinical forms, 123
  Pathogenesis, 121
  Virulence factors, 122
Candids, 123
Cerebral phaeohyphomycosis, 84
Chlamydoconidia, 7
Chromoblastomycosis, 77
  Laboratory diagnosis, 78
  Mycology, 78
    *Cladophialophora carrionii*, 80
    *Fonsecaea compacta*, 79
    *Fonsecaea pedrosoi*, 78
    *Phialophora verrucosa*, 78
    *Rhinocladiella aquaspersa*, 80
  Pathogenesis, 77
  Treatment, 80
Chromomycosis, 77
Chronic mucocutaneous candidiasis (CMC), 124
Citrinin, 197
*Cladophialophora carrionii*, 77
Clamp connections, 12
  Formation of, 12

*Coccidioides immitis*, 109
*Coccidioides posadasii*, 109
Coccidioidomycosis, 109
  Animal pathogenicity, 112
  Disseminated, 110
  Laboratory diagnosis, 110
  Oral manifestations, 110
  Pathogenesis, 109
  Primary pulmonary, 110
  Treatment, 112
Conidia, 7, 10
*Conidiobolus*, 159
*Conidiobolus coronatus*, 165, 166, 167
  Pathogenesis, 166
*Conidiobolus incongruus*, 165
Conidiogenesis, 7
  Method of, 7
    Blastic conidiogenesis, 7
    Thallic conidiogenesis, 7
  Types, 8
Conjunctivitis
  Fungi which cause the disease, 185
Cryptococcosis, 134
  Clinical manifestations, 136
    Central nervous system cryptococcosis, 136
    Cutaneous cryptococcosis, 136
    Ocular cryptococcosis, 136
    Oral cryptococcosis, 137
    Osseous cryptococcosis, 136
    Other foci of infection, 137
    Pulmonary cryptococcosis, 136
  Immune response, 136
  Laboratory diagnosis, 137
  Mycology, 134
  Pathogenesis, 136
  Treatment, 139
*Cryptococcus neoformans*, 134
Culture media
  Assimilation media for yeasts, 204
  Auxanographic plate method, 204
  Enriched media, 202
  For primary isolation of fungi, 201
  Nutritionally deficient media, 202
*Cunninghamella bertholletiae*, 164
*Curvularia geniculata*, 66

## D

Dermatomycosis, 82
Dermatophyte macroconidia
  Generic characteristics, 48

# Index

Dermatophytes
  Characteristics, 52
  Classification, 47
    Anthropophilic species, 49
    Geophilic species, 47
    Zoophilic species, 47
    Grouping on the basis of host preference and natural habitat, 48
  Macroconidia, 48
  Types of lesions and causative species, 49
Dermatophytid, 47
Dermatophytosis, 47
  Immunology, 56
  Laboratory diagnosis, 50
  Treatment, 56
Dimorphic fungus, 5, 73
Disseminated candidiasis, 127

## E

Ectothrix, 49
*Emmonsia*, 187
*Emmonsia crescens*, 187
*Emmonsia parva*, 187
*Emmonsia pasteuriana*, 187
Endophthalmitis
  Fungi which cause the disease, 184
Endothrix, 49
Entomophthorales, 165
  Laboratory diagnosis, 166
  Culture, 166
    *Basidiobolus ranarum*, 166
    *Conidiobolus coronatus*, 167
*Epidermophyton*-1, 47
Ergot alkaloids, 195
Esophageal candidiasis, 125
Eumycetomas
  Diagnostic characteristics of grains, 70
*Exophiala jeanselmei*, 67, 82

## F

Favus, 50
Fluconazole
  Pharmacokinetics, indications and adverse effects, 31
*Fonsecaea compacta*, 77
*Fonsecaea pedrosoi*, 77
  Types of conidial formation in, 79

Fumonisins, 196
Fungal (mycotic) keratitis, 181
  Causative agents, 181
  Clinical features, 182
  Laboratory diagnosis, 182
Fungal antibodies and fungal antigens
  Serological tests for detection of, 25
Fungal endophthalmitis, 183
  Causative agents, 184
  Clinical features, 184
  Endogenous endophthalmitis, 183
  Exogenous endophthalmitis, 183
  Laboratory diagnosis, 184
Fungal infection of ocular adnexa, 184, 185
  Mycotic conjunctivitis, 185
  Mycotic dacryocystitis, 185
  Mycotic infection of eyelids, 184
Fungal keratitis
  Treatment, 185
Fungal sinusitis, 83
Fungi and bacteria
  Distinguishing features, 4
Fungi
  Classification, 7
  Life cycle, 6
  Morphology, 4
  Pathogenesis, 14
    Primary pathogens, 14
  Reproduction, 6
    Asexual reproduction, 6
    Sexual reproduction, 6
Fungus ball, 83
Fungus culture
  Procedure for collection of specimen, 18
*Fusarium*, 194

## G

Germ tube test, 216
GF stain, 20
Giemsa stain, 20, 212
Gilchrist disease, 103
Gliotoxin, 196
Glomeromycota, 9
  Life cycle, 10
GMS staining procedure, 20
Gomori methenamine silver (GMS) stain, 210
Gram staining, 214
Gridley's fungus stain, 212

## H

Haematoxylin and eosin (H&E) stain, 19, 214
Hair infection, 49
  Ectothrix, 49
  Endothrix, 49
  Favus, 50
Heterothallic fungi, 5
*Histoplasma capsulatum*, 95
  Mycelial and yeast phases, 99
*Histoplasma capsulatum* var. *capsulatum*
  Cervical, inguinal lymphadenitis, and papulonodular skin nodules, 97
*Histoplasma capsulatum* var. *duboisii*, 99
*Histoplasma capsulatum* var. *farciminosum*, 100
Histoplasmosis, 95
  Laboratory diagnosis, 97
  Oral manifestations, 97
  Pathogenesis, 96
  Treatment, 101
Homothallic fungi, 5
*Hortaea* (*Phaeoannellomyces*) *werneckii*, 42
  Septate hyphae, 43
Hyalohyphomycetes, 170
Hyalohyphomycosis
  Causative agents of, 170
Hyphae, 5

## I

Id reaction, 47
Interdigital candidiasis, 123
Intrinsic resistance, 35
Invasive fungal sinusitis, 83
Itraconazole
  Pharmacokinetics, indications and adverse effects, 31

## K

Keratitis
  Fungi which cause the disease, 182
Ketoconazole
  Pharmacokinetics, indications and adverse effects, 31
Kingdom Fungi
  Classification of, 9

# Index

## L

*Lacazia loboi*, 89
Lactophenol cotton blue stain, 215
*Leptosphaeria senegalensis*, 67
Lichtheimia, 159, 163
*Loboa loboi*, 89
Lobomycosis, 89
    Laboratory diagnosis, 90
    Pathogenesis, 89
    Treatment, 90

## M

Madura foot, 61
*Madurella grisea*, 65
*Madurella mycetomatis*, 64
Maduromycosis, 61
*Malassezia* species, 41
Mayer's mucicarmine and alcian blue procedures, 20
Mayer's mucicarmine stain for mucin and *Cryptococcus*, 211
Medically important fungi, 12
    Identification of, 24
Microbiological safety cabinets, 23
*Microsporum*-16, 47
Molds, 5
Molecular testing, 23
    In situ hybridization, 23
    Polymerase chain reaction, 23
*Mucor*, 159, 163
Mucorales, 159
Mucormycosis, 159
    Causative agents of, 159
    Laboratory diagnosis, 161
    Pathogenesis, 160
        Cutaneous mucormycosis, 161
        Disseminated mucormycosis, 161
        Gastrointestinal mucormycosis, 161
        Pulmonary mucormycosis, 160
        Rhinocerebral mucormycosis, 160
    Species identification, 162
        *Apophysomyces elegans*, 164
        *Cunninghamella bertholletiae*, 164
        *Lichtheimia (Absidia) corymbifera*, 163
        *Mucor* spp., 163
        *Rhizomucor* spp., 164
        *Rhizopus* spp., 162
        *Saksenaea vasiformis*, 164
        *Syncephalastrum racemosum*, 165
    Treatment, 165, 167
Mucoromycota
    Formation of oospores, 10
Mycetoma
    Causative agents and colour of grains of, 62
    Differential diagnosis, 62
    Epidemiology in India, 69
    Etiology, 62
    Foot, 61
    Hand, 61
    Histological appearance and cultural characteristics
        *Acremonium* spp., 66
        *Actinomadura madurae*, 67
        *Actinomadura pelletieri*, 68
        *Curvularia geniculata*, 66
        *Exophiala jeanselmei*, 67
        *Leptosphaeria senegalensis*, 67
        *Madurella grisea*, 65
        *Madurella mycetomatis*, 64
        *Nocardia asteroides*, 68
        *Nocardia brasiliensis*, 68
        *Nocardia caviae*, 68
        *Pyrenochaeta romeroi*, 66
        *Scedosporium apiospermum*, 66
        *Streptomyces somaliensis*, 68
    Laboratory diagnosis, 63
    Pathogenesis, 62
    Treatment, 69
Mycoses
    Classification, 12
        Opportunistic mycoses, 14
        Subcutaneous mycoses, 14
        Superficial mycoses, 13
        Systemic mycoses, 14
    Epidemiology, 16
        Infection in the community, 16
        Infection in the hospital, 16
        Infection in the laboratory, 17
        Laboratory-acquired mycoses, 17
        Precautions with infected laboratory animals, 17
        Transplacental transmission, 16
        Venereal transmission, 16
    Laboratory diagnosis, 17
        Culture, 20
        Direct microscopic examination of specimens, 18, 19
        Serological tests, 23
Mycotic infection of eyelid, 184
Mycotoxicosis, 194
    Treatment, 197
Mycotoxins
    Mode of acquisition of, 194
    Use as bioweapons, 194

## N

*Nattrassia mangiferae*, 82
*Nocardia asteroides*, 68
*Nocardia brasiliensis*, 68
*Nocardia caviae*, 68
North American blastomycosis, 103

## O

Ochratoxins, 195
Oculomycosis, 181
Onychomycosis, 82, 124
Oospores, 9
Opportunistic fungal pathogens, 14
Oral candidiasis, 124
    Acute pseudomembranous and acute atrophic candidiasis, 124
    Angular cheilitis, 125
    Chronic atrophic and hyperplastic candidiasis or denture stomatitis, 125
Oral thrush, 124
Oropharyngeal candidiasis, 125

## P

*Paracoccidioides brasiliensis*, 114
    Yeast and mycelial phases, 115
Paracoccidioidomycosis, 114
    Clinical features, 114
    Laboratory diagnosis, 115
    Pathogenesis, 114
    Treatment, 116
Paronychia, 124
PAS stain, 20
*Penicilliosis marneffei*, 146
    Clinical findings, 147
    Epidemiology, 146
    Histopathology, 147
    Laboratory diagnosis, 148
    Mycology, 147
    Pathogenesis, 146
    Treatment, 148
*Penicillium*, 146, 194
*Penicillium marneffei*
    Mycelial and yeast-like phases, 147

# Index

Perianal (diaper) rash, 123
Periodic acid-Schiff (PAS) staining, 212
Phaeohyphomycosis, 77, 82
  Cerebral, 83
  Corneal (keratitis), 83
  Cutaneous, 82
  Laboratory diagnosis, 83
  Mycology, 84
    *Alternaria* spp., 86
    *Bipolaris* spp., 85
    *Cladophialophora bantiana*, 84
    *Curvularia* spp., 85
    *Exophiala (Wangiella) dermatitidis*, 85
    *Exophiala jeanselmei*, 86
    *Exserohilum* spp., 87
    *Neoscytalidium dimidiatum (Scytalidium dimidiatum)*, 86
    *Ochroconis gallopava*, 84
  Subcutaneous, 82
  Superficial, 82
  Systemic, 83
  Treatment, 87
*Phialophora verrucosa*, 77
Piedra, 43
  Black piedra, 43
    Treatment, 44
  White piedra, 44
    Laboratory diagnosis, 44
    Treatment, 44
*Piedraia hortae*, 44
*Pityriasis versicolor*, 41
  Laboratory diagnosis, 41
*Pneumocystis*, 141
  Life cycle, 142
  Morphology, 141
  Pathogenesis, 143
*Pneumocystis jirovecii* pneumonia
  Laboratory diagnosis, 143
  Treatment and prophylaxis, 144
Pneumocystosis, 143
Polymorphism, 121
Pseudohyphae, 4
*Pyrenochaeta romeroi*, 66

# R

*Rhinocladiella aquaspersa*, 77
Rhinosporidiosis, 190
  Laboratory diagnosis, 192

Pathogenesis, 191
Treatment, 193
*Rhinosporidium seeberi*, 190, 192
  Life cycle, 192
*Rhinosporidium seeberi* sporangia and *Coccidioides immitis* spherules
  Differences, 192
*Rhizomucor*, 159, 164
*Rhizopus*, 159, 163
Ringworm, 47

# S

Sabouraud dextrose agar (SDA), 22
Sac fungi, 10
*Saksenaea vasiformis*, 164
*Scedosporium apiospermum*, 66
Schizomycetoma, 69
Sclerotic bodies, 78
Selective and differential media, 203
Slide culture, 23, 216
South American blastomycosis, 114
Special stains
  Disadvantages of, 20
Specimens
  Collection and preparation, 206
    Blood for fungal culture, 206
    Blood for serological tests, 207
    Bone marrow, 207
    Cerebrospinal fluid (CSF), 207
    Cutaneous specimens, 208
    Exudates, pus, and drainage, 208
    Fluids, 208
    Sputum, 207
    Stool, 207
    Tissues, 208
    Urine, 208
  Methods for direct microscopic examination, 208, 209
Splendore-Hoeppli material, 166
Sporangiophores, 10
Sporangiospores, 6, 10
Sporangium, 9
Spores, 7
*Sporothrix schenckii*, 73
Sporotrichosis, 73
  Asteroid body in, 75
  Cultural characteristics, 73
  Laboratory diagnosis, 74
  Morphology, 73

Oral manifestations, 74
Pathogenesis, 74
Staining techniques
  Applications and limitations for demonstrating fungi and related pathogens, 21
Stains, 210
  Acid-fast modified Kinyoun stain for *Nocardia* spp., 214
  Alcian blue staining, 213
  Giemsa stain, 212
  Gomori methenamine silver (GMS) stain, 210
  Gram staining, 214
  Gridley's fungus stain, 212
  Haematoxylin and eosin (H&E) staining, 214
  Lactophenol cotton blue stain, 215
  Mayer's mucicarmine stain for mucin and *Cryptococcus*, 211
  Periodic acid-Schiff (PAS) staining, 212
*Streptomyces somaliensis*, 68
*Syncephalastrum*, 159
*Syncephalastrum racemosum*, 165

# T

Taxonomic classification, 8
Tinea, 47
Tinea nigra
  Treatment, 43
*Trichophyton*-24, 47
Trichothecenes, 197

# V

Vaginal candidiasis, 125
Vegetative mycelium, 5
Voriconazole
  Pharmacokinetics, indications and adverse effects, 31

# Y

Yeast-like, 4
Yeasts, 4

# Z

Zearalenone, 196
zygospores, 9